Biochemistry (all blood)	Your laboratory
Alanine aminotransferase	
♂	<45IU/L
♀	<40IU/L
Albumin	34–50g/L
Alkaline phosphatase	35–120IU/L
Alpha-fetoprotein	<10kIU/L
Amylase	<135IU/L
Aspartate aminotransferase	<40IU/L
Bicarbonate	21–25mmol/L
Bilirubin	<19μmol/L
C-reactive protein (CRP)	<5mg/L
Calcium (total)	2.12–2.65mmol/L
Chloride	96–106mmol/L
Cholesterol	3.9–<6mmol/L
High density lipoprotein (HDL)	0.9–1.93mmol/L
Low density lipoprotein (LDL)	1.55–4.4mmol/L
Very low density lipoprotein (VLDL)	0.128–0.645mmol/L
Fasting HDL-cholesterol reference range	
♂	1–1.5
♀	1.2–1.8
Cortisol	
a.m.:	190–650nmol/L
midnight:	<200nmol/L
Creatine kinase	
♂	<190IU/L
♀	<160IU/L
Creatinine	
♂	70–110μmol/L (17–55yrs)
♀	55–95μmol/L (17–55yrs)
Ferritin	
♂	
♀ pre-menopausal	
♀ post-menopausal	

OXFORD MEDICAL PUBLICATIONS

Oxford Handbook of

Genitourinary Medicine, HIV, and Sexual Health

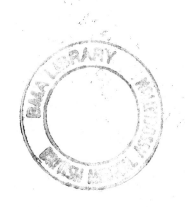

Published and forthcoming Oxford Handbooks

Oxford Handbook of Genitourinary Medicine, HIV, and Sexual Health

Second Edition

Edited by

Richard Pattman

Consultant in Genitourinary Medicine,
NHS Newcastle and North Tyneside Community Health,
Newcastle upon Tyne, UK

K. Nathan Sankar

Consultant in Genitourinary Medicine,
NHS Newcastle and North Tyneside Community Health,
Newcastle upon Tyne, UK

Babiker Elawad

Consultant in Genitourinary Medicine,
NHS Newcastle and North Tyneside Community Health,
Newcastle upon Tyne, UK

Pauline Handy MBE

Lead Nurse in Genitourinary Medicine,
NHS Newcastle and North Tyneside Community Health,
Newcastle upon Tyne, UK

David Ashley Price

Consultant in Infectious Diseases,
Newcastle upon Tyne Hospitals NHS Foundation Trust,
Newcastle upon Tyne, UK

OXFORD
UNIVERSITY PRESS

OXFORD
UNIVERSITY PRESS

Great Clarendon Street, Oxford OX2 6DP

Oxford University Press is a department of the University of Oxford.
It furthers the University's objective of excellence in research, scholarship,
and education by publishing worldwide in

Oxford New York

Auckland Cape Town Dar es Salaam Hong Kong Karachi
Kuala Lumpur Madrid Melbourne Mexico City Nairobi
New Delhi Shanghai Taipei Toronto

With offices in

Argentina Austria Brazil Chile Czech Republic France Greece
Guatemala Hungary Italy Japan Poland Portugal Singapore
South Korea Switzerland Thailand Turkey Ukraine Vietnam

Oxford is a registered trade mark of Oxford University Press
in the UK and in certain other countries

Published in the United States
by Oxford University Press Inc., New York

© Oxford University Press, 2010

The moral rights of the author have been asserted
Database right Oxford University Press (maker)

First edition published as
Oxford Handbook of Genitourinary Medicine, HIV, and AIDS 2005

Second edition published 2010

British Library Cataloguing in Publication Data
Data available

Typeset by Glyph International, Bangalore, India
Printed in China
on acid-free paper through
Asia Pacific Offset Limited

ISBN 978–0–19–957166–6

10 9 8 7 6 5 4 3 2 1

Preface

This handbook provides a wealth of simple and easy to follow information on sexually transmitted infections (STIs), human immunodeficiency virus (HIV), other genitourinary conditions, contraception and sexual health, and the principles of providing a safe, high-quality service. Although designed for the trainee and practitioner in the UK it is envisaged that it will be of global use to all those with an interest in sexual health whatever their level of expertise and wherever they may practice.

The book provides comprehensive practical guidance on genitourinary medicine (GUM) and sexual health, and includes HIV infection in the adult. STIs and related genitourinary problems, contraception, and sexual health together with other areas of practical relevance are also covered (e.g. practice within GUM or sexual health services, medico-legal/ethical issues and frequently asked questions). The chapter on contraception has been enhanced in this edition as the integration of traditionally separate GUM and family planning (now known as sexual and reproductive health—SRH) services gathers momentum.

The continuing rise of STIs has resulted in an extended workforce. This includes the creation of specialist nurses and primary healthcare teams with extended roles. Greater involvement of primary care teams in the provision of both the GUM and SRH aspects of sexual health is essential for promotion of good sexual health. It is intended that the information contained should address the needs of both the generalist and the specialist practitioners in different settings.

The contents start with service development and administration proceeding to medico-legal and ethical issues, routine patient management and flow charts detailing common clinical situations. This is followed by a series of chapters describing STIs and other problems commonly presenting to GUM in a disease-orientated style. Additional material and UK medical eligibility criteria for different contraceptive methods published by the Faculty of Sexual and Reproductive Health are included in the enhanced chapter on contraception. Chapters on HIV infection and the acquired immunodeficiency syndrome (AIDS) follow including an epidemiological overview, basic viral biology, and pathogenesis before proceeding to systematic description of conditions both directly related and opportunistic, their management and concluding with special situations (pregnancy and travel). Commonly used abbreviations are summarized and useful resources provided.

Feedback on errors and omissions would be much appreciated. Please post your comments via the OUP website: ✎ www.oup.com/uk/medicine/handbooks.

Contents

List of colour plates

Contributors

Stephen Bushby
Consultant in Genitourinary
Medicine, Sunderland Royal
Hospital, Sunderland

Babiker Elawad (editor)
Consultant in Genitourinary
Medicine
NHS Newcastle and
North Tyneside Community
Health
Newcastle upon Tyne

Pauline Handy MBE
(editor)
Lead Nurse in Genitourinary
Medicine
NHS Newcastle and North
Tyneside Community Health
Newcastle upon Tyne

Jane Hussey
Consultant in Genitourinary
Medicine, Northumberland
Care Trust, Blyth,
Northumberland

Kathryn Kain
Senior Health Adviser
Newcastle General Hospital
Newcastle upon Tyne

Diana Mansour
Consultant Community
Gynaecologist,
NHS Newcastle and
North Tyneside
Community Health,
Newcastle upon Tyne

Janet McLelland
Consultant Dermatologist,
Newcastle upon Tyne Hospitals
NHS Foundation Trust
Newcastle upon Tyne

Richard Pattman (editor)
Consultant in Genitourinary
Medicine,
NHS Newcastle and North
Tyneside Community Health
Newcastle upon Tyne

David Ashley Price (editor)
Consultant in Infectious Diseases,
Newcastle upon Tyne Hospitals
NHS Foundation Trust,
Newcastle upon Tyne

Jane Richards
Associate Specialist in
Genitourinary Medicine, NHS
Newcastle and North Tyneside
Community Health, Newcastle
upon Tyne

K. Nathan Sankar (editor)
Consultant in Genitourinary
Medicine,
NHS Newcastle and North
Tyneside Community Health,
Newcastle upon Tyne

Jantje Wilken
Associate Specialist in
Genitourinary Medicine,
NHS Newcastle and North
Tyneside Community Health,
Newcastle upon Tyne

Symbols and abbreviations

📖	cross reference
⅋	website
▶	important
▶▶	don't dawdle
❶, ⚠	warning
💣	bomb (controversial topic)
♂	male
♀	female
∴	therefore
~	approximately
≈	approximately equal to
±	plus/minus
↑	increased
↓	decreased
→	leads to
1°	primary
2°	secondary
α	alpha
β	beta
γ	gamma
δ	delta
σ	sigma
3TC	lamivudine
ABC	abacavir
ACOG	American College of Obstetricians and Gynecologists
ACTH	adrenocorticotrophic hormone
AGH	anogenital herpes
AHU	arginine, hypoxanthine, and uracil
AIDS	acquired immunodeficiency syndrome
AIHA	autoimmune haemolytic anaemia
AIN	anal intra-epithelial neoplasia
AIS	adenocarcinoma in situ
ALP	alkaline phosphatase
ALT	alanine aminotransferase
APV	amprenavir
ARS	acute retroviral syndrome

ASCUS	atypical squamous cells of uncertain significance
AST	aspartate aminotransferase
ATV	atazanavir
AZT	zidovudine (see also ZDV)
BAL	broncho-alveolar lavage
BASHH	British Association for Sexual Health and HIV
BCG	Bacillus Calmette-Guerin vaccine
bd	twice daily
BHIVA	British HIV Association
BMA	British Medical Association
BMD	bone mineral density
BSCC	British Society for Cervical Cytology
BV	bacterial vaginosis
BXO	balanitis xerotica obliterans
CAP	chronic abacterial prostatitis
CBP	chronic bacterial prostatitis
CD	cluster differentiation
CDC	Centers for Disease Control
CFT	complement fixation test
CFU	colony-forming unit
CGIN	cervical glandular intra-epithelial neoplasia
CHC	combined hormonal contraceptive
CHOP	cyclophosphamide, hydroxydaunomycin (doxorubicin), oncovin (vincristine), prednisolone
CIN	cervical intra-epithelial neoplasia
CIS	carcinoma *in situ*
CJ	Creutzfeldt–Jakob
CMV	cytomegalovirus
C_{min}	minimum concentration
CNS	central nervous system
COC	combined oral contraceptive
COX-2	cyclo-oxygenase 2
CPAP	continuous positive airway pressure
CRP	C-reactive protein
CSF	cerebrospinal fluid
CT	computed tomography
CYP450	cytochrome P450
D4T	stavudine
DDC	zalcitabine
DDI	didanosine

DEXA	dual-energy X-ray absorptiometry
DFA	direct fluorescent antibody
DGI	disseminated gonococcal infection
DLV	delavirdine
DMPA	depot medroxyprogesterone acetate
DNA	deoxyribonucleic acid
DOH	Department of Health
DSP	distal symmetric polyneuropathy
EBV	Epstein–Barr virus
ED	erectile dysfunction
EFV	efavirenz
EGD	endocervical gland dysplasia
EIA	enzyme immunoassay
EM	erythema multiforme
ENF	enfuvirtide
EPS	expressed prostatic secretions
ERCP	endoscopic retrograde cholangiopancreatography
ESLD	end-stage liver disease
ESR	erythrocyte sedimentation rate
ESRD	end-stage renal disease
EUA	examination under anaesthetic
FBC	full blood count
FGM	female genital mutilation
FI	fusion inhibitor
FPV	fosamprenavir
FSH	follicle-stimulating hormone
FTA	fluorescent treponemal antibody
FTC	emtricitabine
FVU	first voided urine
g	gram
G6PD	glucose-6-phosphate dehydrogenase
GBS	Group B streptococci
GCSF	granulocyte colony-stimulating factor
GI	gastrointestinal
GMC	General Medical Council
GNDC	Gram-negative diplococci
gp	glycoprotein
GUD	genital ulcer disease
GUM	genitourinary medicine
HA	health adviser

HAART	highly active antiretroviral therapy
HAV	hepatitis A virus
HBV	hepatitis B virus
HCC	hepatocellular carcinoma
HCFT	herpes complement fixation test
hCG	human chorionic gonadotrophin
HCGIN	high-grade cervical glandular intra-epithelial neoplasia
HCP	healthcare professional
HCV	hepatitis C virus
hCG	human chorionic gonadotrophin
HDL	high-density lipoprotein
HHV	human herpes virus
HIV	human immunodeficiency virus
HIVAN	HIV associated nephropathy
HLA	human leucocyte antigen
HNIG	human normal immunoglobulin
HPA	Health Protection Agency, hypothalamic–pituitary–adrenal
HPF	high power field
HPV	human papilloma virus
HRT	hormone replacement therapy
HSV	herpes simplex virus
HT	hydroxy tryptomine
HTLV	human T-cell lymphotropic virus
HVS	high vaginal swab
HZ	herpes zoster
IC50	50% inhibitory concentration
ICC	invasive cervical carcinoma
IDU	injecting drug user
IDV	indinavir
Ig	immunoglobulin
IHD	ischaemic heart disease
IIEF-5	International Index of Erectile Function-5
IM	intramuscular
IMB	intermenstrual bleeding
IN	intra-epithelial neoplasia
INR	international normalized ratio
IP	index patient
IRIS	immune recovery inflammatory response
IU	international units
IUD	intra-uterine device

IUS	intra-uterine system
IV	intravenous
KB	keratoderma blennorrhagica
KC	Koerner code
KS	Kaposi's sarcoma
L	litre
LARC	long acting reversible contraception (also known as lasting and reliable contraception)
LCGIN	low-grade cervical glandular intra-epithelial neoplasia
LDH	lactic dehydrogenase
LDL	low-density lipoprotein
LFTs	liver function tests
LGE	linear gingival erythema
LGV	lymphogranuloma venereum
LH	luteinizing hormone
LIP	lymphocytic interstitial pneumonitis
LNG	levonorgestrel
LPV	lopinavir
LS	lichen sclerosis
MAC	*Mycobacterium avium* complex
mcg	microgram
MCV	molluscum contagiosum virus
MHA-TP	microhaemagglutination assay for *Treponema pallidum*
mL	millilitre
MOMP	major outer membrane protein
MOPP	mechlorethamine, oncovin (vincristine), procarbazine, prednisolone
MPC	mucopurulent cervicitis
MRI	magnetic resonance imaging
MRP1	multidrug resistance associated protein 1
MSM	men who have sex with men
MSSU	midstream specimen of urine
MU	mega-unit(s)
NAAT	nucleic acid amplification test
NAM	multi-NRTI associated mutation
NASBA	nucleic acid sequence based amplification assay
NET-EN	norethisterone oenanthate
NFV	nelfinavir
NGU	non-gonococcal urethritis
NHL	non-Hodgkin lymphoma

NHS	National Health Service
NNRTI	non-nucleoside reverse transcriptase inhibitor
NRTI	nucleoside/nucleotide reverse transcriptase inhibitor
NS	necrotizing stomatitis
NSAID	non-steroidal anti-inflammatory drug
NSGI	non-specific genital infection
NSI	non-syncytium-inducing
NSU	non-specific urethritis
NUP	necrotizing ulcerative periodontitis
NVP	nevirapine
OHL	oral hairy leukoplakia
OI	opportunistic infection
p	protein
PACE	probe assay chemiluminescence enhanced
PCB	post-coital bleeding
PCC	post-coital contraception
PCP	*Pneumocystis jiroveci (carinii)* pneumonia
PCR	polymerase chain reaction
PEP	post-exposure prophylaxis
PHI	primary HIV infection
PI	protease inhibitor
PID	pelvic inflammatory disease
PIN	penile intra-epithelial neoplasia
PML	progressive multifocal leukoencephalopathy
PMNL	polymorphonuclear leucocyte
PN	partner notification
POC	progesterone-only contraception
POCT	point-of-care test
POEC	progesterone-only emergency contraception
POP	progesterone-only contraception
PROM	premature rupture of membranes
PUO	pyrexia of unknown origin
RA	rheumatoid arthritis
RCOG	Royal College of Obstetricians and Gynaecologists
ReA	reactive arthritis
RNA	ribonucleic acid
RPR	rapid plasma reagin
RT	reverse transcriptase
RTV	ritonavir
RVVC	recurrent vulvovaginal candidiasis
SARA	sexually acquired reactive arthritis

SCC	squamous cell carcinoma
SCJ	squamo-columnar junction
SDA	strand displacement amplification
SI	syncytium-inducing
SIADH	syndrome of inappropriate secretion of antidiuretic hormone
SIL	squamous intra-epithelial lesion
SIV	simian immune deficiency virus
SJS	Stevens–Johnson syndrome
SQV	saquinavir
SSRI	selective serotonin re-uptake inhibitor
STD	sexually transmitted disease
STI	sexually transmitted infection
TAM	thymidine analogue mutation
TB	tuberculosis
TCA	trichloroacetic acid
TDF	tenofovir
TDM	therapeutic drug monitoring
tid	three times a day
TMA	transcription-mediated assay
TNF	tumour necrosis factor
TOP	termination of pregnancy
TP	*Treponema pallidum*
TPHA	TP haemagglutination assay
TPPA	TP particle agglutination
TV	*Trichomonas vaginalis*
TZ	transformation zone
UPSI	unprotected sexual intercourse
UTI	urinary tract infection
VBU	voided bladder urine
VD	venereal disease
VDRL	Venereal Disease Research Laboratory
VIN	vulval intra-epithelial neoplasia
VL	viral load
VVC	vulvovaginal candidiasis
VZV	varicella zoster virus
WBC	white blood count, white blood cells
WHO	World Health Organization
ZDV	zidovudine (see also AZT)

❶ *All other abbreviations are defined in the text on the page in which they appear.*

The genitourinary medicine service

Service development

Genitourinary medicine

During the 1914–18 World War there was an alarming increase in legally defined venereal diseases (VDs): syphilis, gonorrhoea, and chancroid. A Royal Commission produced the Venereal Disease Regulations (1916) specifying that local authorities should provide clinics which:
- could be accessed directly (without general practitioner referral)
- enabled voluntary attendance
- assured confidentiality
- provided free treatment.

113 clinics were established in 1917.

During the 1939–45 World War there was a concern that troops were being incapacitated by infection, with a core group of individuals acting as a reservoir. Therefore doctors began to question patients about their sexual partners. An individual named by more than one person could be compelled to have treatment, and failure to comply could lead to imprisonment (Defence of the Realm Act 33B 1942). This regulation was subsequently repealed in 1947 but led to the introduction of voluntary partner notification (PN) in the UK, a vital tool in the control of infection. In the UK there are now over 260 clinics led by consultants specializing in genitourinary medicine (GUM) covering a wide range of sexually transmitted infections (STIs) including human immunodeficiency virus (HIV) and other genitourinary conditions or problems. Their name has evolved from 'VD Clinic', 'Special Clinic', or 'Sexually Transmitted Diseases Clinic' to 'Genitourinary Medicine Clinic', 'Sexual Health Clinic', or an eponymous name, and some are integrated with contraceptive services.

STIs and genitourinary conditions present in a variety of guises to different specialties (e.g. dermatology, gynaecology, urology, and infectious diseases). Therefore cross-referral is common and allows for the establishment of multidisciplinary clinics, e.g. for vulval disorders.

Integrated sexual health services

The National Strategy for Sexual Health and HIV (2001) identified wide-ranging differences in the provision of sexual health services throughout England. Concerns that such inequalities might adversely affect the government's attempts to ↓ the number of teenage pregnancies and rates of STIs resulted in the concept of integrated sexual health clinics. GUM and contraceptive services which, in the past, have traditionally operated as separate entities are now working closely together to provide high-quality easily accessible integrated sexual health services for all.

Robust joint training initiatives for both medical and nursing staff have resulted in dual-trained clinicians able to deal with all aspects of routine sexual health care. Specialist clinicians deal with complex STIs and contraception, medical gynaecology, psychosexual problems, erectile dysfunctio,n and HIV care and treatment. Patients now have the opportunity to self-refer for termination of pregnancy (TOP) and information about this service must be made readily available to attendees.

The continued ↑ in infections and unwanted pregnancies may be addressed by the provision of high-quality easily understandable health promotion together with the opportunity to undergo testing in alternative locations. Point-of-care testing allows immediate results and undoubtedly encourages those who may not otherwise attend conventional sexual health services to be screened.

Provision

Aims of genitourinary medicine services

The ultimate goal of GUM is to ↓ STIs within the community. This is achievable by delivering accessible and non-judgemental services that provide free and immediate diagnosis and treatment to those who think they may have, or be at risk of having, an STI. Epidemiological control of infection remains essential to the sexual welfare of the community. However, clinics must reconcile confidentiality with a need for both 1° care and hospital services to be aware of serious chronic health problems in the individual. Health advising with good community links is important for ensuring that PN issues are dealt with efficiently and sensitively, reducing the continued transmission of STIs.

Comprehensive national surveillance programmes are essential when formulating strategies for national screening and treatment policies. Surveillance data inform clinical practice, allow the planning and allocation of resources, and help identify at-risk populations. This is largely achieved by the collection of reliable data from GUM clinics, as information on infection managed elsewhere, including 1° care, is limited.

GUM: core and specialized roles

The core function of GUM is to provide screening, surveillance, diagnosis, treatment, and PN for STIs including HIV. This is combined with sexual health promotion, teaching, training, and research.

In addition some services provide specialized clinics at their main location or outreach venues (e.g. prisons). These are established and resourced to meet local need and may include sessions for:

- chronic or recurrent conditions e.g. HIV, warts, herpes
- problems involving different specialties, e.g. vulval conditions, sexual assault (providing both forensic examination and infection screening), one-stop sexual health (providing contraceptive as well as STI services)
- related problems where service need is identified, e.g. psychosexual and sexual dysfunction
- special groups, e.g. young people, homosexual men and women, ethnic minorities, commercial sex workers.

Doctors

GUM is a consultant-led service with a dedicated higher medical training programme for specialty registrars from specialty training years 3 to 6 (ST3 to ST6). There are also training posts at the more junior levels of foundation year 2 and general practice specialty training years 1 or 2. Many non-consultant career grade doctors, who are known as associate specialists or specialty doctors, are working either exclusively in GUM or in association with contraception and sexual health, 1° care, etc.

Nurse specialists/practitioners

The role of the nurse within GUM has continued to evolve, with specialist (and consultant) nurses now the norm. Nurse-led clinics run alongside conventional medically led services with nursing staff working independently taking responsibility for total patient care, including the examination of new patients under protocol and providing medication through patient group directions. No uniform model of care exists; individual centres implement their own preferred methods.

Health advisers (HAs)

In the UK HAs are employed within GUM in community sexual health advising roles and within the national chlamydia screening programme. The prime public health role of health advisers is the identification and management of partners who may have been exposed to STI(s) in order to prevent onward transmission, i.e. partner notification (PN).

HAs work at community and population levels, identifying local sexual health needs and ensuring that services are accessible to those with the greatest need by effective targeting and the development of innovative practice approaches. They act as advocates for health gain and work collaboratively with others to tackle the wider determinants of health. Their role (Box 1.1) has evolved to encompass a wide range of healthcare issues as recommended in the Manual for Sexual Health Advisers produced by the Society of Sexual Health Advisers (SSHA).

Box 1.1 Role of HAs (varies between clinics)

- Providing a holistic approach to patients, with information, education, treatment, and support.
- Comprehensive needs assessment of index patients (IPs) and other vulnerable groups (e.g. young people, ethnic minorities, those sexually assaulted), including associated social, emotional, or sexual difficulties.
- Effective PN ensuring the attendance and treatment of sexual contacts including settings outside GUM, e.g. 1° care.
- Establishing and maintaining care pathways for patients in primary/ acute care diagnosed with STIs.
- Pre- and post-test HIV discussion.
- Counselling, information, and support to patients, including those with HIV infection and their partners, friends, and relatives.
- Sexual health education provision within GUM and the community, liaising with statutory and voluntary services.
- Research, audit, and service development.
- Support of clinical outreach in non-clinic settings to targeted groups, e.g. increasing the uptake of HIV testing in those most at risk, hepatitis B vaccination for homosexual and bisexual men, STI screening for sex workers.

Availability

Referrals

The majority of patients seen in GUM either self-refer or are seen as a result of PN. 2° referrals are seen, especially from 1° care, contraception services, and rape crisis organizations, with tertiary referrals from gynaecology, dermatology, infectious diseases, urology, etc. These may be formal, with a letter, or based on verbal advice. By common acceptance there is no correspondence unless the patient has been referred by letter. However, in certain situations it may be in the patient's best interests for there to be an exchange of medical information between professionals providing care, but this should have the patient's agreement.

Access

Easy and timely access to the clinic should be available. When the clinic is closed, a pre-recorded telephone message detailing clinic opening hours together with the telephone number for other local GUM services, Accident and Emergency, or NHS Direct is of benefit to anyone with an urgent problem. Appointment availability should be linked to staff numbers and experience. Ideally, patients should be seen within 48 hours. However, testing too soon after an infection risk may produce false-negative results (e.g. 2 weeks for chlamydia); therefore this period should be extended (unless prophylactic treatment is required) or clear information should be given to patients regarding this possibility and re-testing at the appropriate time offered. If this is not possible, careful use of triage may help identify those with urgent problems.

All services should review their location and opening hours to match the needs of the local population. Some clinics provide open access without prior booking, although most utilize some form of appointment system.

Triage

In clinics operating by an appointment system, a robust triage system should be available for urgent situations. Trained staff should be able to assess and prioritize the patient's condition, including advice on optimum screening time intervals following an infection risk, and then arrange the appropriate attendance.

Disability

Any assistance required by the disabled should be highlighted when making an appointment, but accessibility facilities, such as wheelchair access, disabled toilets, minicom systems, etc., should be in place.

Interpreters

Most hospitals are able to provide an accredited interpreting service, but will need time to arrange an interpreter of the appropriate language. Alternatively a telephone system can be used (e.g. Language Line). If possible avoid family friends or relatives acting as interpreters, as information may be withheld by the patient under these circumstances.

The process

Registration

Patients should be allowed privacy during registration by ensuring that they cannot be overheard while providing information or by using of self-completed registration forms. Help must be available to those with difficulties in completing such forms. The amount of information required at registration will differ from clinic to clinic. However, collection of the following data may assist the clinic to contact the patient if required and help with service planning, statistics, and surveillance.

Name	Nationality
Address	Country of birth
Date of birth	Ethnicity
Telephone number(s)	Area of residence
General practitioner	Referral source and documentation
Employment status	Name of partner (if attending)

Patients who refuse to give any information about themselves may attend. The right to anonymity is accepted within GUM. The patient should be issued with an individual clinic identification number that will be used on all specimens and request forms. They should be encouraged to provide at least their date of birth which can be used with the identification number as an additional reference when confirming identity, test results, etc.

Appointment cards showing the patient's identification number and all booked appointments should be issued at the time of registration. Details of the clinic opening times and telephone numbers should be clearly printed on the card.

Waiting areas are inevitably areas of stress for those wishing to remain anonymous. Issuing patients with a welcome leaflet on arrival explaining how the clinic operates will hopefully ↓ anxiety. Those who are acutely distressed should be moved into a private area. The use of a television or music system in the waiting room may help to distract the anxious patient and also reduce the risk of sensitive information being overheard.

Soundex codes

Soundex codes (Box 1.2) together with dates of birth are commonly used within GUM to provide clinical information while protecting individual confidentiality.

Box 1.2 The Soundex code

The Soundex code contains four characters, with the first being the first letter of the surname. The remaining three are numbers derived from the name. When the adjacent letters are from the same category, the second is disregarded. An example is Schmid: since the number 2 represents both S and C, the C is omitted. The letters A, E, H, I, O, U, Y, and W only contribute if they start the name. An empty space is represented by a zero. Once the four-character limit has been reached, all remaining letters are redundant.

Category	Letter
1	B, P, F, V
2	C, S, K, G, J, Q, X, Z
3	D, T
4	L
5	M, N
6	R
No Code	A, E, H, I, O, U, Y, W

Examples: Sankar, S 526; Pattman, P 355; Handy, H 530; Price, P 6200;   Elawad, E 430.

Confirmation of attendance

Letters confirming attendance for a clinic or hospital appointment should be made available for the patient to present to the employer using hospital-headed notepaper without reference to GUM. This letter should state the date and time of the visit together with the date and time of any further appointments.

Reimbursement of travel expenses

Patients attending GUM clinics may reclaim their travel expenses upon receipt of bus/train tickets if the distance travelled is >15 miles from home. Legislation is unclear about those who travel less than this distance. Therefore it is suggested that discretion be used in such cases. This facility is offered to patients irrespective of individual financial circumstances (Department of Health NHS Charges HC11 2002).

Transfer to other GUM clinics

Patients leaving the area can be issued with a summary of investigations and treatments carried out while attending the initial clinic. This allows subsequent clinics to assess the need for further management.

Test results

Various systems are employed throughout the country to provide test results and include:
- returning in person or phoning for all results
- contact by the clinic, (letter, phone, text message, e-mail).

Informing patients that if they are not contacted the results are negative or normal ('no news is good news') is considered poor practice. Some patients, including those working in the sex industry, may request written proof of the test result. When provided, it must be made clear that this may not cover recently acquired infections (e.g. within 'window' periods). Patients must produce a document with photographic identity before issue of such results.

Recall

A computerized system aids the process of recall. Patients are generally reviewed for the following reasons:
- to be given positive test results and treatment
- further management (e.g. ongoing treatment, PN, vaccination, cervical cytology review).

Recall usually takes the form of a letter requesting that the patient contacts the clinic, but may also be by telephone, e-mail, or text-messaging by agreement.

Health advising and partner notification (Table 1.1)

The concept of PN in the UK was first introduced in the 1940s with the aim of identifying, diagnosing, and treating the contacts of people with VD. This now extends to all STIs and is an essential part of infection control, and has led to the establishment of health advisers (HAs).

The Department of Health (DoH) (2003) *Effective Commissioning of Sexual Health and HIV Services* recommends that:

- every GUM department should have health advisers
- there should be no single-handed health adviser posts
- there should be at least one whole time equivalent health adviser for every consultant-led site in GUM.

As part of a drive to ensure that all HAs are accountable and registered a guidance document, *Sexual Health Advising – Developing the Workforce* (DoH/SSHA/Unite 2008), has been produced. This document recognizes the need to have a robust preparation programme in place to prepare the future HA workforce and to strengthen the public health role of HAs. this was also an aim of the National Strategy for Sexual Health and HIV (DoH 2001).

Table 1.1 Partner notification

Infection	PN method		Trace period s = symptomatic as = asymptomatic
	Patient	Provider	
Cervicitis (mucopurulent), PID, epididymitis	✓	✓	Current sexual partners
Chancroid	✓	✓	10 days from disease onset
Chlamydia	✓	✓	4 weeks (s) 6 months (as) or last partner if longer
Donovanosis	✓	✓	40 days from disease onset
Gonorrhoea	✓	✓	2 week (s) males 12 weeks (as) males and all females or last partner if longer
Hepatitis A	✓	✓	2 weeks prior to and 1 week after onset of jaundice
Hepatitis B	✓	✓	2 weeks prior to onset of jaundice or based on risk
Hepatitis C	✓	✓	Assessment if asymptomatic and for hepatitis B until surface Ag negative.
Anogenital herpes	✗	✗	Offer advice and STI screening
HIV	✓	✓	Risk assessment informs PN for asymptomatic cases (If 1° infection – 3 months)
Lymphogranuloma venereum	✓	✓	30 days from disease onset
Non-gonococcal urethritis	✓	✓	4 weeks (s) 6 months (as) or last partner if longer
Pediculosis	✓	✗	12 weeks: current partner
Scabies	✓	✗	8 weeks: current partner, household members
Syphilis (early)	✓	✓	12 weeks (1°) Up to 2 years (2°, early latent)
Syphilis (late)	✓	✓	10 years. Vertical transmission possible for a decade post-infection; therefore includes children born to infected mothers
Trichomoniasis	✓	✗	Current partner
Anogenital warts/ molluscum	✗	✗	Offer to screen current partners

The World Health Organization (WHO) 2003: notification and management of sexual partners

Contacting the sex partners of clients with an STI, persuading them to present themselves at a site offering STI services, and treating them promptly and effectively are essential elements of any STI programme. However, these actions should be carried out sensitively and with consideration of social and cultural factors to avoid ethical and practical problems such as rejection and violence, particularly against those who are vulnerable.

Aim of PN

The ultimate aim is to break the chain and transmission of STIs and rates of infection by:
- Stressing the importance of PN to those diagnosed with certain STIs.
- Providing them with information on the nature, exposure, and risk of infection. The need to have sexual partners appropriately managed before sexual intercourse resumes must be emphasized.
- Identifying, contacting, and screening sexual partners of the IP, providing information and offering treatment if appropriate.

Description of terms and methods used in PN

PN should be conducted so that all information remains confidential and the process is voluntary and non-coercive. Consultation with the HA should take place in a non-clinical soundproofed environment free from interruption. Arranging for medication to be provided to patients by HAs via patient group directives emphasizes the importance of PN.

Patient referral: IPs with an STI are encouraged to notify their sexual partner(s) of any infection risk. HAs can help the IP to decide what information should be passed on to partners and how best to do this.

Contact slips: Issue of contact slips to IPs is a widely used method of notifying sexual partners. Passed onto sexual contacts, they detail:
- IP identification number
- Department of Health diagnostic (KC60) code or the name of the infection (with the IP's permission) and date of diagnosis
- name and address of the issuing clinic.

When presented at any GUM, clinic slips inform staff of the IP's infection, thus initiating appropriate screening and treatment of the sexual contact. Information can be communicated back to the issuing clinic to confirm that PN has taken place and indicate infection(s) found, which may be important for the care of the IP. Patient referral may also take place without issuing contact slips, e.g. when the contact is only accessible by telephone or lives abroad. KC60 codes are not applicable outside the UK. WHO codes are available but are not widely used.

Provider referral: These are offered to those IPs who do not wish to inform their sexual partner(s) themselves. The IP provides partner details to the HA after reassurance that confidentiality will not be compromised. HAs make direct contact with at-risk sexual partner(s) based on information provided by the IP. Evidence demonstrates that provider referral is more effective than partner referral.

Contract referral: This allows the IP and HA to negotiate an acceptable time span in which the IP will attempt to contact sexual partner(s). If unsuccessful, provider referral may follow by agreement.

No referral: Where PN is impractical (involves careful risk–benefit analysis), e.g. when there is insufficient information or a threat of violence to the IP or HA.

While partner notification remains a voluntary activity within the UK, countries such as Sweden and certain states of the USA have made it a legal requirement.

Sexual health promotion

Definition

Sexual health promotion is an activity which proactively and positively supports the sexual and emotional health and well-being of individuals, groups, communities, and the wider public, and reduces the risk of HIV transmission. The key aim is to ↓ inequalities in sexual health.

Specific aims

- ↓ transmission of HIV and STIs (advice on safe sex)
- ↓ prevalence of undiagnosed HIV and STIs by encouraging testing
- ↓ unintended pregnancy rates
- Education to ↓ stigma of STIs and HIV

Objectives include raising awareness, education and provision of information, and service-provider development.

Methods of sexual health promotion

These should be carefully chosen to match the needs of the target group. They can be divided into direct and indirect methods.

Direct methods

- National and local media health campaigns to ↑ public awareness
- Individual one-to-one work in a sexual health setting (health advisers, nurse specialists)
- Condom distribution, e.g in youth clinics, family planning clinics and primary care
- Screening for STIs and HIV in a variety of easily accessible settings
- Promoting self-care, e.g. over-the-counter emergency contraception, pregnancy testing, advice on testicular self-examination
- Targeted community work, particularly with marginalized and vulnerable groups (outreach, street, and group work)
- Dissemination of materials such as leaflets, posters, and magazines which also inform clients about local sexual health services
- Peer education programmes
- Sex and relationship education in formal and informal educational settings

Indirect methods

- Training courses and workshops for those involved in sexual health work
- Conferences where research and best practice can be shared
- Development of policies and strategies including local needs assessment
- Inter-agency working, especially within the voluntary and community sector (e.g. Terrence Higgins Trust)
- Support and advice to groups developing sexual health services
- Engaging in research
- Discussion with health commissioners to enable funding and provision of services.

Settings for sexual health promotion

Can be widespread in diverse settings by trained staff from different disciplines, including:

- schools
- further education, training colleges, and universities
- pubs, clubs, and recreational settings (e.g. gyms), including poster and leaflet displays, condom machines in toilets, etc.
- Residential care: for people with disabilities or learning difficulties, older adults, hostels for people seeking asylum, refuge from abuse, and people lacking permanent accommodation
- prison and young offenders' institutions
- drug and alcohol services: needle exchanges and methadone clinics
- sex venues such as saunas and cruising areas
- community centres including youth clubs and faith groups
- workplaces including armed services (barracks etc.), pharmacies, NHS
- clinic settings: GUM, 1° care, family planning, TOP clinics.

Good practice in health promotion

Accurate information should be provided that is clear, easily accessible, and up to date. It should be offered in a non-judgemental way, sensitive and respectful to the diversity of individual and community beliefs and attitudes. Misconceptions should be challenged, and stigma and prejudice should be actively discouraged. This information should empower individuals to make responsible decisions about their sexual health. Information should be evidence based. Discussion should be encouraged to explore ideas, thoughts, and feelings. Support should be available to all, but particularly those who are vulnerable and marginalized.

Performance targets

Department of Health Sexual Health Strategy (2001)

Hepatitis B vaccination

- All homosexual/bisexual men, sex workers, and injecting drug users attending GUM should be offered hepatitis B immunization at their first visit.
- Uptake of the first dose of vaccine in those not previously immunized should be 90%.
- Uptake of three doses of vaccine in those not previously immunized should be 70%.

HIV

All GUM attendees should be offered an HIV test on their first screening for STIs (and subsequently according to risk) with a view to:

- Increasing the uptake of the test by those offered it to 60%.

Specialty specific standards for physicians in GUM

Standard 1

The physician shall ensure that a sexual history is obtained and document-ed in all persons presenting to a GUM service with a new clinical problem. This shall be done in accordance with the current national guidelines for obtaining such a history. The physician should ensure that a sexual history is re-taken and documented at least every 6 months for persons being followed up for infectious conditions.

Standard 2

Physicians should offer an HIV antibody test to all persons attending a GUM clinic on the occasion of their first screening for STIs, unless the person is already known to be HIV antibody positive. The test shall be offered in accordance with current national guidelines.

Physicians should offer an HIV antibody test to all persons attending a GUM clinic on the occasion of their first screening for STIs, unless the person is already known to be HIV antibody positive. The test shall be offered in accordance with current national guidelines.

Ethical and medico-legal issues

Introduction

This section deals with some of the ethical and medico-legal aspects specific to HIV infection and GUM. Most medico-legal problems arise from:

- failure to appreciate legal responsibilities
- problems in clinical management
- medication errors
- administrative errors
- failure of communication and inadequate clinical records.

Awareness and adherence to relevant law and General Medical Council (GMC) guidance is essential. If in doubt seek advice from experienced colleagues, professional bodies, or medico-legal defence organizations.

Confidentiality

Common law and the Data Protection Act 1984 protect personal health information. Confidentiality is central to the trust between patient and healthcare professional (HCP). Without its explicit assurance the patient may not volunteer a full history and medical care may be compromised. It is particularly important for those dealing with sexually transmitted infections (STIs) where patients provide highly sensitive information. This is formally recognized by the NHS Trusts and Primary Care Trusts (Sexually Transmitted Diseases) Directions 2000 🕮 see p. 38. These apply to any healthcare setting and not just GUM clinics.

To maintain confidentiality the following practices should be adopted:

- anonymize patient data on records/forms/specimens by using identification (ID) numbers, dates of birth, or soundex codes (🕮 see p. 7)
- offer the patient a choice on how they would like to be called from the waiting room
- do not discuss patients outside the health team or where the conversation can be overheard by others
- ensure that any consultations are in private e.g. triage patients in a separate room, not at reception
- disclose information to general practitioner only following consent from the patient (unless it falls within the STD Directions 2000).

Public interest

There are some situations when confidentiality may be broken, however, it may be necessary to justify any decisions in accordance with GMC guidance. These include disclosures to protect both the patient or others. For example victims of knife crime, child abuse or domestic violence. Specific regulations apply to 'serious communicable diseases' including HIV, Hepatitis B and C, the latter two (and also hepatitis A) being notifiable. Problems may also be encountered if the patient is unable to take responsibility for his/her management (e.g. prisoners, mental health patients). Before breaching any confidential information this should be discussed and explained to the patient and with senior colleagues. Up to date GMC guidance should also be sought.

Consent

It is good practice and a legal requirement to obtain consent from a patient before treatment. Failure to do so can result in complaints to the individual's employing authority or relevant professional body, criminal proceedings for assault or indecent assault, and civil proceedings (e.g. if injuries arise following treatment without informed consent). To be valid, consent must be given voluntarily by a competent fully informed patient. A detailed discussion, clearly recorded in the notes, is required.

Consent is required for investigations, treatment, disclosure of information, research, photography/video recording, and teaching (e.g. medical students observing a consultation). In certain situations the use of a signed consent form is required. It must be made clear that refusal to participate in such activities will not compromise clinical care.

The person obtaining consent must be fully aware of the situation, ideally directly involved in it, and able to answer any queries. To help understanding, and therefore the ability to give valid consent, information should be provided clearly, using written or visual aids. If the patient cannot understand English, an interpreter, accredited if possible, should be provided and additional time set aside. In certain situations it is helpful to involve another member of the health team such as a health adviser. It may be necessary to provide time, over a number of sessions, to allow the patient to reach their informed decision.

To obtain consent for a screening test the patient should be aware of the following:
- description of the test
  - why the test is being taken
  - what it involves
- the likelihood of receiving positive or negative results
- implications of a positive result to the person and partner(s)
- any medical, social, or financial implications
- requirement for follow-up tests/treatment.

Mental Capacity Act 2005 (enacted October 2007)

Applies to England and Wales (similar principles apply in Scotland).

Statutory framework, largely based on common law, to empower and protect vulnerable people who may be unable to make their own decisions. It clarifies who can decide when and how to proceed. It also enables people to plan for a time when they may loose capacity through Lasting Powers of Attorney and Advanced Decisions. It only applies if the person is shown to lack capacity. When capacity to decide is lacking, the doctor should provide treatment in the patient's best interests under the common law doctrine of necessity, unless limitations apply.

Key principles
- A person must be assumed to have capacity unless it is established that he/she lacks capacity.
- A person is not to be treated as unable to make a decision unless all practical steps to help him/her to do so have been taken without success.
- A person is not to be treated as unable to make a decision merely because he/she makes an unwise decision.

- An act done, or decision made, under the Act for or on behalf of a person who lacks capacity must be done, or made, in his/her best interests.
- Before the act is done, or the decision is made, regard must be had to whether the purpose for which it is needed can be effectively achieved in a way that is less restrictive of the person's rights and freedom of action.

Capacity

For the purposes of the Act, a person lacks capacity in relation to a matter if at the material time he/she is unable to make a decision for him/herself in relation to the matter because of an impairment of, or a disturbance in, the functioning of the mind or brain. It does not matter whether the impairment or disturbance is permanent or temporary (e.g. symptoms of alcohol or drug use). Therefore capacity can fluctuate and the assessment made is relevant to the person's state at that time.

Capacity assessment

A person is unable to make a decision for him/herself if he/she is unable:
- to **understand** the information relevant to the decision (if information is given by simple language, visual aids, etc., may still be regarded as able to make the decision)
- to **retain** that information (if only for a short time, may still be regarded as able to make the decision)
- to **use or weigh** that information as part of the process of making the decision, or
- to **communicate** his/her decision (whether by talking, using sign language or any other means).

It is good practice for professionals carrying out a proper capacity assessment to record the findings in the relevant professional records. Ultimately the Court of Protection can make a decision about capacity.

Best interests

No statutory definition but:
- consider
  - whether (and if so, when) person will have capacity
  - if practicable, encouraging participation
  - if possible, the person's past wishes, beliefs, values, etc.
- take into account (if practicable and appropriate) the views of anyone named by the person to be consulted, e.g. carer, anyone interested in person's welfare, donee of a Lasting Powers of Attorney, Court Deputy
- when in relation to 'life-sustaining treatment' not to be motivated to bring about death when considering whether the treatment is in the best interests of the person concerned.

Exceptions:
- where the person has made a valid advance decision to refuse treatment
- in specific circumstances the involvement of a person who lacks capacity in research.

Ultimately the Court of Protection can be asked to make a decision. Always ensure that a written record is made of the process followed.

Consent: children

The age of consent for medical treatment in England, Scotland, Wales, and Northern Ireland is 16.

Competence

England and Wales

Any competent person, regardless of age, can give consent for medical treatment. A patient is competent if they can understand the choices and their consequences, including the nature, purpose, and possible risk of any treatment or non-treatment. Although parental support should be encouraged, if the patient does not wish the parent's involvement this view should not be overridden. When establishing if a patient under the age of 16 years is competent the Fraser Ruling (Gillick competence) should be followed. The Gillick case (*Gillick v West Norfolk and Wisbech Health Authority* [1985], 3 All ER 402 HL) established the current legal position in England and Wales. Although this ruling is directed towards contraceptive services, it can be extrapolated to include the management of STIs and details of the following points:

- the patient should be encouraged to inform his/her parents of the consultation
- the patient understands the potential risks and benefits of the treatment and advice
- the healthcare provider (HCP) must take into account whether the patient will engage in sexual activity without contraception
- the HCP must assess whether the patient's physical or mental health, or both, are likely to suffer if he/she does not receive contraceptive advice or supplies
- the HCP must consider whether the patient's best interests would require the provision of contraceptive advice or methods, or both, without parental consent.

Guidance published in 2004 highlights that where a request for contraception is made by a person under the age of 16, doctors and other HCPs should establish a rapport with the young person and give him/her the time and support to make an informed choice. They should do this by discussing:

- the emotional and physical implications of sexual activity, including the risks of pregnancy and STIs
- whether the relationship is mutually agreed or whether there may be coercion or abuse
- the benefits of informing their GP
- encouraging discussion with a parent of carer.

Any refusal should be respected. In the case of abortion, where the young woman is competent to consent but cannot be persuaded to involve a parent, every effort should be made to help her find another adult to provide support.

Scotland

Gillick competency is not relevant in Scotland. The Age of Legal Capacity (Scotland) Act 1991 gives statutory power to the minor to consent to medical or dental treatment. This act goes beyond the Fraser Ruling, stating that children <16 years have the legal capacity to consent to any surgical, medical, or dental treatment or procedure so long as that child is capable of understanding the nature and consequences of the proposed treatment or procedure. In England and Wales if a child refuses treatment, this can be overruled by a person with parental responsibility for the child or by the court. This is not the case in Scotland where the above Act protects the child's right to refuse examination or treatment, presuming the child has the capacity under the legislation.

Immature patients

GMC guidelines state that if a doctor does not consider the patient to be capable of giving consent because of immaturity, the relevant information may be disclosed to an appropriate person or authority if it is thought to be in the best interests of the patient. However, the following conditions should be met:

- the patient does not have sufficient understanding to appreciate the implications of advice or treatment
- the patient cannot be persuaded to involve an appropriate person in the consultation
- the doctor believes it is in the best medical interests of the patient.

Child protection issues

There is a duty of confidentiality to all patients, irrespective of their age. The exception is when disclosure of information is in their best medical interests or the patient or other vulnerable persons are at risk of harm. The HCP must be prepared to justify his/her decision to his/her professional body. Under such circumstances, if the patient cannot be persuaded to make a voluntary disclosure, the HCP should explain to the patient that confidentiality cannot be preserved. However, confidentiality is important for young people and it is important to ensure that there is no breach when that young person is not at risk.

The age of a 'child' for child protection purposes has been raised from 16 years to 18 years by the Sexual Offences Act 2003, applicable in England and Wales and, in part, in Northern Ireland (📖 Legislation pertinent to GUM p. 42).

Although legislature varies throughout the UK, the principles of care are similar. Key legislations relevant to safeguarding children are:

- The Children Act 1989
- Children (Scotland) Act 1995
- Education Act 2002
- Homelessness Act 2002
- Sexual Offences Act 2003
- The Children Act 2004.

- Key guidance documents underpinned by legislation are:
- England and Wales: *Working Together to Safeguard Children—A Guide to Inter-agency Working to Safeguard and Promote the Welfare of Children*
- Scotland: *Protecting Children—A Shared Responsibility*.

Social services are the lead agency for child protection with statutory responsibilities and the police have powers to intervene when there are concerns about a child's welfare. Local authorities are charged with establishing Local Safeguarding Children Boards (England and Wales) and Child Protection Committees (Scotland) which are the key statutory mechanisms for agreeing how relevant organizations will cooperate to safeguard and promote the welfare of children and ensure that this is done efficiently.

Child abuse is almost always committed by a perpetrator known (and often trusted) by the child. Abuse may be:
- physical
- emotional
- sexual
- neglect—this also includes the abuse of an unborn child (e.g. drug misuse during pregnancy) which may lead to inclusion on the Child Protection Register after the 20th week of pregnancy.

Sexual activity and abuse

Although the legal age of consent for sex is 16 years for both heterosexual and homosexual sex in the UK (except for Northern Ireland where it is 17 years), an estimated 25% of boys and girls are sexually active below this age.

Under 13 years

Not legally capable of consenting to sexual activity, and penetrative sex is classed as rape. Any offence under the Sexual Offences Act 2003 is very serious and should be taken to indicate a risk of significant harm to the child. All cases should be discussed with the child protection lead within the organization with the presumption that the case is then reported to social services. There may be situations where reporting is not considered to be necessary, but all must be fully documented including the reasons where a decision is taken not to share information.

The age of criminal responsibility in the UK is 10 years (except Scotland where it is 8 years).

13–15 years

Sexual activity with a child aged under 16 years is an offence. Where consensual it may be less serious than if the child were under 13, and the law is not intended to prosecute mutually agreed sexual activity between young people of a similar age unless it involves abuse or exploitation. However, it may have serious welfare consequences. In every case of sexual activity involving a child aged 13–15 consideration should be given as to whether there should be a discussion with other agencies and whether a referral should be made to social services. The professional should make this assessment using the considerations detailed in Box 2.1. Where confidentiality needs to be preserved, a discussion can still take place as long as the child is not identified. All cases should be fully documented and include detailed reasons where a decision is taken not to share information.

16 and 17 years

It is an offence for a person to have a sexual relationship with a 16- or 17-year-old if that person holds a position of trust or authority in relation to them. Otherwise, although sexual activity is unlikely to involve an offence, it may still involve harm or the risk of harm.

Box 2.1 Child assessment for risk (from *Working Together* 2006)

The following considerations should be taken into account when assessing the extent to which a child (or other children) may be suffering or at risk of harm, and therefore the need to hold a strategy discussion in order to share information:

- the age of the child – sexual activity at a young age is a very strong indicator that there are risks to the welfare of the child (whether boy or girl) and, possibly, others
- the level of maturity and understanding of the child
- what is known about the child's living circumstances or background
- age imbalance—in particular where there is a significant age difference
- overt aggression or power imbalance
- coercion or bribery
- familial child sex offences
- behaviour of the child, i.e. withdrawn, anxious
- the misuse of substances as a disinhibitor
- whether the child's own behaviour, because of the misuse of substances, places him/her at risk of harm so that he/she is unable to make an informed choice about any activity
- whether any attempts to secure secrecy have been made by the sexual partner, beyond what would be considered usual in a teenage relationship
- whether the child denies, minimizes, or accepts concerns
- whether the methods used are consistent with grooming
- whether the sexual partner(s) is known by one of the agencies.

Sexual offences

These include both ♂ and ♀ and apply irrespective of the relationship between those involved, e.g. a ♂ can be convicted of raping his wife.

Rape
- In law, rape can only be committed using the penis; it cannot be committed with an object.
- Penetration has to be proven in order to show that intercourse has taken place.
- It is not necessary for ejaculation to have taken place in order to prove the offence of rape.

In England and Wales a ♂ commits rape if he intentionally penetrates with his penis the vagina, mouth, or anus of another person, ♂ or ♀ without that person's consent or if they are under 13.

In Scotland rape is defined as vaginal penetration and is covered by common law. Anything else is the crime of indecent assault. Rape of a ♂ is treated under the common law offence of aggravated assault.

In Northern Ireland rape includes vaginal or anal intercourse with a ♂ or ♀ without their consent.

Women cannot be charged with rape, but in England and Wales may be charged with sexual assault by penetration.

Sexual assault by penetration (England and Wales)
It is an offence for someone ♂ or ♀ intentionally to penetrate the vagina or anus of another person with a part of their body or anything else without their consent. The purpose also has to be sexual defined as follows:
- a reasonable person would always consider it to be so, or
- if a reasonable person may consider it to be sexual, depending on the circumstances and intention.

NB: Excludes practitioners who legitimately conduct intimate searches or medical examinations.

Indecent/sexual assault
In England and Wales any unwanted sexual behaviour or touching of another person without reasonable belief that they consented. Touching covers all physical contact of a sexual nature (as defined above), whether with a part of the body or anything else, or though clothing. It may include forced acts of oral sex and forcing someone to watch pornography or masturbation.

In Scotland indecent assault on a ♂ or ♀ is a common law offence. In Northern Ireland indecent assault on a ♀ is a common law offence but in a ♂ it is provided for in the Criminal Justice (N. Ireland) Order 2003.
- Gross indecency: includes situations where a person tries to persuade a child under the age of 14 to touch them indecently.
- Buggery (sodomy): anal intercourse with someone who does not consent or is not yet 16 or where the intercourse is not done in private.

Causing a person to engage in sexual activity without consent

This offence covers non-consensual activity not within the definition of rape or sexual assault. It applies when a person intentionally causes another to engage in sexual activity without consent. Examples: person A forces person B to masturbate, A forces B to manually stimulate a third person, A compels B to penetrate her/him.

Indecent exposure

In England, Wales, and Northern Ireland it is an offence for someone, ♂ or ♀, to expose their genitals if they intended another person to see them and to be caused alarm or distress. In Scotland this is covered by common law.

Incest

Sexual abuse between a ♂ and his mother, sister, half-sister, daughter, or granddaughter, as well as between a ♀ and her father, brother, half-brother, son, or grandson, irrespective of consent.

Consent: specific issues

Epidemiological studies

Testing for epidemiological purposes (e.g. for HIV, hepatitis C virus) is important for planning disease management, but raises ethical issues. It generally involves screening surplus material (e.g. serum) taken for other tests to allow meaningful epidemiological data to be obtained, ensuring that it cannot be linked to the anonymous individual. However, it is acknowledged that the information gained will not directly benefit that person. It is generally agreed that the benefit to public health outweighs the ethical dilemma of testing without consent to avoid biased sampling. Written information explaining the nature of this testing should be available to patients within the clinic as leaflets or posters which must highlight the option to refuse without prejudice.

Testing in error

GMC guidance states that mistakes should be acknowledged, with apology, and appropriate support offered. The patient must be given the choice as to whether he/she is given the result of the test. If the patient refuses to receive a positive result (with health implications for that individual, partners, and others), advice should be obtained from professional bodies.

Occupational exposure to infection

In the case of a needlestick injury or other occupational exposure to a HCP it may be important to determine if the patient has a blood-borne infection such as HIV. If unconscious, the GMC advises that such testing should not be requested until consciousness has been regained and agreement obtained. In the event of a patient being unable to give consent for any reason, testing should not be carried out for the sole benefit of the healthcare worker. If the source's status is not known, this should be discussed with occupational health and legal advice sought.

Post-mortem testing for sexually transmitted blood-borne infections (HIV, hepatitis B and C, syphilis)

If a member of staff has been exposed to the blood or body fluids of a deceased patient, screening is permitted, although the agreement of a close relative or next of kin should be sought. Any person who is brainstem dead and being considered for organ donation requires screening for such infections, and this should be explained to the relatives.

Where a post-mortem is required, the deceased may be screened for these infections if relevant to the cause of death. Information should be disclosed regarding a positive diagnosis to any persons known to be at risk of the infection, e.g. sexual contacts; otherwise it must remain confidential.

Intimate examinations and chaperones

In 2001 the General Medical Council produced guidance on the use of chaperones (Box 2.2), which was reinforced in the Ayling Report published in 2004 recommending that trained chaperones are made available for all intimate examinations. The GMC issued revised guidance in 2006 under *Maintaining Boundaries*. It stresses the importance of patient perception as to what may be construed as being intimate. This is most likely to include examination of the breasts, genitalia, or rectum, but could also include any examination where it is necessary to touch or even be close to the patient (e.g. fundoscopy).

Chaperones

The GMC advises that, wherever possible, the patient should be offered the security of having an impartial observer (a 'chaperone') present during an intimate examination. This applies whether or not the examiner is the same gender as the patient. A chaperone does not have to be medically qualified but ideally should:

- be sensitive and respectful of the patient's dignity and confidentiality
- be prepared to reassure the patient if he/she shows signs of distress or discomfort
- be familiar with the procedures involved in routine intimate examinations
- be prepared to raise concerns about a doctor if misconduct occurs.

In GUM the use of friends and relatives (as endorsed in the Ayling Report) is not advised, as their use could compromise either the disclosure of important information which may only be volunteered during the examination or the personal relationship with the chaperone. In addition, it is unlikely that such a person will be familiar with the procedures involved and the doctor could be at risk of malicious accusations through collusion.

In GUM it is standard accepted practice to provide a chaperone when ♀ patients are examined by ♂ doctors. In all other situations a chaperone should be offered, although the acceptance rate is low. A report from an Australian sexual health clinic published in 2007 records that only 7.3% and 6% of ♂ patients expressed a desire for a chaperone when being examined by ♂ and ♀ practitioners, respectively. The equivalent figures for ♀ patients were 26.8% and 5.5%.

In 2002, the Royal College of Nursing produced guidance on *Chaperoning: The Role of the Nurse and Rights of Patients*, which largely related to the nurse acting as a chaperone and the availability of one for any examination or procedure. However, it states that 'nurses and other health care professionals should also consider being accompanied by a chaperone when undertaking intimate examinations and procedures to avoid misunderstanding and, in rare cases, false accusations of abuse'.

Box 2.2. The intimate examination and conduct
(GMC guidance)

Before conducting an intimate examination you should:
- explain to the patient why an examination is necessary and give the patient an opportunity to ask questions;
- explain what the examination will involve, in a way the patient can understand, so that the patient has a clear idea of what to expect, including any potential pain or discomfort;
- obtain the patient's permission before the examination and record that permission has been obtained;
- give the patient privacy to undress and dress and keep the patient covered as much as possible to maintain their dignity. Do not assist the patient in removing clothing unless you have clarified with them that your assistance is required.

During the examination you should:
- explain what you are going to do before you do it and, if this differs from what you have already outlined to the patient, explain why and seek the patient's permission;
- be prepared to discontinue the examination if the patient asks you to;
- keep discussion relevant and do not make unnecessary personal comments.

Chaperones
You should record any discussion about chaperones and its outcome. If a chaperone is present, you should record that fact and make a note of their identity. If the patient does not want a chaperone, you should record that the offer was made and declined.

HCP–patient relationship

Patients attending GUM clinics can be both physically and emotionally vulnerable because of the intimate details they often have to reveal. Staff must not allow themselves to be influenced by any personal or professional relationship with the patient. It is important for the HCP to explain to the patient precisely what is involved during an examination. Complaints of indecent assault have been made by patients against HCPs irrespective of the gender of either. Therefore all patients should be offered a chaperone for any intimate examination and this should be documented. The use of friends and relatives is not advised, as their presence could compromise the disclosure of important information. As in any medical setting, courtesy and good communication are essential. Should a complaint be made an explanation with a simple apology, if appropriate, may be sufficient to resolve the issue.

Guidelines

National management guidelines are available (📖 Useful resources p. 615). However, departmental or regional guidelines may be produced to reflect local variations in clinical practice. Guidelines, whether national or local, must be available to all staff and updated regularly in line with clinical evidence-based expert opinion. Demonstrating that guidelines were followed and therefore a recognized standard of care was provided can refute a clinical complaint. As guidelines are updated, it is also important to archive old versions which may be required for a retrospective review.

Staff meetings should be used to highlight any guideline changes and discuss any issues regarding them. Where possible services within geographical areas should follow the same or have similar guidelines to allow consistency in patient management. This can be achieved through regional GUM networks which may also help with funding issues over certain management options if regional guidelines advise on them.

Prescribing

Medication errors account for a high level of complaints and claims. This is usually due to errors that can be avoided by simple checking procedures and a clear explanation to the patient. The following are common causes of error: badly transcribed instructions, illegible prescriptions, miscalculation of dosage, prescribing contraindicated drugs, not checking for potential drug interactions, not reviewing repeat prescriptions, and failure to act on laboratory results. Good prescribing practice should involve clear verbal and written instructions to the patient, checking for drug interactions and taking a history for any possible contraindications.

In unusual or complex situations or when the treatment advised is unfamiliar, check with an experienced colleague or pharmacist before prescribing or dispensing.

Patient records

It is a requirement of professional organizations and good medical practice to keep clear, accurate, and legible notes. They are also essential in dealing with complaints and claims. Records should contain information on how a diagnosis was reached and information given to the patient. At all times care must be taken to ensure that there is no unintentional disclosure of third-party information. The use of a clinic pro forma sheet for general consultations and screening and for more specialized situations such as sexual assault can greatly improve clinical record keeping, by ensuring all essential information is sought and detailed. Notes must be dated and clearly signed by the individual who should also indicate their status.

The Data Protection Act 1984 and the Access to Medical Records Act 1990 allow patients the right to see their medical records. In order to protect third-party confidentiality, it is wise to record ID numbers rather than names in a patient's case notes when referring to sexual contacts. If patients obtain formal access to their records all third-party information must be removed.

Storage of patient's records should be in a secure part of the GUM clinic. Records should be retained for a minimum of 8 years (Public Records Acts 1958 and 1967). In the case of children and young people they should be retained until the individual's 25th birthday (26th if the notes were made when the patient was aged 17). Records of patients attending with syphilis or HIV may be held for the period of time dictated by locally agreed policy, and prolonged storage may be required for the case records of those enrolled in research.

Electronic technology

The use of computer records, e-mails, faxes, and text messages has the potential for breaching patient confidentiality. The GMC has guidelines for the security of personal information by electronic processing. If necessary, specialist advice should be sought on the security of such information.

To maintain patient confidentiality and confidence in the service, computerized medical record systems must overtly exhibit a high level of security. Many clinics have stand-alone systems, but if linked to a network, robust systems must be in place to ensure that sensitive patient information cannot be accessed by any unauthorized personnel including HCPs working in other services. Individual computers should be password protected, especially for patient-related information, with the level of information accessible appropriate to the staff member involved. As with written records, patients have the right of access to all electronically held material with the exclusion of third-party information.

Computers and fax machines should be kept in a secure setting, computer passwords should be changed regularly, and any information sent by e-mail should be encrypted as it may be intercepted. The use of pre-arranged codes can help protect confidentiality.

Partner notification issues

If a person infected with an STI is reluctant to inform sexual partners, you may disclose information about a patient, whether living or dead, in order to protect a person from risk or serious harm. For example, you may disclose information to a known sexual contact of a patient with HIV where you have reason to think that the patient has not informed that person and cannot be persuaded to do so. In such circumstances you should tell the patient before you make the disclosure and you must be prepared to justify a decision to disclose information. In such circumstances clear documentation and discussion with colleagues is vital.

This situation is more difficult. The patient must be counselled that they have the duty to inform any sexual partners of their infection. This is especially relevant to someone who continues to carry a chronic infection such as HIV or hepatitis B and C viruses and remains infectious. It is also essential to document such advice in the patient's case records.

Ethically, the same principles apply to the other STIs although the consequences compared with HIV infection are generally less serious.

Numerous prosecutions have taken place for the 'reckless' transmission of HIV. These have been based on Section 20 of the Offences against the Person Act, which was not designed for HIV transmission. Guidance from the Crown Prosecution service recommends the following.

- The defendant needs to have known they were infectious to others and how the infection is transmitted.
- The defendant needs to know they were infectious at the time of transmission, or have good reason to believe they were infected, without actually being tested.
- They will need to show that they disclosed their HIV status to their partner prior to consensual sex.
- Phylogenetic analysis of the HIV in both must be used to show that they are the likely source of infection
- Transmission must take place for a 'reckless' charge. However, there is a charge of 'attempted intentional transmission' (to date no one has been prosecuted with this).
- Prosecutions are unlikely to take place for one-off sexual encounters.
- Guidance on condom use is not clear. However, it is likely that a condom would have to be absent or inadequate for a prosecution to take place.

The Terrence Higgins Trust can be contacted by patients for advice on 0845 1221 200, if they are concerned about the possibility of prosecution. Guidance is available on ℘ www.cps.gov.uk/legal/section7/chapter_h.html

Asylum seekers and refugees

It is important that no individual is discriminated against when establishing their right to free NHS care. To avoid this all patients need to be asked where they have lived for the last 12 months; this cannot be judged on their appearance, nationality, or language. To assist with patients who may not be entitled, every trust should have an overseas manager.

One of the following documents is required to confirm refugee or asylum seeker status:

• a letter from the Home Office stating the patient is a refugee
• a letter from the Home Office confirming that the patient has made an application for asylum
• a travel document issued in the UK in accordance with the convention on the status of refugees.

Definitions

Ordinary resident: living lawfully in the UK voluntarily and for settled purposes. (often taken to be for last 12-month period, but this is a guideline for screening questions rather than the true definition).

Asylum seeker: an individual who has made a formal application to the Home Office for recognition as a refugee under the 1951 UN Convention.

Refugee: any person who 'owing to a well founded fear of being persecuted for reasons of race, religion, nationality, membership of a particular social group or political opinion, is outside the country of his nationality and is unable, or owing to such fear, is unwilling to avail himself of the protection of that country' (1951 UN Convention relating to the status of refugees).

Illegal immigrant: person in the UK without proper permission; usually entered on visitors' visa and not returned or application for asylum refused.

Failed asylum seeker: when application has been rejected after an initial decision and appeal. They are either deported or leave voluntarily.

Indefinite leave to remain: given to people recognized as refugees, allowing them to remain in the UK without a time limit.

Exceptional leave to remain: a discretionary status usually granted to someone who does not qualify as a refugee, but has genuine humanitarian reasons for staying in the UK.

Confidentiality

Sometimes, for administrative purposes, health information is requested by third parties. Patients need to know this and that information concerning HIV status can be useful when planning appropriate care if relocated. However, no information can be passed on without the patient's prior consent.

Exception from medical charge

Refugees, anyone who has formally applied for asylum, and those with exceptional leave to remain are exempt from charges for medical treatment under the NHS. (Statutory Instrument No 306, NHS Regulations 1989). The DoH Guidance *Implementing the Overseas visitors Hospital Charging Regulations* (January 2007) provides a full list of exemptions for charging. There is separate guidance for Scotland and Wales. Northern Ireland has no charging arrangements. Treatment for STIs should be available free of charge to any patient, as are family planning services. The exception is HIV and AIDS, where only the initial test and counselling are free of charge to those not entitled to full NHS treatment (except in Scotland where HIV care is free), and termination of pregnancy (National Health Service Act 1977, Schedule 12, Section 77). However, withholding proper medical care from someone with a serious illness could contravene Article 2 (Right to Life) or Article 3 (Freedom from Torture) of the Human Rights Act 1998. The DoH guidance states that the decision whether treatment is immediately necessary is a clinical judgement and not to be undertaken by administrative staff. Any charge for such treatment will still stand, but if it proves to be unrecoverable then it should be written off. HIV treatment can be considered to be always immediately necessary (life saving and to prevent the condition becoming life threatening). Those unsuccessful in asylum application can continue with treatment for a condition free of charge (continue their HIV care including starting antiretrovirals) as long as they have completed 12 months residency. If they develop a new condition, this will be chargeable. Treatment for many infectious diseases, including TB, is free to all; a full list of these is available in the DoH guidance.

Details of those entitled to full NHS hospital treatment are available at ℘ www.doh.gov.uk/overseasvisitors.

Mental health patients

Mental Health Act 2007

This only refers to treatment for the mental condition itself and not any physical condition. However, the two may be closely linked, e.g. in advanced HIV or late syphilis. Sometimes the courts may be called upon to determine what is and is not 'treatment of the psychiatric condition'.

Consent

Any competent mental health patient attending for STI screening or treatment must be consenting. Even if the patient is sectioned under the Mental Health Act consent is still required, unless the STI is directly related to the mental condition. The exception is when the patient is not mentally competent to make a decision, when testing or treatment may be performed in the patient's 'best interests' under common law. In such circumstances it is advisable to seek a second opinion from an experienced colleague and document the reasons clearly.

Confidentiality

If the patient attends with a mental health nurse, offer an alternative chaperone – the patient may be uncomfortable in discussing sexual health issues in the company of staff responsible for his/her mental health. Only relevant information relating to the mental health or treatment of the patient should be passed on, with the patient's consent. The exception would be a condition causing potential harm to others, e.g. a positive HIV result in a violent mental health patient.

Prisoners

HCPs, whether working in clinics within or outside the prison, should not disclose anything about the prisoner's state of health to security guards. The prisoner is entitled to be examined in private. An exception (thereby allowing prison guards to be present in the same room) should only be made to prevent any disorder or crime, or for protection of the HCP's rights and freedoms (Article 8(1) of the European Convention on Human Rights).

HIV-positive HCPs

The GMC advises that doctors or other HCPS with a serious communicable disease, such as HIV, are entitled to the same level of confidentiality and support as every other patient. However, if there is knowledge or good reason to believe that the HCP is practising, or has practised, in a way which places patients at risk, an appropriate person in the HCPs' employing authority, e.g. an occupational health physician, or a relevant regulatory body must be informed. Wherever possible the HCP concerned must be advised before such information is passed on to an employer or regulatory body. The Public Interest Disclosure Act 1998 protects any employee who discloses concerns about a colleague in the public's best interests.

Death

Living wills

These allow competent people to give instructions about what is to be done if they subsequently lose the capacity to decide or communicate.

Advance statements These are not legally binding. They are a statement written on preferences of care, such as type of diet preferred (e.g. vegetarian) and type of bathing preferred. They can be overridden in the individual's 'best interests'.

Advance decisions These are legally binding. They document decisions to refuse certain treatments should they lose capacity. However, strict formalities are required when that treatment would be required to sustain life.

Lasting power of attorney A person can appoint another to act on their behalf if they should lose capacity in the future. The attorney is able to make both health and welfare decisions.

Death certificates

GMC guidance states that if HIV or any other STI has contributed to the death it is unlawful to omit this from the death certificate.

Release of information after death

Any information recorded after 1 November 1991 is subject to the Access to Health Records Act 1990. This states that a deceased patient's representative has a statutory right of access to health information which is directly relevant to a claim. However, no information can be provided if the patient has requested non-disclosure and this is recorded in their records. Results of investigations that the deceased believed to be confidential may not be disclosed. Therefore it is important to counsel patients on such matters, especially with sensitive diagnoses like HIV. Problems may arise when an insurance company refuses payment under a life insurance policy if a doctor refuses to disclose information. Despite this, any information that the doctor believed the patient would have wished to remain confidential should not be disclosed. Information recorded before November 1991 cannot be disclosed, as the duty of confidentiality extends beyond death. If further advice is required this should be sought from the medical ethics committee via the BMA.

Writing statements and court appearances

Statements may be required for a variety of reasons – from insurance companies, solicitors, or a police statement.

Before writing a statement the following should be established:

- *What questions the enquirer wants answered.* Exclude irrelevant information.
- Whether the information provided is as a *professional witness* (a factual report concerning a patient to whom the doctor has provided care) or an *expert witness* (to give an opinion concerning a patient who may not have been under the care of that individual).
- *Has the patient given consent?* Always check that the patient understands what the information is for and that they have consented to it being passed onto a third party, even if the person requesting the information states that the patient has given consent. However, consent is not required for a coroner's statement or if demanded by an order of the court.
- *Is the statement required to deal with criticism regarding the medical management of the patient?* Always consult defence organizations prior to sending any completed statement.

Doctors are usually only required in court if there is dispute as to the contents of any statements provided. If called to court because of the medical management of a patient, the doctor involved should contact his/her defence organization for advice.

Legislation pertinent to GUM

▶ Although there are differences in the legal systems and instruments within the countries constituting the UK, the general principles affecting the management of patients are similar.

NHS Trusts and Primary Care Trusts (Sexually Transmitted Diseases) Directions 2000

These came into force on 1 April 2000 replacing the NHS Trusts (Venereal Diseases) Regulations and apply only to England.

Confidentiality of information

Every NHS Trust and Primary Care Trust shall take all necessary steps to secure that any information capable of identifying an individual obtained by any of their members or employees with respect to persons examined or treated for any sexually transmitted disease shall not be disclosed except:

- for the purposes of communicating that information to a medical practitioner, or to a person employed under the direction of a medical practitioner in connection with the treatment of persons suffering from such disease or the spread thereof; and
- for the purpose of such treatment or prevention.

National Health Service Act 1977 (Schedule 12, Section 77)

The Act states that no charge is to be made to patients in relation to any medication or investigation required in the treatment of venereal diseases. Treatment for sexually transmitted infections (referred to as venereal disease in the text) should be available free of charge. The exception is HIV and AIDS where only the initial test and counselling is free to those not entitled to full NHS treatment.

Addendum HM (68) 84, section 27 accompanying the 1968 NHS (VD) Regulation SI 1624 Article 3

This states that medical and other staff involved in contact tracing are not liable to defamation.

The Aids Control Act 1987

This Act relates to the collection and annual reporting of statistics relating to HIV and AIDS. It further addresses the availability of facilities and staff for testing, consultation, treatment, and health education. Note that HIV and AIDS are not notifiable diseases.

The Sexual Offences Act 1967

This Act permits male homosexual practices by two consenting adults in private. The age of consent for sex between men was lowered from 21 to 18, and more recently further reduced to 16 in England, Wales, and Scotland, and 17 in Northern Ireland.

Sexual Offences Act 2003 (enacted May 2004)

This act more closely defines 'consent' and the abuse of trust, especially with regard to children. The age of a 'child' set in the Protection of Children Act 1978 has been raised from 16 to 18 years. Although it should not alter normal practice, clinic staff need to be aware that 'children' up to the age of 18 years fall within its protection. It redefines 'sexual' with, for example, attention to 'grooming', use of the Internet, child pornography, prostitution, administration of a substance with intent to commit a sexual offence, and other miscellaneous offences including voyeurism and bestiality.

It protects the public, especially children, from sexual harm. Sexual offences prevention orders replace sex offenders and restraining orders. In addition, new sexual harm and foreign travel orders have been created.

In view of concerns expressed by those providing sexual healthcare and advice to young people, a statute has been introduced to ensure that a person does not commit an offence if the action taken is to:

- protect the child from STIs
- protect the physical safety of the child
- prevent the child from becoming pregnant
- promote the child's well-being with advice.

This is conditional that such action does not cause or encourage a child's participation and is not for the purpose of obtaining sexual gratification.

Anyone who acts to protect a child (e.g. teachers, relatives, friends), and not just HCPs, are now covered.

The Prohibition of Female Circumcision Act 1985

This makes female genital mutilation an offence except on specific physical or mental health grounds. A local authority may exercise its responsibility to make enquiries under section 47 of the Children's Act 1989 if it has reason to believe that a child is likely to be or has been the subject of female genital mutilation.

The Public Health (Infectious Diseases) Regulations 1988 SI 1988/1546 (England and Wales)

Modification of section 38 of the Act as it applies to AIDS states that 'justice of the peace may on application of any local authority make an order for the detention in hospital of an inmate of that hospital suffering from AIDS… if the justice is satisfied that on his leaving hospital proper precautions to prevent the spread of that disease would not be taken by him, (a) in his lodging or accommodation or (b) in other places to which he may be expected to go if not detained in hospital.'

The Public Health Regulations (Notification of Infectious Diseases) (Scotland) Regulations 1988 SI 1988/1550:

These Regulations make no reference to AIDS.

Public Health (Control of Diseases) Act 1984 or Public Health (Infectious diseases) Regulations 1988

These Acts list notifiable diseases. Among the many infections, it should be remembered that hepatitis A, B, and C are all notifiable. Any doctor who makes the diagnosis is required by statute to notify the proper officer of their local authority.

The standard clinic process and sexual health in primary care

The genitourinary medicine (GUM) patient

It is estimated that 1 in 7 adults over the age of 16 in the UK has attended a GUM clinic at least once. Many who attend may not harbour an active sexually transmitted infection (STI) but wish to exclude one. The 'GUM patient' does not fit a single stereotype. While it may be more common for young people to attend, a wide age range from <16 to >60 are seen. Their demographic characteristics vary, depending on the risk factors of the local and commuting population and the acceptability and accessibility of GUM services to potential users. Slightly more ♂ than ♀ attend, with sexuality and ethnicity varying geographically. The following groups of people are more likely to attend:

- ♂ aged 25–34
- ♀ aged 16–24
- those who have changed sexual partners recently
- those having multiple sexual partners
- those single, separated, or divorced.

Special situations

The distressed or aggressive patient

While most patients attending may feel anxious and embarrassed, some are intensely distressed. The psychological responses to STIs or risk of such include severe anxiety, depression, a strong sense of stigma, shame, feelings of guilt, low self-esteem, and anger. Strong negative responses such as these may hamper communication and lead to apparently irrational behaviour. It is necessary to understand and appraise the emotional state of the patient when providing optimum care. If a patient is aggressive, the priority should be safety while attempting to de-escalate the situation.

Under-age patient (📖 Chapter 5, Children p. 108)

Adolescents <16 years attending GUM have a high incidence of STIs and report a low use of reliable contraception. Some may also have suffered sexual abuse.

Survivors of sexual assault or rape (📖 Sexual assault: general principles p. 102)

May attend for sexual health screen and STI risk assessment and due consideration should be given to any post-traumatic stress that may dominate the patient's mood and emotions.

Risk factors

Social and demographic

The following risk factors have been noted in various epidemiological studies. They are likely to vary over time and across different geographic regions but are useful in planning local service provision and targeting specific sexual health promotion. Clinically they are useful in risk assessment.

- Age <25 years: the highest rates of gonococcal and chlamydial infections occur in age groups 16–19 years in ♀ and 20–24 years in ♂.
- Being single: separated, divorced, or not in a stable relationship (compared with marital, stable relationship, or widowed status) are associated with higher rates of STIs.
- ≥2 partners in preceding 6 months.
- Use of non-barrier contraception.
- Residence in inner city.
- Symptoms in partner.
- History of previous STI.
- Ethnicity or migration: prevalence of several infections, notably syphilis, gonorrhoea, and HIV infection, is higher in certain ethnic minority groups and immigrants
- Sexual orientation: for example, syphilis, gonorrhoea, HIV, and hepatitis B virus infections are more prevalent among ♂ who have sex with ♂ (MSM).

Sexual

Certain types of physical contact carry higher risks for certain infections, e.g. penetrative sex and HIV, orogenital contact and anogenital herpes.

Types of sexual practice

Knowledge of the wide range of sexual practices and the vocabulary in use is of value in advising those at risk of STIs.

Sexuality and relationship

- Heterosexuality (opposite sex): (heterophilia, 'straight')
- Bigynist (sex between 1 ♂ and 2 ♀), bivirist (sex between 1 ♀ and 2 ♂).
- Homosexuality (same sex): general (homophilia, 'gay', iterandria, uranism).
- Cruising describes searching for MSM partners in public places, e.g. common land, saunas, bath-houses, toilets (cottaging).
- ♀ homosexuality: lesbianism, cymbalism, gynecozygous.
- Bisexuality (both sexes): ambisexual, amphisexual, androgynophilia, sexoschizia.
- Cybersex: use of the Internet to deliver sexual pleasure.

'Safe sex' (no penetration by penis into vagina, anus, or mouth)

Arousal from kissing (basoexia), manual genital stimulation (mutual masturbation and heavy petting), body rubbing (frottage and 'dry rooting'), rubbing buttocks (pygotripsis), feet (podophilia), kneading flesh (sarmassophilia); tickling (titillagnia), lap dancing (squatting above a sitting person and non-genital rubbing).

Penile positioning into the axilla (axillism), between breasts (coitus a mammilla and mazophallate), between legs (coitus interfermoris), between knees (genuphallation).

Genital stimulation using the mouth

- Insufflation: blowing air into a body cavity, usually the vagina).
- Penile oral sex: fellatio, 'blow-job', corvus, irrumation, penosugia.
- ♀ genital oral sex: cunnilingus, gamahucheur, clitorilingus (clitoral tongue stimulation).

Anorectal stimulation

- General terms for anal sex: anocratism, arsometry, buggery, coitus analis, pederasty, proctophallism, sodomy, sotadism.
- Oral stimulation: analinctus and hedralingus (anal licking), anophilemia (anal kissing), analingus and rimming (anal penetration with tongue).
- Specific penile anal sex: androsodomy (with ♂), anomeatia (with ♀).
- Manual: fisting, brachioprotic eroticism (fist/arm into anorectal canal).

Arousal with body fluids

- Urine: golden enema/douche/shower (urine deposited into anus/vagina/over body), urolagnia, urophilia, water sports.
- Faeces (scat): coprolagnia and coprophilia (arousal), coprophagy (consumption).
- Miscellaneous: hygrophilia (body fluids), blood sports (blood), mucophage (ingestion of mucous secretions), salirophilia (ingestion of sweat or saliva), felching (ingestion of semen from vagina or anus), emetophilia and Roman shower (vomit and vomiting over partner).

Sadomasochism

- Sadism:arousal by inflicting pain.
- Masochism (pain translated to erotic feelings).
- Algophilia and doleros (arousal from pain).

Examples: caning/flagellation (using cane/whip), bondage/strangulation (physical restraint/constriction), electrophilia (arousal from electricity), meatotomy (urethral dilation).

Sex with animals

Bestiality, zoophilia. Specific examples include cynophilia (dogs), entomophilia (insects), ophidiophilia (snakes), felching (inserting animals into vagina or anus).

Use of sex toys and piercings

- Arousal enhancers: penis substitutes (dildos, vibrators, olisbos, anal, butt plugs) and genital piercings (rings, bars, beads, wires, etc).
- Erection sustainers: rings and bands (e.g. cock ring).

Use of drugs during sex

- Amyl nitrite for euphoria and sphincter relaxation.
- Crack cocaine ↑ desire.
- Alcohol and some tranquillizing drugs (sometimes used illicitly, e.g. 'drug rape') remove inhibitions.

The sexual history

Taking a sexual history and discussing sexual health issues are vital elements of the consultation, eliciting essential information on the STI risk. It must be non-judgemental and empathic, thereby promoting effective patient participation. When taking a sexual history:

- Put the patient at ease with proper initial introduction and positioning.
- Reassure regarding confidentiality.
- Explain why a sexual history is needed.
- Check if patient agrees to be asked personal questions.
- Ideally interview the patient alone but respect the patient's desire to have a third person present which may help to ↓ anxiety.
- Avoid distractions during the consultation.
- Display a non-judgemental attitude.
- Do not make assumptions about patient's sexuality or sexual behaviour.
- Listen actively and maintain adequate eye contact, observing non-verbal communication.
- Use language the patient understands, avoiding jargon, with appropriate intonation, pauses, and cues to gain information.
- Reflect what patient says to clarify and confirm.

Pro formas ensure a systematic approach to history-taking (Algorithm 3.1). Asking when last sexual intercourse took place is a useful way to start the sexual history (details of sexual partners, contraception, and sexual risks). Presence of a third person, especially sexual partner, may inhibit this. Types of sexual practices reported can help in planning which specimens to obtain. Obtain any information patient has on the nature of sexual partner's infection(s). Where mother-to-child transmission is relevant enquire about clinical presentations in the children.

Conducting the consultation through an interpreter or when cross-cultural issues are relevant may be difficult. It is preferable to use an unrelated interpreter but sometimes this may not be possible.

1. Introduce yourself and your position to the patient. He/she may be anxious or feeling guilty and therefore it is important to put him/her at ease as soon as possible.

2. Determine the presenting problem or concern. There may be information available to you (e.g. contact information) which should be accessed before and not in the presence of the patient.

| Personal concern | Concern arising because of STI contact |

Obtain information about presenting problem or concern (its nature, duration, other relevant symptoms, etc).

Obtain information as to the patient's knowledge of his/her contact and nature of the infection. Do not divulge any sensitive 3rd party information. It may be necessary to explain in some detail the rationale for partner notification and potential benefit to your patient. Enquire about any relevant symptoms etc.

Obtain relevant background information
- Past STIs and other relevant present and past medical history
- For ♀, contraceptive, gynaecological, and obstetric history
- Current/recent drug history and drug allergies
- Drug misuse

Sexual history
- Last sexual contact—date, relationship (regular/casual), sex (male/female), country (if relevant). More detailed information may be obtained such as the type of contact and use of protection (condoms) though the latter merely ↓ risk and should not alter immediate clinical practice except for HIV post-exposure prophylaxis.
- Other contacts in last 3 months (incubation/ latent period for most symptomatic STIs) and last 12 months (helpful in risk assessment).

Finally
- Thank patient for providing this information (often embarrassing to them).
- Discuss and explain further recommended investigation and management plans based on the information available.

Algorithm 3.1 Taking a sexual history

Routine examination: general principles

Prior to the examination the patient should be given an explanation and his/her agreement obtained. Certain procedures require written consent (e.g. local anaesthesia, minor surgery, and clinical photography).

The examination room should be warm and comfortable with a screened area allowing privacy while the patient undresses. An examination couch with good lighting is required (with stirrups/leg rests for ♀ to allow examination in the semi-lithotomy position).

The patient should undress below the waist and be provided with drapes or gowns. Irrespective of the gender of the patient or the examiner, a chaperone must be offered (◻ GMC Guidance 2001, p. 25), who may also be able to assist in the collection of specimens and reassure the nervous patient. The acceptance or refusal of a chaperone should be documented in the patient's notes. Chaperones should sign to confirm their attendance during the examination. Although the GMC suggests that a patient's friend or relative could act as a sole chaperone, this is not advised in GUM as it may compromise confidentiality and the provision of relevant information to the healthcare professional (HCP).

The examination trolley should be set up prior to the examination. Specula should be pre-warmed in water, which also acts as a vaginal lubricant. Lubricating gels should be avoided whenever possible as they may inhibit the growth of *Neisseria gonorrhoeae*. The use of lubricants cannot be avoided for proctoscopy, but care should be taken to ensure that swabs are not contaminated. During examination the patient should be kept informed of progress, but unnecessary or facetious comments must be avoided. Convenient facilities should be available to obtain urine specimens.

Serology

A venous blood sample for syphilis and HIV should be taken with consent from patients at risk of an STI. Because of the sensitivity arising from HIV testing and the implications of a positive result, additional discussion may be required to ensure fully informed consent (◻ HIV pre-test discussion p. 436). Testing for hepatitis B and C virus may also be required.

Examination

General

Skin rashes/lesions, generalized lymphadenopathy, hair loss, jaundice, mucosal lesions (orogenital), conjunctivitis/uveitis, and arthritis may arise from STIs, and genital problems may be features of dermatological or systemic diseases.

Women (Fig. 3.1)

- Inspect the entire pubic and anogenital area ensuring that the labia are parted and the clitoral hood gently retracted.
- Palpate the inguinal area for lymphadenopathy.
- Urethral specimens. There is doubt about the value of routine urethral samples for Gram staining and culture for *N.gonorrhoeae*; however, they have been shown to be useful on occasions. Urethral sampling may be deferred until the end of the examination as it may cause discomfort. The addition of a urethral swab to an endocervical specimen ↑ the detection of chlamydial infection.
- Introduce a speculum lubricated with warm water.
- Inspect the vagina and cervix for atypical discharge, mucosal lesions, and signs of inflammation.
- Take vaginal material from the posterior vaginal pool/vaginal walls using a loop or swab and prepare a suspension in normal saline on a slide protected with a cover-slip. An additional swab should be prepared as a Gram-stained smear.
- If cervical cytology is required it is best taken at this stage.
- Before microbiological sampling clean the cervix using a cotton ball held in a sponge-holder to remove vaginal material
- Take an endocervical swab to prepare a Gram-stained smear and to plate onto selective medium for *N.gonorrhoeae* (or send in transport medium, e.g. Amies, Stuart).
- Take an endocervical swab for *Chlamydia trachomatis*, rotating it within the walls of the cervical canal. Although cervical specimens are not essential with nucleic acid amplification tests (NAATs), it is important to inspect the cervix (especially for mucopurulent cervicitis) and to take swabs for *N.gonorrhoeae*. Hence it is also reasonable to screen this site for *C.trachomatis*.
- If there are any signs or symptoms to suggest lower abdominal or pelvic pathology offer a bimanual pelvic and abdominal examination.
- Urine specimens should be obtained if pregnancy testing is required or a urinary tract infection (mid-stream sample) suspected. They can also be used for chlamydia testing (1st 20mL) by NAAT and for certain enzyme immunoassays (EIAs).

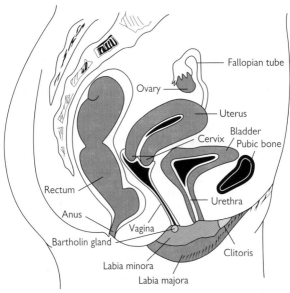

Fig. 3.1 Female genital anatomy

Men (Fig. 3.2)

- Inspect the entire pubic and anogenital area for skin lesions, masses, discharges, and signs of infestation. This includes the glans penis and sub-preputial sac by retracting the prepuce.
- Palpate the inguinal area for lymphadenopathy and scrotal contents for masses, tenderness, and other anomalies.
- Examine the urethral meatus for discharge and skin lesions, especially warts. If there is urethral exudate, any symptom of urethritis, or history of penile sexual contact with gonorrhoea, a gentle scraping from the urethra should be taken using a small plastic loop and smeared onto a microscope slide for Gram-staining. It may be necessary for the urethra to be gently massaged to obtain a specimen. Ideally samples should be taken 3–4 hours after last micturition.
- The same loop can then be used to plate directly onto selective medium for *N.gonorrhoeae* even if there is no material to prepare a slide. If a transport medium (e.g. Amies or Stuart) is used, a separate swab is required which the laboratory should ideally receive within 48 hours for plating provided that it is kept refrigerated.
- Urethral sampling for *C.trachomatis* can be undertaken at this time using an NAAT (or EIA). It is recommended that a fine urethral swab is inserted 1–4cm into the urethra and rotated once against the urethral wall, although in clinical practice this is often not possible. Alternatively, urine can be tested by NAAT or EIA licensed for urine specimens.
- Finally, the patient should provide a first voided 20mL urine specimen (ideally having retained their urine for 3–4 hours before testing). As well as providing a test sample for *C.trachomatis* it can also be examined for threads, a possible indicator of urethritis. A second, mid-stream sample can be obtained especially if urinary tract infection needs to be excluded. Samples can also be tested by dipstick for blood, protein, glucose, nitrites, and leucocytes as required.

Extra-genital infection

Rectum In those at risk, especially MSM, proctoscopy and screening for *N.gonorrhoeae* and *C.trachomatis* (if NAAT is available) should be offered, remembering that infection may occur without penile penetration. The anal canal and distal 5cm of the rectum should be examined with a proctoscope to check for pus (which can be sampled and prepared as a Gram-stained smear) and other lesions (e.g. warts). This also minimizes faecal contamination when taking swabs. Lubricants should be used with care around the anal sphincter to avoid rectal contamination as they may impair the isolation of *N.gonorrhoeae*.

Rectal testing for *N.gonorrhoeae* should also be offered to ♀ at risk (e.g. with symptoms, urogenital gonorrhoea, contacts of gonorrhoea, and following sexual assault). Chlamydia screening may also be considered.

Pharynx Swabs for *N.gonorrhoeae* should be offered to those at risk especially if symptomatic, gonorrhea found at other site(s), contacts of gonorrhoea, MSM, and those sexually assaulted.

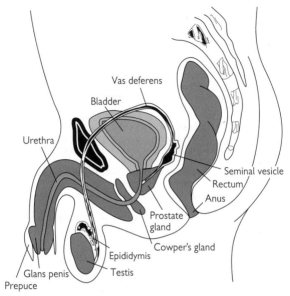

Fig. 3.2 Male genital anatomy

Principles of management and review

General

At the end of the consultation the patient will require further advice and information on their condition or situation, its management, and the need, when relevant, for further follow-up which may include repeat or additional tests. It is important to make these recommendations clear and explicit with the provision of written information.

Treatment

- If specific treatment is required it should:
  - be based on regularly reviewed local or national guidelines
  - recognize individual factors (e.g. other medical conditions, allergies, pregnancy, etc.)
  - meet individual patient needs to maximize adherence (especially long-term HIV treatment).
- Treatment dispensed by a nurse must be provided under local Trust ratified patient group directions.
- Any medicine dispensed and advice given must be documented in the patient's records.

Management points

- Confirm that any test results relate to the patient and that complete information is available (e.g. antibiotic sensitivity).
- Explain the nature of the condition and its implications.
- Discuss rationale for treatment including a risk–benefit analysis and specific information on the treatment recommended, and obtain patient's agreement.
- Ensure full STI screening is offered (explaining possibility of coexisting infections).
- Provide additional advice that may include:
  - avoidance of sexual intercourse even with condoms (until infection cleared and partner treated)
  - possible effects on combined hormonal contraception
  - additional self-help information
  - general sexual health promotion.
- Consider sexual partner(s) and partner notification issues when indicated (with health adviser).
- Agree arrangements for obtaining results and/or further review (which may include tests of cure).

Pharmacy arrangements

Ideally medication should be dispensed, free of charge, to the patient while he/she is in the clinic.

Free treatment

Treatment of STIs excluding HIV/AIDS (but including initial diagnosis of and counselling support for HIV) is free without any prescription charge to all attendees at GUM clinics irrespective of their nationality. HIV/AIDS management after the initial diagnosis and counselling is subject to the standard regulations concerning entitlement to NHS hospital treatment (🕮 Asylum seekers and refugees p. 36).

Sexual health in primary care

Primary Care Trusts (PCTs) have principle responsibility for:
- ensuring that the National Strategy for Sexual Health and HIV is implemented at local level
- coordinating local sexual health planning and commissioning
- ensuring appropriate capacity and resources are available to deliver these standards.

Levels of service provision

Sexual health services are divided into levels as outlined in the National Strategy for Sexual Health and HIV (Box 3.1).

Box 3.1 Level 1 services

- Sexual history and risk assessment
- STI testing for women
- HIV testing and counselling
- Pregnancy testing and referral
- Contraception information and services
- Assessment and referral of men with STI symptoms
- Cervical cytology and referral
- Hepatitis B vaccination

If a primary care practice is unable to provide Level 1 service it should be made clear in the practice information and explicit arrangements made for their patients through other practices or community services. PCTs should identify and support primary care teams with special interests in sexual health which can provide locally enhanced services to a high standard. GPs and nurses need to undertake specific training to develop and maintain skills required. These services can be offered to unregistered patients or those registered with other practices. PCTs should develop provision of a full range of Level 2 services (Box 3.2) in collaboration with GUM and Community Family Planning to meet local needs and fill gaps in existing service provision.

Box 3.2 Level 2 services

- Intra-uterine device insertion.
- Testing and treatment for STIs.
- Contraceptive implant insertion.
- STI partner notification.
- Invasive STI testing (until non-invasive tests are available).

A pragmatic guide to STI testing in general practice

For extensive testing refer to local GUM service and contact local laboratories regarding test methods and arrangements.

Asymptomatic patients

Test patients at high risk (under-25s and new partner in preceding 12 months).

- Test for *C.trachomatis and N.gonorrhoeae* (the latter is particularly important if local outbreak or in a high-prevalence area). If positive for gonorrhoea refer to Level 2 or 3 service for culture and sensitivities.
- MSM: urine NAAT test for *C.trachomatis* and *N gonorrhoeae*, rectal swab for *N.gonorrhoeae* and *C.trachomatis*, pharyngeal swab for *N.gonorrhoeae*.

Symptomatic patients

- Women
  - Vaginal discharge: trichomonas, candida, and bacterial vaginosis (high vaginal swabs). If at high risk, test for chlamydia, gonorrhoea (endocervical swabs). If trichomoniasis is suspected, consider GUM referral for immediate microscopy. If over 25 and no new partner since last tested, assess symptoms and pH paper test. If pH ↑ (i.e. >4.5) treat for bacterial vaginosis; if pH normal treat for candidiasis. If symptoms fail to resolve investigate/refer to GUM.
  - Urinary symptoms ± abdominal pain: STI needs to be excluded.
- Men
  - Urethral discharge ± dysuria: test for chlamydia and gonorrhoea.
  - Testicular swelling: exclude STI and request MSU (especially if over age 35).
- Anogenital ulceration: consider early referral to GUM. If this is not possible and herpes suspected start antiviral treatment immediately.

HIV testing

If local prevalence exceeds 2 in 1000 (local PCT data) all men and women registering with a general practice should be offered an HIV test. Otherwise a risk assessment should be performed (📖 Chapter 38, p. 436). Positive test: refer to GUM.

Syphilis and hepatitis B testing

Consider sexual and contact history. If positive syphilis serology, refer to GUM. If positive hepatitis B serology, refer to gastroenterology. If patient at risk of hepatitis B administer hepatitis B vaccination (📖 Chapter 24, p. 296).

Investigations and microscopy

Laboratory testing

Introduction

Certain infections can be detected or diagnosed within clinics or surgeries but others require microbiological services, also essential for confirmatory and antimicrobial sensitivity testing. If on-site microscopy is unavailable, the use of air-dried swabs sent for laboratory staining and microscopy should be considered. This is applicable for vaginal discharge (e.g. bacterial vaginosis, candidiasis) and also for ♂ urethral discharge for polymorphonuclear leucocytes (PMNLs) indicating urethritis and Gram-negative intracellular diplococci, which are highly suggestive but not diagnostic of gonorrhoea.

The optimum minimum time to take swabs for screening from asymptomatic patients following a specific incident has not been established. It will depend on the type of test used, the site screened, and the presence/absence of infected secretions. However, 7–14 days after a sexual risk is suggested (and is compliant with sexual assault guidelines).

The timing of serological tests should take into consideration the 'window periods' of the respective infections. Final exclusion tests must be advised at the end of this time. Baseline assays soon after the incident may be useful, especially if subsequent repeat tests are positive.

Chlamydia trachomatis

Nucleic acid amplification test (NAAT)

♂ urethra, endocervix, first voided 20mL of urine (especially ♂), vagina, vulva. Although not essential, urethral samples from ♀ enhance the detection rate when combined with endocervical specimens. In addition, rectal samples (although unlicensed) have been shown to be useful in ♂ who have sex with ♂ (MSM). Important to take if MSM present with anorectal symptoms because of recent outbreaks of lymphogranuloma venereum (recently reported in W. Europe). If confirmed, genotype for L1, L2, or L3.

Not licensed for oropharyngeal specimens.

Enzyme immunoassay (EIA)

Still widely used but are at least 30% less sensitive than NAAT. Not suitable for urine and vulvo-vaginal testing in ♀ and certain kits are not recommended for urine testing in ♂.

Culture

Not widely available now but still considered important in medico-legal situations (e.g. assault and rarely if antibiotic resistance is suspected).

Transport and storage

Specimens for culture should be kept refrigerated at all times. Storage of NAAT and EIA specimens for >24 hours at room temperature may result in sample degradation, although absolute data are lacking. If delays are anticipated, storage at 4°C is recommended. Manufacturer's instructions should be followed.

Neisseria gonorrhoeae

Culture

Routinely from ♂ urethra and endocervix. Although not essential, urethral samples from ♀ enhance the detection rate when combined with endocervical specimens.

Rectal and pharyngeal specimens should also be considered if at risk, remembering that rectal gonorrhoea may occur without peno-anal penetration. If a carbon dioxide incubator is available specimens can be plated directly onto selective growth medium (e.g. modified New York City culture medium), although they will require to be transported to the laboratory in a carbon dioxide enriched environment (e.g. in candle jars).

Otherwise specimens must be sent in a transport medium (e.g. Amies, Stuart). Their use only reduces sensitivity by ~10% (compared with direct inoculation) provided that the specimens are refrigerated and received by the laboratory within 48 hours.

Nucleic acid amplification test

Limited availability but more sensitive compared with culture. From urogenital sites only, positive results need culture for confirmation and antibiotic sensitivity testing.

Bacterial vaginosis (BV)

Swab from posterior fornix. Prepare air-dried smear from the swab or send in transport medium (Amies, Stuart) requesting a Gram stain for bacterial flora and clue cells. A result suggestive of BV does not necessarily indicate the need for treatment, which must be assessed clinically.

Herpes simplex virus (HSV)

Swabs of vesicular fluid or from ulcers

Culture

Must be sent in transport medium. Standard viral transport systems should be kept refrigerated but some commercial systems (e.g. Virocult®) can be maintained at ambient temperature as HSV will survive for up to 12 days at up to 23°C. Local laboratory or manufacturer's instructions should be consulted.

Real-time polymerase chain reaction

Highly sensitive (detects 11–88% more cases than culture), specific, allows typing, and is rapid. Manufacturer's instructions should be consulted for transport.

Others

- Immunofluorescent antigen detection: provided by some laboratories using material (sample in viral transport medium).
- Type-specific serology: of little diagnostic value.

Trichomonas vaginalis

Swab from posterior fornix or urethra/sub-preputial sac (if indicated) in growth medium (e.g. Feinberg–Whittington incubated at 37°C) or transport medium (Amies, Stuart), refrigerated, and received within 24–48 hours. Although some laboratories provide a culture service, most diagnose on slides prepared from the swabs.

Candida spp.

Swab from vaginal wall or vulva, glans penis, prepuce, anus, etc. if indicated in transport medium (Amies, Stuart) without any special precautions. *Candida* spp. are common skin and genital commensals and therefore the need to treat must be based on clinical findings.

Serology

Clotted blood is required with no special arrangements needed for transport. Baseline assays are useful, especially if subsequent repeat tests are positive.

- Syphilis and HIV: seroconversion usually occurs within 2–6 weeks but may take up to 3 months, when repeat or initial testing should be recommended.
- Hepatitis B surface antigen and hepatitis C antibody: can usually be detected within 3 months of infection although occasionally may take longer. In high-risk situations a further test at 6 months is advisable.

More detailed information on testing in specific situations and less common infections can be found in the relevant chapters.

Frequently asked questions

Will the tests hurt?

♂: You will feel some discomfort but it should not be painful. The swabs only take a few seconds to take. You may notice slight discomfort on urinating the first time after the swabs have been taken.

♀: We use a speculum inserted into the vagina to take the swabs, similar to when having a smear taken. We also take swabs from the urethra (urinary passage).

Are you going to use the umbrella?

No. This is an old instrument used for ♂ >40 years ago. Modern swabs are taken with very fine swabs.

Will I get the result today?

No. You will not get all your results today.

If you are ♀, microscopy at the time of your appointment may show thrush, bacterial vaginosis, or trichomoniasis. We can also sometimes detect gonorrhoea, but this needs to be confirmed by swabs taken at the same time and sent to the laboratory. Swabs are also taken for chlamydia at the same time. The results for chlamydia and gonorrhoea are available within a week.

In ♂ we can diagnose NSU or gonorrhoea on the day if microscopy is performed (usually if there is a urethral discharge). Gonorrhoea needs to be confirmed by swabs taken at the same time and sent to the laboratory. We also send swabs to the laboratory for chlamydia and the results of all swabs are available within a week.

Blood tests results take up to 7 days. However, if there is a particular concern we can obtain a preliminary result within 24 hours.

Do they need repeating?

We rarely need to do tests of cure nowadays. You will be told if you need a test of cure. Swabs do not need repeating unless the first tests were taken too soon after a risk (within 1 week), there is a high infection risk, symptoms persist, or there is a risk of reinfection/new infection.

I'm on my period. Can you still do the tests?

Yes. We can still take swabs whilst you are menstruating. However some prefer to wait until their period has finished.

The microscope

Two microscopes are usually required, one for direct light and phase contrast illumination and the other for dark ground microscopy.

Objective lenses

- 10×, 40× (low power): provide overall magnification of 100× and 400×. Suitable for screening for clue cells, trichomoniasis and candidiasis, and fungal infection although may require high power to confirm. Also used to identify scabies mites and threadworm ova.
- 100× (high power): provides overall magnification of 1000×. Must be used with immersion oil.

Used to examine specimens for PMNLs, gonococci, and other bacteria, including treponemes. Separate objectives required for direct light/phase contrast and dark ground illumination.

Condensers (Fig. 4.1)

- Direct light
- Phase contrast (must match with the same Ph code on the objective)
- Dark ground (used with immersion oil between lens and under surface of the slide).

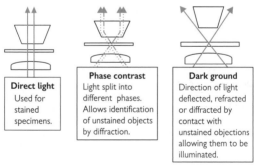

Fig. 4.1 Condensers

Microscopy: general points

- Ensure lenses are wiped clean of immersion oil and dust with a lens tissue after use.
- To avoid lens damage ensure that high-power objective lens is not aligned when slides are moved to and from the microscope.
- When using dark ground microscopy place a drop of oil on the condenser and raise until it just touches the slide.
- When using phase contrast ensure that the Ph codes on the condenser and objective match.
- Start with low power to identify a good wide field, and approximate focus before moving to high power.

Slide preparation

Gram stain
- Fix the smear by heating the slide or submerging it in 95% methanol for 2 minutes.
- Apply crystal violet, methyl violet, or gentian violet (a combination of the first two) for 15 seconds.
- Apply an aqueous solution of iodine for 15 seconds.
- Decolorize slide with acetone for 3 seconds.
- Rinse slide with water.
- Apply red counterstain (e.g. carbol fuchsin, basic fuchsin, or neutral red) for 15 seconds.
- Rinse slide in water.
- Carefully dry the slide.

Preparation of ulcer fluid for dark ground microscopy for *T.pallidum* (📖 Chapter 6, Diagnosis: regular investigations p. 122)
- Clean the ulcer with a swab soaked in sterile saline.
- Squeeze the lesion gently to release serum.
- Collect serum with the edge of a cover-slip and mount in normal saline.
- Gently press the cover-slip onto the slide.

Clinic-based tests

Examination by microscopy

Gram-stained smear

- ♂ urethra/urine threads: PMNLs, Gram −ve intracellular diplococci.
- Glans penis/sub-preputial sac: yeast spores ± hyphae, mixed Gram +ve and −ve cocco-bacilli ± curved rods (generally anaerobes).
- ♀ urethra and cervix: PMNLs, Gram −ve intracellular diplococci.
- Vagina: lactobacilli (Plate 1), PMNLs, mixed Gram +ve and −ve cocco-bacilli ± curved rods (generally anaerobes), Gram +ve cocci, yeast spores ± hyphae.
- Rectum: PMNLs, Gram −ve intracellular diplococci.
- Ulcers: Gram −ve coccobacillus in shoals (*Haemophilus ducreyi*) – unusual finding.

Saline suspension

- Phase contrast:
  - vagina or sub-preputial sac/glans penis—clue cells/motile curved rods, *T.vaginalis*, yeast spores ± hyphae
  - urethra: *T.vaginalis*.
- Dark ground
  - Ulcers – *T.pallidum*
  - Vagina or sub-preputial sac/glans penis—clue cells/motile curved rods, *T.vaginalis*, yeast spores +/− hyphae
  - urethra: T.vaginalis.

Skin samples

- Burrow material for scabies mite
- Skin scales in 10% potassium hydroxide for mycelia (tinea/ringworm)
- Perianal transparent adhesive tape strip—threadworm ova

Vaginal discharge

- 'Whiff test'—addition of 10% potassium hydroxide releases pungent amines
- pH >4.5

Both are indicators of bacterial vaginosis. Unnecessary if Hay–Ison diagnostic criteria used (Chapter 14, Diagnosis p. 208).

Urine

Inspection

Urine haze in ♂ (not cleared by addition of 5% acetic acid) ± threads in first pass suggests anterior urethritis. A second specimen (MSSU) may be of value in suggesting posterior urethritis or UTI (if turbid) and is essential for culture and sensitivity. Urine may also be required for pregnancy testing.

Urinalysis

- Sugar, ketones—diabetes (recurrent candidiasis, balanitis).
- Protein, leucocytes, blood, nitrites—UTI.
- Persistent proteinuria/haematuria—refer to nephrology.

Pregnancy test (immunoassay), urine, and serum

First documented in Egypt (1350BC) when ♀ who suspected that they were pregnant urinated on wheat and barley seeds over a 7 day period. Germination of either seed (probably due to ↑ levels of oestrogen) indicated pregnancy (70% accuracy demonstrated in 1963).

Pregnancy testing can be performed on urine or serum samples. Both tests detect β human chorionic gonadotrophin (hCG), a glycoprotein hormone produced by the placental trophoblastic cells shortly after implantation. A positive result indicates secretory activity of trophoblastic tissue normally associated with the presence of a viable fetus.

Urine (qualitative test)

Urine sampling kits give only a positive or negative result. Samples can detect hCG levels above 25–50mIU/mL. Levels of urinary hCG average 100mIU/mL following the first missed menstrual period and ↑ up to 200,000mIU/mL at 10–12 weeks of pregnancy. There is a dramatic fall in levels after this time. Test read after 3 minutes.

Limitations of urine test
- Unable to distinguish between uterine and ectopic pregnancy.
- Occasional false-negative results in ectopic pregnancy.
- Inability to distinguish between pituitary luteinizing hormone (LH) and hCG. Positive result may be obtained in the presence of a hydatidiform mole, chorioadenoma, or choriocarcinoma.
- Conditions such as trophoblastic disease and certain non-trophoblastic neoplasms can cause higher levels of hCG.
- 10% of pregnancies are undetectable on the first day of missed menses.
- False-positive results estimated at up to 10%.
- False-negative results may be due to dilute urine.

Serum

More accurate and should be considered if urine testing is negative but there is a pregnancy risk. Tests can detect hCG levels above 5–10mIU/mL. Positive results may be obtained within 7–10 days of conception. Qualitative (just positive or negative) and quantitive tests are available. The latter allow exact measurement of the amount of serum hCG, useful in assessing the stage of pregnancy. Serum hCG doubles every 36–48 hours in the early stages. A subnormal response may indicate miscarriage or ectopic pregnancy. Extremely high levels of hCG may suggest multiple pregnancy.

Routine female microscopy

Vaginal Gram-stained smear

1. Are there bacteria present and what are they like?

Grade 0	Grade I	Grade II
Epithelial Cells only	*Lactobacilli only*	*Reduced lactobacilli and mixed bacteria*
• Post-menopause	• Normal flora	• intermediate transitional phase
• Pre-menarche		
• Antibiotics		
• Intra-vaginal gels		

Grade III	Grade IV
Mixed bacteria/no lactobacilli and 'clue cells'	*Gram +ve cocci only (often in chains)*
• Indicates bacterial vaginosis	• Usually irrelevant

Treatment for bacterial vaginosis required for Grade III (and occasionally Grade II) with symptoms/signs.

2. Are there any yeast spores and/or hyphae?

Usually associated with vaginal PMNLs if symptomatic.		
Hyphae +/– spores	*Usually*	*Candida albicans*
Spores alone	*Probably*	*Candida glabrata*

3. Are there vaginal PMNLs?

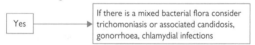

Yes → If there is a mixed bacterial flora consider trichomoniasis or associated candidosis, gonorrhoea, chlamydial infections

Urethral and cervical Gram-stained smears

Are PMNLs present?

- Urethra: ↑ risk of gonorrhoea. Therefore check urethral and cervical smears especially carefully for gonococci.
- Cervix: variable depending on menstrual cycle, sexual activity, and contraception (often ↑ with hormonal methods). >30 per high-power field correlates best with gonococcal or chlamydial infections.

Are Gram-negative diplococci (GNDC) present?

Examine urethral and cervical smears for intracellular GNDC. Urethral smear of doubtful value if cervix examined. Finding extracellular GNDC ↑ sensitivity by 20% but ↓ specificity by 4%.

Vaginal preparation in saline protected by a cover-slip

- Switch light source to phase contrast (or dark ground).
- Screen slide (low power) for motile protozoa, spores ± hyphae.
- If necessary switch to high power. Place a drop of immersion oil on to cover-slip before examining. Can also be used to identify clue cells and motile vibrios (*Mobiluncus* spp.) often found in bacterial vaginosis.

Routine male microscopy

Urethral Gram-stained smear

Are PMNLs present?
Non-gonococcal urethritis diagnosed by finding:
- ≥5 PMNLs per high-power field (averaged over 5 fields with the greatest concentration of PMNLs)
- no GNDC.

Are GNDC present (with intracellular organisms)?
If seen allows a working diagnosis of gonorrhoea. Generally associated with numerous PMNLs.

Gram-stained smear from urine

Useful if urine threads in first voided urine (FVU) specimen and no urethral material to sample directly. The slide can be prepared from threads or centrifuged FVU. Ideally, urine should not be passed for at least 3–4 hours before assessment.

Are PMNLs present?
Non-gonococcal urethritis diagnosed by finding:
- ≥10 PMNLs per high-power field (averaged over 5 fields with the greatest concentration of PMNLs)
- no GNDC.

Are GNDC present (with intracellular organisms)?
Allows a working diagnosis of gonorrhoea.

Saline suspension of sub-preputial, glans penis, or urethral material

Sub-prepuce and glans
If balanitis/balanoposthitis check for:
- yeast spores ± hyphae
- clue cells (anaerobic balanitis)
- T.vaginalis.

A Gram-stained smear can also be used.

Urethra
T.vaginalis (may occasionally be seen with urethritis).

Accuracy of microscopy

Infection and site	Sensitivity (%)	Specificity (%)
Gonorrhoea		
Urethral Gram stain from symptomatic ♂	90–95	95–99*
Urethral Gram stain from asymptomatic ♂	50–75	
Rectal Gram stain from MSM	35–80†	95–100*
Urethral Gram stain from ♀	20	Unknown
Cervical Gram stain	23–65	88–100*
Bacterial vaginosis (Hay–Ison criteria)		
Vaginal Gram-stained specimen	97.5	96
Trichomoniasis (saline suspension)		
Suspension of vaginal discharge	40–80	If motile protozoa seen 100
Suspension of male urethral/ sub-preputial material	30	
Candidiasis		
Vaginal Gram stain if symptomatic	65	No data
Vaginal saline suspension	40–60	
Primary syphilis		
Dark ground examination of ulcer material in saline	79–86	77–100

*This excludes *Neisseria meningitidis* which rarely may be found (indistinguishable morphologically from *N.gonorrhoeae*).
† Higher level if rectal pus.

Rapid point of care tests (POCTs)

Rationale

Useful in resource-limited settings where expensive laboratory facilities are not available. Some may also be used by the patient at home.

Also useful and practical in situations where decisions for treatment or further investigation is required while the patient is still present. Studies have demonstrated that POCTs can lead to the treatment of a greater number of infected patients as they often do not re-attend for results assuming that results will be negative.

Properties of an ideal POCT

- Easy to perform and read (minimal training required)
- Inexpensive
- Rapid results
- Easy to store (equipment as a single unit, no specific storage requirements, long shelf life)
- Sampling acceptable to the patient
- Able to be used by both sexes
- Reproducible
- Incorporate a test control
- High sensitivity and specificity
- Undergone quality assurance tests (i.e. CE marked)

Chlamydia POCTs

Immunoassays for chlamydial antigen (usually lipopolysaccharide) using anti-chlamydial monoclonal antibody. A number are commercially available.

- Clearview® Chlamydia MF: ♂ first-catch urine (sensitivity 77.8%, specificity 97.5%) and ♀ endocervical swabs (sensitivity 93.8%, specificity 99.8%), lateral flow immunoassay, result in 30min.
- Clearview® Chlamydia: only for endocervical swab (sensitivity 87%, specificity 98.8%), result in 15min.
- Biostar® OIA® Chlamydia: endocervical swab (sensitivity 83.6%, specificity 100%), optical immunoassay, result in 19min.
- Quidel® Quickvue® Chlamydia: endocervical swab (sensitivity 92%, specificity 98.6%), cytology brush, lateral flow immunoassay, result in 12 min.
- Chlamydia Rapid Test (Diagnostics for the Real World Ltd): enzyme immunoassay for chlamydial lipopolysaccharide using signal amplification to increase sensitivity. Dipstick test on vaginal swab or male urine using FirstBurst® collection system.

Because of the low sensitivities of tests it is important to obtain a confirmatory sample for NAAT testing if facilities are available.

Gonorrhoea POCTs

Some commercially available e.g. Biostar® Optical Immunoassay and the double-sandwich immunoassay OneStep Rapicard™ Instatest (Cortez Diagnostics), others are in the development stage. The Biostar® OIA®

Gonorrhoea test identifies the L7/L12 ribosomal protein marker which only occurs in the gonococcus and not other Neisseria species (sensitivity 87.8%, specificity 98.5%). Uses endocervical swab in ♀ and urine in ♂, result in 24 minutes.

Confirmatory swab for culture to determine antibiotic sensitivities prior to treatment essential.

HIV POCTs

Used widely in clinical practice. Over 60 different products are produced. Recommended in the following settings:
- community
- source testing in exposure/needlestick incidents
- high-risk situations in which venepuncture is refused
- when rapid results are required.

There are three types of rapid assay.
- Particle agglutination: HIV antigen coated on latex particles. Requires 10–60min for result. Often comes with a reader to help with a weak agglutination result
- Immunoconcentration (flow-through): uses solid phase capture technology involving the immobilization of HIV antigens on a porous membrane. Several stages with addition of specimen, wash buffers, and signal reagent; control on the membrane as a coloured dot. Performed in 5–15min. Examples include *INSTI*™ *HIV1/HIV2 Rapid Antibody Test* (BioLytical Laboratories)
- Immunochromatographic (lateral flow) strips: specimen diluted in buffer and the test strip applied to solution. Specimen migrates through the strip and combines with signal reagent(s). Positive reaction appears as a line on the strip where HIV antigen or antibody has been applied. Control line appears beyond the HIV antigen line. Performed in less than 20min. Examples include *Determine* ® *HIV1/2* (Inverness Medical) which incorporates both antigen and antibody and shows reactivity to each in a separate line in addition to a control line that validates the test.

Antigens vary with individual assay, often from viral envelope (gp41, 120, 160). Some include p24 core antigen. Tests have been developed which, in addition to HIV-1, will identify HIV-2 (using gp36 antigen), appearing positive at a different location on the strip or membrane. Difficulty in some tests identifying Group O subtypes and certain HIV-2 strains.

POCTs allow plasma, whole-blood or finger-prick to be used, but alternatives such as oral fluid samples, e.g OraQuick *ADVANCE*® Rapid HIV1/2 Antibody Test (OraSure Technologies Inc.), and urine tests have been developed.

Documented concerns over the rates of false positives in low-prevalence settings because of the poor positive predictive value of some tests. Recommended that all positive results be confirmed by serological tests. These tests may not be reliable if the patient is still within the 'window period'.

A variety of other POCTs have been developed for syphilis (e.g. *Determine*® *TP* assay) and for hepatitis B and C.

Commensals and confounders

Genital specimens include various micro-organisms which may not be pathogenic. These include hydrogen peroxide producing *Lactobacillus* spp. which indicate normality and other organisms, usually commensal but pathogenic under certain conditions. Therefore results of routine genital specimens should be interpreted in the clinical context and inappropriate antibiotic treatment should be avoided.

Leptothrix

Elongated chain of lactobacilli that may be mistaken for *Candida* spp. on microscopy. Usually not clinically significant but may be associated with vaginitis.

Group B β-haemolytic streptococci: *Streptococcus agalactiae*

Vaginal carriage rates in ♀ attending GUM clinics 12–36%; usually not clinically significant except in late pregnancy (📖 Chapter 31, Group B β-haemolytic streptococci p. 346).

Actinomyces israelii

Found in 3% of ♀ genital specimens – 4% if using intrauterine device (IUD). Detectable on cervical cytology or vaginal wet mount and Gram-stained smears. If asymptomatic, no intervention is required. However, removal (and culture) of IUD and treatment with penicillin or erythromycin may be indicated if otherwise unexplained symptoms, e.g. intermenstrual bleeding, dyspaerunia, and pelvic pain.

Actinomycosis (suppurative upper-genital tract infection) is a rare complication, especially associated with long-term use of plastic IUDs (📖 Chapter 10, Aetiology p. 168).

Neisseria meningitidis

↑ rates of nasopharyngeal carriage in MSM and those practising orogenital sex, reporting multiple sexual partners, or diagnosed with anogenital gonococcal infection (>20% in these groups compared with a general rate of 5–15%). High rates also found in university students (up to 34%). Anogenital carriage in up to 2% of MSM, 0.2% of heterosexual ♂, and 0.1% ♀. May rarely cause urethritis in ♂.

Other micro-organisms

- *Gardnerella vaginalis*, *Prevotella melaninogenica*, *Peptostreptococci*, and other anaerobic organisms may be detected in genital specimens because of low-level colonization without bacterial vaginosis.
- *Ureaplasma urealyticum*, *Bacterioides urealyticum*, and *Mycoplasma hominis* may also be found without any clinical manifestations.
- *Corynebacterium species*, *Escherichia coli*, and coagulase-negative staphylococci in genital specimens are usually of no clinical significance but rarely may be implicated in vaginitis.
- Spirochaetes: *Brachyspira aalborgi* and *Brachyspira pilosicoli* colonize colo-rectal epithelium in up to 30% of people in some developing countries and a similar proportion of MSM or those with HIV infection in the developed countries. In addition, *Treponema denticola*, *Treponema vincentii*, and other similar treponemes associated with periodontal infections and *Treponema refringens*, *Treponema phagedenis*, and *Treponema minutum*, found as commensals in the genitalia, need to be distinguished from *T.pallidum* in rectal, oral, or genital specimens.

Specific genitourinary situations

Men with symptoms suggesting urethritis

Factors suggesting sexually acquired cause
- Presentation: ↑ likelihood if new sexual risk/suspicion about a partner with urethritis arising within 4 weeks (usually).
- Age: most commonly found in ♂ from late teens to 50 years.
- Symptoms: usually prominent dysuria and/or urethral discharge (may just be found on examination).↑ urinary frequency and systemic symptoms unusual.

Management
- Urethral smear: ≥5 polymorphonuclear leucocytes (PMNL) per high-power field (HPF) and/or urinary thread from first voided urine (FVU): ≥10 PMNL per HPF. Consider sending air-dried smear to lab if on-site microscopy unavailable.
- Urethral swab (culture or nucleic acid amplification test (NAAT)) or FVU (NAAT) for *Neisseria gonorrhoeae (NAAT should be supported by culture)*; FVU or swab using NAAT for *Chlamydia trachomatis*.
- Consider:
  • mid-stream sample of urine (MSSU) to exclude urinary tract infection (UTI), if relevant.
  • exposure to other STIs—consider screening, e.g. syphilis and HIV serology.
- Treat on microscopy findings or clinical assessment if microscopy unavailable (while awaiting lab results).
- Partner notification/contact tracing must be arranged. Contacts of gonorrhoea, Non-specific urethritis (NSU) / chlamydia should be treated epidemiologically
- Abstain from sex until treatment completed and partner(s) treated.

Factors suggesting non-sexually acquired cause: consider underlying UTI
- Sexual history: long-standing stable sexual relationship/not sexually active
- Age: >50 years (prostatism with UTI more common)
- Symptoms: ↑ frequency, loin pain, pyrexia, malaise

Management
- Consider/exclude STI:
  • urethral smear for Gram stain, specimens for *N.gonorrhoeae* and *C.trachomatis*.
  • offer syphilis and HIV serology.
- FVU and MSSU typically both opaque, failing to clear on acidification (e.g. 5% acetic acid). Dip-stick usually shows leucocytes, nitrites, protein, and blood. Send MSSU for microscopy, culture, and sensitivity.
- If suspected, manage as UTI.

Balanitis and balanoposthitis

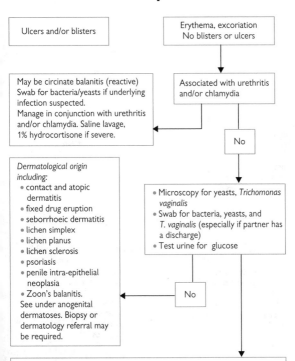

Ulcers and/or blisters

Erythema, excoriation
No blisters or ulcers

May be circinate balanitis (reactive)
Swab for bacteria/yeasts if underlying
infection suspected.
Manage in conjunction with urethritis
and/or chlamydia. Saline lavage,
1% hydrocortisone if severe.

Associated with urethritis
and/or chlamydia

No

*Dermatological origin
including:*
- contact and atopic
  dermatitis
- fixed drug eruption
- seborrhoeic dermatitis
- lichen simplex
- lichen planus
- lichen sclerosis
- psoriasis
- penile intra-epithelial
  neoplasia
- Zoon's balanitis.
See under anogenital
dermatoses. Biopsy or
dermatology referral may
be required.

- Microscopy for yeasts, *Trichomonas
  vaginalis*
- Swab for bacteria, yeasts, and
  T. vaginalis (especially if partner has
  a discharge)
- Test urine for glucose

No

- Candida: azoles, offer check to ♀ partner
- Trichomoniasis: oral metronidazole, treat ♀ partner
- Anaerobes: saline lavage, oral metronidazole if severe
- Aerobes: often found as commensals so only treat if symptomatic.
  - *Staphylococcus aureus*—antibiotics dependent on sensitivity.
  - Group A and B streptococci—as above.
  - *Gardnerella vaginalis*—usually found with anaerobes; manage accordingly.

Vulval irritation/discomfort/pain

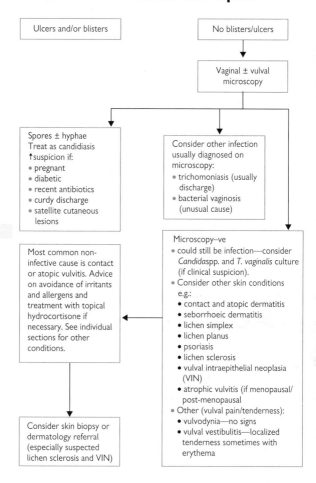

Ulcers and/or blisters

No blisters/ulcers

Vaginal ± vulval microscopy

Spores ± hyphae
Treat as candidiasis
↑suspicion if:
- pregnant
- diabetic
- recent antibiotics
- curdy discharge
- satellite cutaneous lesions

Consider other infection usually diagnosed on microscopy:
- trichomoniasis (usually discharge)
- bacterial vaginosis (unusual cause)

Most common non-infective cause is contact or atopic vulvitis. Advice on avoidance of irritants and allergens and treatment with topical hydrocortisone if necessary. See individual sections for other conditions.

Microscopy–ve
- could still be infection—consider *Candida* spp. and *T. vaginalis* culture (if clinical suspicion).
- Consider other skin conditions e.g.:
  - contact and atopic dermatitis
  - seborrhoeic dermatitis
  - lichen simplex
  - lichen planus
  - psoriasis
  - lichen sclerosis
  - vulval intraepithelial neoplasia (VIN)
  - atrophic vulvitis (if menopausal/post-menopausal
- Other (vulval pain/tenderness):
  - vulvodynia—no signs
  - vulval vestibulitis—localized tenderness sometimes with erythema

Consider skin biopsy or dermatology referral (especially suspected lichen sclerosis and VIN)

Altered vaginal discharge

The normal physiological discharge will alter with the time of the menstrual cycle, pregnancy, and sometimes hormonal contraception. Finding lactobacilli without other anomalies provides reassurance pending swab results.

Remember that it is common for infections to coexist.

Primary vaginal conditions

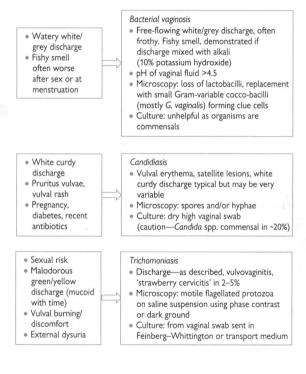

- Watery white/grey discharge
- Fishy smell often worse after sex or at menstruation

Bacterial vaginosis
- Free-flowing white/grey discharge, often frothy. Fishy smell, demonstrated if discharge mixed with alkali (10% potassium hydroxide)
- pH of vaginal fluid >4.5
- Microscopy: loss of lactobacilli, replacement with small Gram-variable cocco-bacilli (mostly *G. vaginalis*) forming clue cells
- Culture: unhelpful as organisms are commensals

- White curdy discharge
- Pruritus vulvae, vulval rash
- Pregnancy, diabetes, recent antibiotics

Candidiasis
- Vulval erythema, satellite lesions, white curdy discharge typical but may be very variable
- Microscopy: spores and/or hyphae
- Culture: dry high vaginal swab (caution—*Candida* spp. commensal in ~20%)

- Sexual risk
- Malodorous green/yellow discharge (mucoid with time)
- Vulval burning/discomfort
- External dysuria

Trichomoniasis
- Discharge—as described, vulvovaginitis, 'strawberry cervicitis' in 2–5%
- Microscopy: motile flagellated protozoa on saline suspension using phase contrast or dark ground
- Culture: from vaginal swab sent in Feinberg–Whittington or transport medium

Other causes commonly seen in **GUM**

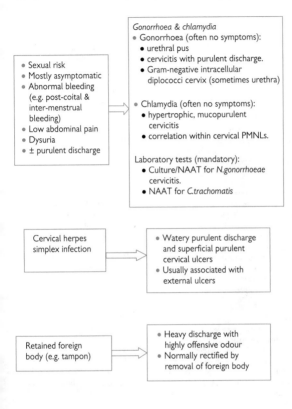

- Sexual risk
- Mostly asymptomatic
- Abnormal bleeding (e.g. post-coital & inter-menstrual bleeding)
- Low abdominal pain
- Dysuria
- ± purulent discharge

Gonorrhoea & chlamydia
- Gonorrhoea (often no symptoms):
  - urethral pus
  - cervicitis with purulent discharge.
  - Gram-negative intracellular diplococci cervix (sometimes urethra)

- Chlamydia (often no symptoms):
  - hypertrophic, mucopurulent cervicitis
  - correlation within cervical PMNLs.

Laboratory tests (mandatory):
- Culture/NAAT for *N.gonorrhoeae* cervicitis.
- NAAT for *C.trachomatis*

Cervical herpes simplex infection

- Watery purulent discharge and superficial purulent cervical ulcers
- Usually associated with external ulcers

Retained foreign body (e.g. tampon)

- Heavy discharge with highly offensive odour
- Normally rectified by removal of foreign body

Anogenital ulceration

Traumatic
- Timing—immediately after incident
- Appearance (often irregular—as dermatitis artefacta)

Management
Exclude STI cause
Bacterial swab (if 2° infection)
General STI screen
Advise
- Saline lavage
- Antibiotics for secondary infection if necessary

Possible STI
- Herpes: multiple, painful, preceded by vesicles. Most common infective cause
- Syphilis: 1° chancre—typically single and painless (multiple painful ulcers now more common):2°—'snail track', usually with skin rash
- Tropical: (suspect if travel history or exposure). Typical presentations:
  - chancroid—multiple, soft, painful ulcers
  - lymphogranuloma venereum (LGV)—usually bilateral inguinal lymphadenopathy (preceded by transient, small, painless ulcer)
  - granuloma inguinale—pruritic papule followed by granulomatous ulcer

Investigations
- Herpes—swab for herpes simplex virus
- Dark-ground examination for treponemes. Consider repeating on 3 separate days if clinically suspicious. Ensure full syphilis serology requested
- Swab for *Haemophilus ducreyi*
- Swab ulcer/bubo pus for *C.trachomatis*; blood for LGVCFT
- Biopsy for Donovan bodies

Other
- Neoplastic: progressive over weeks or months (age usually over 50 years)
- 'Dermatological', e.g. aphthous ulcers/Behçet's disease—usually chronic, relapsing associated with oral ulcers and if Behçet's other systemic symptoms

Management
Urgent urology referral if carcinoma suspected.
Dermatological referral may be required for other conditions

The most common infective cause in GUM is genital herpes

First episode

- Diagnosis
  - Swab – in viral transport medium
  - Diagnostic confirmation important although treatment should commence on clinical grounds
  - Full STI screen advised. Internal examination in ♀ may be deferred until acute symptoms resolved.
- Management
  - If clinically suspected, start oral antiviral treatment.
  - Analgesia may be required (e.g. 30–60mg codeine phosphate 4–6 times a day)
  - Recommend saline lavage
  - Suggest micturition in warm bathwater if severe dysuria. Suprapubic catheterization may be required if urinary retention.

Recurrence

- Supportive treatment (e.g. saline bathing) unless unusually severe when oral antiviral treatment is justified.
- STI screen only if new risk.

Frequent recurrence (>6 per year)

- Anticipatory episodic treatment.
- Suppressive treatment.

Genital lumps and bumps

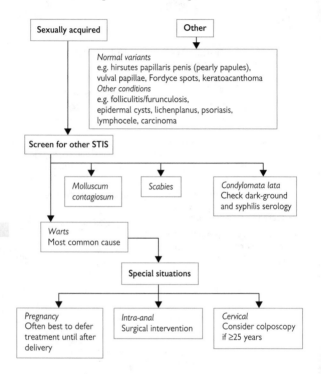

Proctitis

Passive anal sex +/– symptomatic proctitis (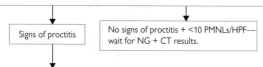 see Chapter 19
Proctocolitis and entric infections p. 247).
Examine with proctoscope and:
swab for Gram stain, *Neisseria gonorrhoeae* (NG) + *Chlamydia
trachomatis* (CT) – with LGV typing if +ve.
Serology: advise syphilis (STS) and HIV for all—STS crucial if syphilis
considered, chlamydial serology (for LGV) if available.

Signs of proctitis

No signs of proctitis + <10 PMNLs/HPF—
wait for NG + CT results.

Suspected NG (Gram –ve intracellular diplococci) on smear:
Treat: ceftriaxone or cefixime, consider CT prophylaxis
(doxycycline or azithromycin). Review and revise on receipt
of test results.

>10 PMNLs and no evidence of NG—consider CT
Treat: start doxycycline 21 day course pending LGV
genotyping.
Stop after 7 days if no LGV genotype detected. Review and
revise on receipt of test results.
Test of cure recommended if azithromycin used.

If ulcerative mucosa +/– perianal lesions—consider herpes +/–
syphilis. Dark ground samples for *Treponema pallidum* (TP),
swabs for TP and herpes PCR (and/or herpes simplex virus
culture).
Treat: cover for herpes with aciclovir. Review and revise
on receipt of test results.

Management of sexual contacts

Table 5.1 Epidemiological treatment for contacts of STIs

Infection of index case	Treatment need	Contact treatment
♀ candidiasis	✗	
♂ candidiasis	✓	Antimycotic treatment often required
Chancroid	✓	Ciprofloxacin 500mg twice daily for 3 days Ceftriaxone 250mg single dose, IM
Chlamydia	✓	Azithromycin 1g stat., doxycycline (100mg twice daily for 7 days (recommended if likely rectal infection), erythromycin 500mg twice daily for 14 days
Donovanosis	✓	Azithromycin: to current contacts and those from 30 days prior to onset of symptoms
Epididymitis (if non-gonococcal)	✓	Azithromycin, doxycycline, erythromycin (as chlamydia)
Gonorrhoea	✓	Single doses of cefixime 400mg; ciprofloxacin 500mg; amoxicillin 3g + probenecid 1g; ceftriaxone 250mg IM
Hepatitis A	✓	Hepatitis A vaccine HNIG* – close contacts <2 weeks
Hepatitis B	✓	Specific hepatitis B immunoglobulin (<7 days). Super-accelerated active immunization
HIV	✗/✓	If <72 hours, consider post-exposure prophylaxis (PEP) with highly active antiretroviral therapy for 1 month
Lymphogranuloma venereum	✓	Doxycycline: to current contacts and those from 30 days prior to onset of symptoms
Non-gonococcal urethritis	✓	Azithromycin, doxycycline, erythromycin (as chlamydia)
Mucopurulent cervicitis and PID	✓	Azithromycin, doxycycline, erythromycin (as chlamydia). Consider anti-gonorrhoea treatment
Pediculosis	✓	Permethrin or malathion to sex contacts
Scabies	✓	Permethrin or malathion to sex and household contacts
Syphilis – early	✗/✓	Consider benzathine benzylpenicillin 2.4MU IM stat or oral doxycycline 100mg twice daily for 14 days
Syphilis – late	✗	
Trichomoniasis	✓	Metronidazole 2g single dose or 400mg twice daily for 7 days

* Human normal immunoglobulin

Table 5.2 No partner treatment required

Infection	Need	Contact treatment
Bacterial vaginosis	×	Not required
Hepatitis C	×	
Anogenital herpes	×	
Anogenital warts/molluscum contagiosum	×	

NB: Tables 5.1 and 5.2 only provide information about epidemiological treatment. They do not cover the requirement to offer contacts at risk STI screening, information, and advice.

Oral sex

- Oro-penile: fellatio
- Oro-vulval: cunnilingus
- Oro-anal: anilingus (also spelt analingus)

Lifestyle reports suggest an increase in oral sex, especially among adolescents and ♂ who have sex with ♂ (MSM). Factors include a younger age at sexual debut, avoidance of pregnancy, and reducing HIV risk (in MSM). Oral sex is often not regarded as sex, or as relevant to the transmission of infection, so direct questions regarding its practice must be asked when relevant (Box 5.1).

Non-infective

Idiosyncratic reports of genital lesions arising from trauma, usually from the teeth, but also related to the use of piercings. Underlying medical conditions may aggravate, e.g. vulval haematoma in ♀ with essential thrombocytopenia. Oral injuries arising from fellatio have been reported, with the typical lesion appearing as a circular area on the soft palate consisting of erythema, petechiae, dilated blood vessels, and vesicles. A case of accidental condom inhalation has been reported in a ♀ presenting with a chronic cough, sputum, and fever with a collapse-consolidation of the right upper lobe. Videobronchoscopy revealed the presence of a condom in the right upper lobe bronchus. Case reports have associated vaginal insufflation (blowing into the vagina) with venous air embolism (through the uterine veins or subplacental sinuses) during pregnancy, and pneumoperitoneum (presenting with acute severe abdominal pain) in any ♀, including those who have undergone hysterectomy, independent of operative procedure.

Infective

Adenovirus

A probable cause of non-gonococcal urethritis (NGU) associated with receiving oral sex. Adenovirus infection has also been implicated in cervicitis and genital ulceration as well as keratoconjunctivitis. Seasonal clustering of cases is reported. Types identified in studies are 4, 8, 9, 35, 37, and 49, and NGU typically presents with marked dysuria, mucoid urethral discharge, and meatitis. Extragenital manifestations include conjunctivitis, pharyngitis, and constitutional symptoms.

Bacterial vaginosis (BV)

There is a lack of clear reproducible evidence of an association with oral sex in general. However, a significant association has been reported with receiving oral sex in lesbians. *Mycoplasma hominis*, associated with BV, has been isolated from the throats of partners of ♀ who carried BV vaginally, and a history of having ever performed fellatio is significantly associated with *M.hominis* throat carriage.

Candidiasis

Symptomatic culture-proven recurrent vulvovaginal candidiasis (VVC) is associated with cunnilingus, although it appears that isolated episodes are not. Although *Candida* spp. are found in the mouth, saliva may have an important role in recurrent VVC as other associated factors include recent ♀

masturbation with saliva and ♂ masturbation with saliva in the past month. It has been postulated that antimicrobial products in saliva could clear local bacteria, providing an advantage to resilient candida spores provoking recurrent VVC, have a direct irritant effect or otherwise alter the local immunological state.

Chancroid
Isolated case reports alleging orogenital transmission.

Chlamydia trachomatis
Chlamydial throat infection has been reported in 3.7% heterosexual ♂, 3.2% ♀, and 1.4% MSM, with a significant association in ♀ to ever having performed fellatio. It has also been found in patients with eye infection which in turn could be caused by contact with infected semen or genital secretions. Symptoms arising from isolated throat infection are extremely unusual and currently there are no data on infections transmitted from the throat.

Cytomegalovirus
Found in saliva, semen, genital secretions. ↑ infection rates associated with a history of sexually transmitted infections. Considered to be transmitted by kissing; therefore spread by oral sex is feasible.

Epstein–Barr virus (EBV)
Cause of infectious mononucleosis (glandular fever). Classically spread by infected saliva through kissing, EBV has also been detected in semen, cervical secretions, and vulval ulceration. Although unproven, sexual transmission including oral sex is a possibility.

Enteric infection
Shigella spp, *Salmonella* spp, *Campylobacter* spp, *Cryptosporidium* spp, *Entamoeba histolytica*, cytomegalovirus, *Giardia duodenalis*, and *Enterobius vermicularis* are all widely reported in MSM as being spread by oro-anal sex or fellatio after insertive anal intercourse (📖 Chapter 19). *Isospora belli* enteritis has been reported in immunocompromised MSM following oro-anal sex.

Gonorrhoea
Oral infection usually involves the pharynx (asymptomatic in >90%), but stomatitis is also reported (following cunnilingus). In patients with gonorrhoea pharyngeal infection is found in 10–30% MSM, 5–15% ♀, and 3–10% heterosexual ♂. Disseminated infection from a pharyngeal source has been reported. There is clear evidence supporting the transfer of *N.gonorrhoeae* from the throat to the male urethra and case reports alleging throat infection from oro-anal sex or kissing. Gonococcal conjunctivitis can arise following contact with infected semen or genital secretions during oral sex.

Granuloma inguinale
Rare case reports of oral manifestations suggest that the mouth may be an infection reservoir but no evidence of orogenital transmission.

Herpes simplex virus (HSV)

There has been an ongoing national and international increase in the incidence of new genital infections caused by HSV1, predominantly in ♀, compatible with the reports of greater rates of oral sex. HSV1 seroconversion in young ♀ has been shown to be directly associated with receiving oral sex and vaginal intercourse. Genital HSV1 infection is associated with receiving oral sex, with a weaker association with vaginal sex, suggesting that it is the partner's mouth which is the infection source. HSV2 infection can also be transmitted during oral sex causing oro-pharyngeal infection. However, unlike HSV1 infection, oral reactivation and viral shedding are uncommon.

As well as typical herpes infection both HSV1 and HSV2 can cause NGU without visible lesions, with HSV1 more common, and a positive association with the latter, NGU, and oral sex.

Hepatitis (viral)

Hepatitis A

RNA (ribonucleic acid) virus found in faeces and typically spread through the oro-faecal route. Studies suggest a link between oro-anal sex and hepatitis A in MSM with some outbreaks clearly associated with this practice. In addition, hepatitis A may also be acquired by ingesting infected urine.

Hepatitis B

Hepatitis B virus antigen has been found in semen, saliva, cervical fluid, and faeces although much higher levels are found in blood. Anus-to-mouth transmission during oro-anal sex is considered to be an important factor, especially if there is any local bleeding. Although population studies have shown an association between oro-anal sex and hepatitis B infection, others have failed to confirm it.

Hepatitis C
Although sexually transmissible, its rate of transmission through this route is very small and much less than for HIV and hepatitis B. However, it is associated with HIV infection in MSM, especially those engaging in un-protected receptive and insertive anal sex, fisting, use of sex toys, and oro-anal sex.

Human herpesvirus 8 (HHV8)—cause of Kaposi's sarcoma (KS)
Studies in MSM have shown that oro-anal sex is a risk factor for KS and HHV8 infection is associated with both insertive and receptive oro-anal sex.

Human immunodeficiency virus (HIV)
Found in saliva at much lower concentrations than in semen and vaginal fluid, but probably ↑ infection risk if local oropharyngeal or ano-genital inflammation, ulceration, or bleeding (even after tooth brushing or dental flossing). However, anti-HIV inhibitory factors in saliva, especially secre-tory leucocyte protease inhibitor from the parotid glands, have protec-tive properties against HIV infection, contributing to the low rates of oral transmission. Potentially the greatest danger for an uninfected person is the oral reception of infected ejaculate irrespective of swallowing or spitting it out. However, HIV transmission to both ♂ and ♀ has been reported during fellatio without ejaculation and HIV has been detected in pre-ejaculatory fluid. Most data relate to MSM with studies from London and San Francisco suggesting that 6% and 8%, respectively, believed that they had acquired HIV through oral sex alone. These figures are probably overestimates, as from previous studies other risk factors were later ad-mitted. Although giving oral sex carries the most risk, new infections have been reported in men receiving oral sex from an infected ♂ or ♀. The transmission of HIV infection by cunnilingus has been reported between ♀ although a 3-month study following serodiscordant lesbian couples practising cunnilingus showed no seroconversions.

Human papillomavirus (HPV)
The development of oropharyngeal warts is uncommon, but when found is usually caused by types 6, 11, 16, and 18, i.e. those most commonly caus-ing genital infection. The development of an oral condyloma attributed to cunnilingus with an infected partner has been reported. High-risk (most commonly type 16) HPV infection is associated with HIV infection (espe-cially CD4 counts <200cells/mL, oral mucosal abnormalities, and >1 oral sex partner. The natural history of oral HPV infection is similar to genital infection. In patients with oropharyngeal cancer there is a significant as-sociation with HPV type 16 (and oral infection with any of 37 HPV types) with or without the established risk factors of tobacco and alcohol use. The data on the role of oral sex are unclear. Associations with a high life-time number of vaginal or oral sex partners (with a 250% increased risk for those with >5 oral sex partners) and concurrent oral infection in a sexual partner have been reported. However, other studies have failed to show an association between oral sex and oral or genital HPV infection.

Lymphogranuloma venereum (LGV)

There are no data associating the recent development of LGV proctitis in MSM with oral sex. However, oral lesions and cervical adenopathy due to LGV have been reported following oral sex. Ocular inoculation can give rise to a follicular conjunctivitis, often accompanied by pre-auricular lymphadenopathy.

Molluscum contagiosum

May be found on the cutaneous lip and peri-oral skin, usually in clusters, especially when immunocompromised. When extensive often signifies advanced HIV disease.

Non-chlamydial non-gonococcal urethritis (NGU)

Although the sexually transmitted nature of non-chlamydial NGU has been demonstrated, an association with oral sex has not been confirmed.

Pediculosis

Pthirus pubis may be transmitted from pubic hair to facial hair (i.e. beard, moustache, eyebrows, and eyelashes) during orogenital sex.

Respiratory tract organisms

- Neisseria meningitidis—case reports and series. Most common—anal infection in MSM, usually asymptomatic. Case reports of urethritis associated with fellatio and cervicitis, vulvovaginitis, and salpingitis in ♀ although asymptomatic carriage more common than with urethral infection in ♂.
- Moraxella catarrhalis—less common than N.meningitidis. Urethritis reported in ♂.
- Streptococcal infection—isolated case reports of acute balanitis following fellatio caused by group A streptococci. Balanitis due to group B infection appears to be related to vaginal coitus.

Haemophilus influenzae—case reports of H.influenzae-associated septic abortion related to recent oral sex.

Syphilis

The resurgence of syphilis in the UK, W. Europe, and N. America has largely arisen in MSM and their partners. Studies have shown that over a third reported oral sex as the only risk factor, frequently not considering this to be a risk. Oral sex is much less likely to be condom protected compared with anal sex. The reporting of oral sex (often anonymous) among MSM is extremely common, and there is a significant association with higher numbers of oral sex partners although not with particular oral practices. Kissing as a means of transmission has also been implicated.

Box 5.1 Receptive oral sex or receiving oral sex

Descriptions of oral sex can be confusing because of variable interpretation. 'Receptive oral sex' has been used in the same sense as receptive anal sex, i.e. accepting the sexual partner's penis into one's mouth. Insertive oral sex has similarly been used to describe the act of inserting one's penis into the partner's mouth. On the other hand 'receiving oral sex' has been used to describe male or female genital stimulation by the sexual partner's mouth. 'Giving or (performing) oral sex' is the opposite of 'receiving', i.e. stimulating the partner's genitals by one's mouth. In view of the greater applicability, the descriptions used in this book are:

- 'receiving oral sex' to indicate genital stimulation by the sexual partner's mouth
- 'giving oral sex' to indicate stimulating the sexual partner's genitals.

Pregnancy

Bacterial vaginosis (BV)

Increased bacterial production of cytokines and prostaglandins and amniotic fluid/chorioamniotic infection leading to:

- chorioamnionitis
- low birth weight
- preterm birth (relative risk 1.5–2.3) from preterm labour and premature rupture of membranes
- 2nd trimester miscarriage (up to 3–6-fold risk)
- endometritis (pre/post delivery including Caesarean section).

History of previous premature delivery ↑ risk of further preterm birth 7-fold with BV. Risk of preterm birth higher with BV in early rather than late pregnancy.

Data from clinical trials screening for and treating BV during pregnancy have produced conflicting results. Therefore current UK (BASHH guidelines recommend:

- Symptomatic ♀ should be treated (as if non-pregnant).
- There is insufficient evidence to recommend routinely screening and treating asymptomatic ♀ attending GUM for BV.

Candidiasis

Vaginal prevalence rate doubles in pregnancy to ~40% (↑ circulating oestrogens and vaginal glycogen). Although not usually associated with chorioamnionitis or preterm delivery, there is limited evidence that eradicating vaginal candidiasis during pregnancy may ↓ risk of preterm delivery.

Chlamydia

Associated with preterm delivery, low birth weight, premature rupture of membranes (PROM), intrapartum pyrexia, endometritis, neonatal infection (Ⓐ Chapter 8, p. 152) and post-abortal pelvic inflammatory disease. Screening is advised for those at risk, including those having surgical termination of pregnancy (rates of 2–30% reported). Tetracyclines, fluoroquinolones, and co-trimoxazole are contraindicated during pregnancy.

Gonorrhoea

In view of the ↑ risks of preterm delivery, low birth rate, PROM, endometritis, and neonatal infection (Ⓐ Pregnancy and the neonate, p. 140), and post-abortal pelvic inflammatory disease, screening for gonorrhoea is advisable in PROM, septic abortion, intra/postpartum fever, or those considered to be at risk. Quinolone and tetracycline antibiotics are contraindicated during pregnancy.

Group B streptococcal infection

Ⓐ See Chapter 31, *Streptococcus agalactiae*, p. 346.

Hepatitis B virus (HBV)

Pregnancy does not ↑ maternal morbidity or mortality from HBV infection or ↑ the risk of fetal complications, although preterm labour increases with acute HBV infection. In acute maternal infection the neonatal risk depends on gestational age with 10% transmission risk in the 1st trimester rising to

80–90% in the 3rd trimester. With chronic HBV infection, i.e. hepatitis B surface antigen (HBsAg) positive, transmission risk depends on maternal infectivity with 90% of infants born to hepatitis B e antigen (HBeAg) ♀ becoming chronic carriers compared with <5% if HBeAg negative and HBsAg positive. Maternal screening in pregnancy is important as neonatal passive immunization (hepatitis B immunoglobulin) given within 24 hours of birth combined with active vaccination ↓ the 90% chronic carriage rate with HBeAg +ve infection to 10–15% and with HBeAg –ve infection to <1%.

Hepatitis C virus (HCV)

~5% of infants born to HCV-infected ♀ become infected, i.e. serum HCV-RNA detected in at least two samples and/or HCV antibody reactive when the infant is at least 15 months old. Maternal HIV co-infection ↑ the risk of transmitting HCV 2–3-fold. As only 30–50% of infected infants have HCV-RNA detected at birth, it seems that the majority acquire infection at delivery. However, several studies have shown no difference in the neonatal incidence rate with regard to mode of delivery. Although there are contradictory data on breastfeeding it need not be avoided in mono-infected pregnant ♀.

Herpes simplex virus (HSV)

85% of neonatal infections are acquired perinatally (exposure from infected birth canal), with 5% due to intrauterine exposure (usually ascending lower genital tract infection) and 10% postnatally (contact with family and staff). Risk of neonatal herpes is very low (probably <1%) for ♀ with recurrent herpes. Highest risk is when the mother has not seroconverted by delivery, with a 40–50% risk of neonatal herpes if primary infection is acquired in the 3rd trimester and a 20% risk for initial HSV-2 infection with previous HSV-1 infection.

Oral aciclovir should be prescribed as indicated for initial episodes and intravenous aciclovir for severe genital or disseminated infection, with case reports demonstrating significantly improved survival of the neonate. It is rarely indicated for the treatment of recurrences during pregnancy. For further information see ☐ Chapter 21, p. 270.

HIV

Most HIV transmission risk occurs during delivery and postpartum (breastfeeding), with antepartum (transplacental) spread uncommon. Pregnancy does not ↑ maternal morbidity or progression of infection. In ♀ with asymptomatic infection there is no ↑ in fetal malformations or antenatal mortality and only a small ↑ in spontaneous abortion, possible ↑ in low birth weight and preterm delivery. With optimized antenatal/postnatal care and antiretroviral treatment transmission rates are ↓ from 10–40% to <2%.

Sexually acquired reactive arthritis

This is uncommon in pregnancy, but if treatment is required select appropriate antibiotic (📖 Chapter 8, p. 156), try to restrict use of non-steroidal anti-inflammatory drugs and avoid methotrexate, gold salts, and tumour necrosis factor (TNF) blockers (📖 p. 201).

Syphilis

Syphilis can be transmitted at any stage of pregnancy. In early untreated maternal syphilis preterm delivery or perinatal death will occur in 50% of all maternal 1° or 2° syphilis and 40% of those with early latent infections. With late untreated infection up to 20% prematurity/perinatal death 10% of infants develop congenital syphilis. Therefore all pregnant ♀ should be screened for syphilis at the initial booking visit.

Early syphilis is treated with procaine benzylpenicillin G 750mg IM daily for 10 days or benzathine benzylpenicillin, single dose in 1st and 2nd trimester with a second dose if treated during the 3rd trimester after 1 week. Second-line treatments include oral amoxicillin 500mg with oral probenecid 500mg 4 times a day for 14 days, IM ceftriaxone 500mg daily for 10 days (limited data) and oral macrolides (erythromycin 500mg 4 times a day for 14 days or azithromycin 500mg daily for 10 days). However, there are case reports of congenital infection with macrolides, so if used neonatal treatment is required after delivery. Late syphilis is treated as for non-pregnant patients but excluding doxycycline. See also (📖 Syphilis management: early and late p. 126).

Trichomoniasis (TV)

There is an independent association in pregnancy with premature rupture of the membranes, preterm delivery, and low birth weight. Although treatment (with metronidazole) is advocated for symptomatic ♀, there is no value in providing antenatal screening and treatment for asymptomatic ♀. There is no evidence that treatment will ↓ the risk of preterm birth and in one trial the treatment of asymptomatic ♀ with metronidazole appeared to be associated with preterm birth. The reason is unclear, and it has even been postulated that it may be due to an immune reaction elicited by the dying TV or virus released from its cytoplasm.

Urinary tract infection (UTI)

More common during pregnancy with 2–10% of ♀ having asymptomatic bacteriuria. Without treatment this persists with a third progressing to acute pyelonephritis. Complications include low birth weight/prematurity, pre-eclampsia, maternal anaemia, amnionitis, and intra-uterine death with risks reduced by treating asymptomatic bacteriuria.

Symptomatic UTI most commonly occurs towards the end of the 2nd trimester because of hormonal changes, although progression to pyelonephritis is uncommon.

All pregnant ♀ should be screened for bacteriuria, ideally by urine culture although reagent strip testing, although less effective, is cheaper. Asymptomatic and symptomatic bacteriuria should be treated for 7-10 days (📖 Chapter 20, Management p. 258) avoiding aminoglycosides, quinolones, tetracyclines and trimethoprim (1st trimester). ♀ with acute pyelonephritis should be assessed in hospital as hydration is crucial.

Warts

Commonly appear, proliferate, or enlarge rapidly during pregnancy, probably related to relative immunosuppression. There is no known association of human papilloma infection with pregnancy complications and they do not usually obstruct vaginal delivery. Occurrence of Buschke–Lowenstein tumours has been reported occurring during pregnancy.

Treatment options are limited as podophyllotoxin and podophyllin are contraindicated and imiquimod is not licensed in pregnancy although its use has been reported. As risks are low and regression after delivery is usual, information and reassurance are appropriate for most ♀ affected.

Sexual assault: general principles

Definitions (see 📖 Sexual offences, p. 26)

Statistics

Sexual assault is common: worldwide 1 in 4 women experience sexual violence by an intimate partner in their lifetime. The British Crime Survey 2008/9 shows that 2.8% of adults between 16 and 59 had experienced serious sexual assault since age 16. 36% of people told no one and only 13% reported to police. Only 6% of those reporting rape see their assailant convicted.

Myths/misconception

♂ who are anally raped may have an erection and ejaculate as a normal physiological response. It does not mean that they are homosexual, or have enjoyed or consented to it. The absence of physical trauma does not exclude rape. Many victims are too afraid to fight off an attack for fear of further assault or loss of life. A victim can appear calm and even smile following a rape, but this does not mean the rape accusation is false—it is a normal coping mechanism. Rape is not committed because of an overwhelming sex-drive with a sexual motivation. It is usually an act of violence and power with the vast majority premeditated.

Drug-facilitated sexual assault

Alcohol is the drug most commonly associated with sexual assault. Other drugs implicated include cannabis, benzodiazepines, cocaine, antidepressants. The use of Rohypnol® (flunitrazepam) has been reported widely in the media but research has not confirmed this.

Presentation

May be within hours or years after an attack to a variety of services including GUM or sexual health clinics. It is important to ensure that there are sensitive links with the police and support agencies (e.g. sexual assault referral centres). The patient should be offered a choice of ♂ or ♀ experienced staff if possible. A suitable appointment with minimum waiting time and private waiting area should ideally be provided if distressed. It is crucial to explore the person's needs and wishes and ensure that arrangements are in place for anonymous reporting of incidents to the police for those not wanting to make a formal charge.

Early priorities

in acute situations treatment of serious physical injury following assault takes precedence over obtaining forensic evidence. Timed samples of blood and urine are important (for alcohol and drug assays), together with oral samples (mouth washings/swabs) which should be taken as soon as possible after the attack to avoid the loss of potentially useful evidence.

Forensic testing

No attempt to perform a forensic examination should be made unless forensically trained and in a suitable environment with the correct equipment to perform it. Forensic examination can be useful up to 7 days following an assault. Local police services should give advice on where this is performed. Currently there are 29 sexual assault referral centres in England and Wales. The person should be advised to retain all clothing involved unwashed, retain sanitary wear and not to bathe/wash prior to the forensic examination.

Sexual assault: history checklist

▶ Always inform the patient that he/she need only give as much information as he/she feels comfortable with. Asking a patient to give full details of an assault can be very distressing.

- *Date of assault:* essential for determining when STI screening should occur and the use of emergency contraception.
- *Location of assault:* needed to assess the background prevalence of certain STIs, especially if the attacker is a stranger.
- *Attacker(s) details:* assessing the risk of the acquisition of STIs:
  - number
  - known or stranger
  - if known—any risk factors for blood-borne viruses.
- *Was assault reported to police? / Does the patient want to report? / Has a forensic examination been performed?* Important as forensic examination should be performed prior to STI screening.
- *Were alcohol/drugs taken prior to attack?* To establish the possibility of 'drug rape'.
- *Is the GP aware of the assault and/or has the patient contacted a rape support agency?* To assess any treatment given and psychological support arranged.
- *Details regarding type of attack:* to determine the exact nature of the attack for legal purposes and the risks/sites of possible STIs or injury:
  - physical injury
  - vaginal penetration
  - anal penetration
  - oral penetration
  - digital penetration
  - was a condom used?
  - ▶ Those assaulted may be too upset to recall this information or may have blanked out the detail as a means of coping. Therefore it is wise to offer screening from all sites and this may provide additional assurance to the patient.

Sexual assault: forensic assessment

Purpose

To establish:
- exact documentation of injuries
- identification and retrieval of any possible evidence
- relevant illnesses/previous trauma which may affect the interpretation of injuries/evidence.

Consent

Must cover both non-genital and genital examination and the recording of findings (including photography), the retention of relevant items of clothing, the collection of forensic evidence, and disclosure to police, Crown Prosecution Service, and Crown Court (rather than being subject to medical confidentiality).

Forensic assessment

Timing

- Ideally within 72 hours of the incident (although examination after >72 hours may be appropriate) and within 7 days (for DNA evidence), although examination after this may still be useful to document injuries.
- In adults spermatozoa persist in:
  - the vagina for 7 days
  - the mouth for 2 days
  - the anus for 3 days

Azoospermic samples can be identified.

Evidence

- Account of events, from both complainant and police officer, including the possible use of alcohol and drugs
- Activities subsequent to the incident, including cleansing (body, teeth, hair), eating and drinking, and change in sanitary protection
- Timing of consensual sex within 10 days of the assault (before or after)
- Relevant medical, surgical, gynaecological, and psychiatric history (can affect interpretation of examination)
- Medication (including non-prescribed) in preceding days
- Relevant social information
- General examination for injuries (or their absence)
- Genital (and/or anal, oral) examination, details of instruments used, vaginal (speculum) examination, colposcopy (to magnify any suspicious lesions), proctoscopy
- Reaction of complainant to general and oro-anogenital examination
- Retrieval of alleged assailant's body fluids or other material for DNA analysis (e.g. genital, anal swabs, swabs from unwashed skin which have been in intimate contact with the assailant, pubic hair cuttings
- Identification and recovery of other material (e.g. fibres, hair, skin particles)
- Control swabs from uncontaminated skin
- List forensic specimens taken

Injuries

In post-pubertal ♀, anogenital injury is found in up to a third of those sexually assaulted. Severity of assault is a poor predictor of anogenital injury. However, presence of anogenital injury is considered to carry more weight in obtaining a conviction.

Record site (anatomical terms may require definition) using a 'clock-face' for anogenital lesions.

- Bruise. Leakage of blood into skin due to blunt trauma:
  - petechiae—bruises <2mm due to increased pressure (strangulation etc.), oblique blunt trauma, suction, blunt trauma through fabrics, medical causes (infection, coughing, medication, blood disorders)
  - purpura—larger haemorrhages within the skin
  - haematoma—blood collection beneath the skin.

Bruising may be difficult to interpret in hairy skin, affected by skin colour and medication/drug abuse, and exaggerated with skin fragility (e.g. in the elderly). It may not correlate with the size of the object inflicting injury, the severity of the blow, or the site of impact (due to tracking of blood), and will vary according to site (related to underlying bone). It is impossible to age bruises with precision. Appearances may assist in the interpretation of its cause (e.g. bruising from finger-tips).

- Abrasions (scratches—linear, grazes—broad)—involve only outer skin layers
- Lacerations (tears)—full-thickness splitting of skin, usually irregular and often associated with bruising
- Others—incision, stab wounds, thermal (dry heat or moist heat (scald)), electrical, friction, cigarette, fracture
- Record of injury should include, as appropriate, its nature, dimensions, colour (if bruising), pattern, site, associated injuries, pre- and coexisting injury, depth, active bleeding, suturing/dressing, presence of foreign material in wound.

Interpretation of findings

Normal/abnormal; scaled evaluation of certainty about likely cause of the injuries, their causal consistency with other information available. This is an opinion and therefore should be provided by an expert to the court. Take care never to step outside your clinical expertise.

Sexual assault: management

▶ **If the patient wishes to report the assault to the police examination and screening for STIs should be deferred until forensic tests have been taken as evidence may be lost. The patient may also wish to have a forensic examination without police involvement (self-referral) which is possible in some centres.**

The management of victims of sexual assault can appear complex and should include screening for STIs, emergency contraception, and psychological support. Occasionally, medical evidence may be required in court and well-written clear notes are vital for this. The use of a pro forma for sexual assault cases can help to ensure that no vital areas of management are missed and all necessary information is recorded.

History taking

The history should be taken with a degree of flexibility, depending on the emotional state of the patient, and be performed in a calm and sensitive manner. In addition to the standard history, detailed information should be taken regarding the assault.

Examination

In recent assault cases the presence or absence of visible trauma should be clearly documented with the use of diagrams. If any injury requires medical treatment, this should be provided before any further examination. The absence of any injuries does not exclude rape. In cases of recent forced oral penetration examine for haemorrhages on the palate. Offer proctoscopy if recent forced anal penetration for signs of trauma.

Investigations

It is rare for the presence of an STI to legally reinforce a case of rape. As people who have been assaulted may have pre-existing STIs, it is advisable to do a full screen at presentation. However, it is recommended that swabs are repeated 2 weeks after the assault as early sampling may miss recently acquired infection. Ensure that patients fully understand what tests are recommended and their implications. Where possible the 'chain of evidence' should be implemented (i.e. every handover of the specimen is signed, dated, and timed). As well as the standard STI screen and microscopy, additional specimens should be considered. If the patient does not want serological testing at presentation a serum specimen can be stored. This may help to clarify the timing of any subsequent seroconversion.

Management

Offer treatment for any infection found. Assess mental state and suicide risk. A health adviser can reinforce information given, provide links for psychological support, and clarify the follow-up arrangements. Ensure that the patient leaves the clinic with contact numbers of agencies able to provide further emotional support.

Sexual assault: investigations checklist

NB: Swabs should only be taken after forensic samples have been taken, if relevant.

- *Microscopy:* urethral, cervical and rectal smears (if relevant) for *N.gonorrhoeae*, vaginal preparations for yeasts, bacterial vaginosis, and *T. vaginalis*.
- *NAAT for C.trachomatis:* urethra and cervix. May also detect rectal infection.
- *Culture for N.gonorrhoeae:* urethra, cervix, throat, and rectum (advised in ♀ even in the absence of forced anal penetration). NAAT for screening can be considered as highly sensitive but should be confirmed by culture for medico-legal purposes.
- *Culture for T. vaginalis:* vagina.
- *Serology:*
  - syphilis
  - HIV
  - hepatitis B virus
  - hepatitis C virus (if patient has risk factor, assailant unknown, or if assailant known to have risk factor)
  - storage (if patient does not wish baseline testing).

Sexual assault: management checklist

- *Treat any infection found*
- *Emergency contraception:* if indicated (📖 Reversible contraception: emergency contraception p. 386).
- *Prophylactic antibiotics:* consider for chlamydia and gonorrhoea if the patient cannot tolerate an examination or requires an intra-uterine device for emergency contraception.
- *Hepatitis B immunization:* may have a protective effect if given within 6 weeks following an assault.
- *HIV prophylaxis:* individual risk assessment needed, including type and location of assault and assailant risk factors.
- *Support:* may be provided by a health adviser, specialist nurse, or other agencies.
- *Consent to write to general practitioner:* helpful to provide comprehensive care.

Review: for follow-up of any infection detected, repeat investigations (to cover 'window periods'), hepatitis immunization, and psychological support.

Children

Sexual abuse involves forcing a young person to take part in sexual activities whether or not the young person is aware of what is happening. If suspected, screening for STIs should be considered. If infection is found in a child aged <3 years, vertical transmission from the mother is possible so she should be offered STI screening. This may be extended to the siblings and others in the household.

All GUM clinics should have:

- Guidelines for the management of children.
- A nominated consultant physician to take the lead for children as part of a multidisciplinary team, access to formal child protection training.
- Details of local child protection policies and procedures.
- Chain of evidence procedures (Sexual assault: management p. 106).
- Regular audit of adherence to child protection guidelines.

Sexually transmitted infections

▶ The significance of an STI in children requires careful interpretation. It may be used as corroborative evidence to indicate sexual abuse. If infection is found, test and treat any consensual or non-consensual sexual contacts (with consent), and test (and treat if appropriate) parents when there is a chance of vertical transmission.

STI testing

This should be performed at baseline with tests for gonorrhoea and chlamydia repeated 2 weeks after the last penetrative contact (if necessary) and serology for HIV, syphilis, and hepatitis B and C after 12 weeks. If post-exposure HIV prophylaxis has been given or the child is at a high risk of exposure to hepatitis B or C repeat serology after 6 months is advised.

NAATs are generally accepted as the gold standard for chlamydia, although they are unlicensed for oropharyngeal, rectal and urogenital specimens in children. Any positives should be confirmed by a different NAAT (although culture is considered to be the most specific test for chlamydia, it is rarely available). Culture for gonorrhoea is still the gold standard though a NAAT can be done in addition or if urine is being tested. Any positive NAAT should be confirmed by culture.

When testing pre-pubertal girls (usually <11 years) introital swabs should be used from inside the labia minora but avoiding the hymen. A trans-hymenal (ENT) swab may be used if the hymenal orifice is large enough to allow the passage of a swab without distress. First voided urine for chlamydia and gonorrhoea NAAT should be undertaken in boys (and girls if other tests not feasible). In post-pubertal girls endocervical swabs should be used in preference to vulval or trans-hymenal swabs provided that a speculum is tolerated.

Specimens

Girls: urogenital
- Essential—vulval or trans-hymenal (pre-pubertal), endocervical if post-pubertal (providing speculum tolerated):
  - culture for *N.gonorrhoea* ± microscopy
  - NAAT for *C.trachomatis* ± *N.gonorrhoeae*
  - culture for *C.trachomatis* (if available)
- Optional
  - If discharge present—microscopy (if available) for *T.vaginalis*, *Candida* spp, bacterial vaginosis, and swab (in Amies medium) for *T. vaginalis* and *Candida* spp. culture and microscopy for clue cells.
  - If examination declined—urine NAAT for *C.trachomatis* ± *N.gonorrhoeae*

Boy: urogenital
- If urethritis (meatal swab—pre-pubertal; urethral swab – post-pubertal):
  - microscopy for pus cells and Gram-negative intracellular diplococci
  - culture for *N.gonorrhoeae*
  - culture for *C.trachomatis* (if available)
- Urine for *C.trachomatis* ± *N.gonorrhoeae*.

Extragenital samples
- Consider as routine but essential if oral or anal assault disclosed or suspected. Pharyngeal and rectal swabs for:
- NAAT for *C.trachomatis* ± *N.gonorrhoeae*
- culture for *N.gonorrhoeae*
- culture for *C.trachomatis* (if available).

Anogenital blisters or ulcers
- Swab for herpes simplex virus (HSV)—NAAT or culture
- HSV serology for IgM and IgG (paired sera at 3 week interval)
- Consider dark ground microscopy for *Treponema pallidum*
- Consider swab for *Haemophilus ducreyi* (culture or NAAT).

Anogenital warts
HPV typing is currently controversial. It may be considered in specific cases but not justified for routine use.

Serology
Consider testing for HIV, syphilis, hepatitis B and C in all cases, depending on risk factors. Check at presentation and 12 weeks after the assault. Repeat serology advised 6 months after the assault for HIV infection (if post-exposure prophylaxis supplied) and for hepatitis B and C if considered to be at high risk.

Management

Wherever possible treatment for children should be prescribed within the terms of the product licence. However, some conditions may require drugs not specifically licensed for paediatric use. If in doubt, discuss with local pharmacist.

Specific infections

Bacterial vaginosis (BV)

Garderella vaginalis has been isolated from the vagina in 4–14% (as for adults) and may be part of the normal flora. The relevance of finding BV in children is unclear as BV is not classified as a STI. Variable rates of BV, from 7% to 34%, have been demonstrated in sexually abused girls. (However, it has been shown to be related to ↑ in sexual partners in adolescent girls).

Chlamydia

Found in the rectum, vagina, conjunctiva, or nasopharynx of infants. Estimated risk of perinatal transmission 50–70%, mostly conjunctivitis, but up to 15% have infection of the vagina and rectum (which can persist up to 3 years). Genito-rectal chlamydial has been reported in 0.4–17% of sexually abused children. Asymptomatic presentation is common, especially girls with cervicovaginal infection.

Gonorrhoea

Estimated risk of perinatal transmission resulting in gonococcal ophthalmia of 30%. In studies since 1988 gonorrhoea infection has been found in 1–4.6% of sexually abused children. Gonococci can survive for up to 24 hours on toilet seats and longer on swabs, but (apart from one report from an aeroplane toilet) there is no evidence of transmission. However, historically, outbreaks of infection have been reported in children living in overcrowded conditions.

Most common symptom is vaginal discharge, but ~45% is asymptomatic.

Herpes

Prevalence in pre-pubertal children unknown but uncommon. Genitals are the most likely source of HSV type 2 infection (as an uncommon cause of oral infection) but its detection in a child does not prove sexual contact. Auto-inoculation from the mouth is possible (rare in adults), and transmission from a maternal recurrent whitlow and following metzitzah (the sucking of the circumcision wound by the circumciser to promote healing following religious circumcision) has been reported.

HIV

Most children have acquired infection non-sexually, although transmission following assault has been reported and is likely to increase.

Syphilis

Pre-pubertal children presenting with 1° or 2° stages of syphilis occurring beyond the neonatal period should be considered to be victims of sexual abuse. Congenital syphilis is now uncommon in the UK.

Trichomoniasis

Found in ~5% of infants born to infected mothers and may persist for 3–6 weeks in oestrogenized vagina and longer in the urinary tract, although it is unlikely to persist beyond the 1st year. In children being investigated for sexual abuse, 1–4% have been found to be infected. *T.vaginalis* does not survive for long in the alkaline pre-pubertal vagina and its presence suggests recent abuse. Although considered rare, non-sexual transmission is possible as *T.vaginalis* may survive on damp towels or flannels for several hours. Girls usually present with vulvovaginitis although asymptomatic infection may occur.

Warts

Peak age incidence is between birth and 4 years with reports of anogenital warts twice as common in girls. Vertical transmission of human papilloma virus (HPV) can occur at birth and rarely *in utero*, with an incubation period ranging from months to years, so warts developing within the first year of life are likely to be acquired perinatally. The most common types causing warts in adult are HPV types 6 and 11, with both, especially type 11, found in laryngeal papillomas. Approximately 2% of children aged 1–12 years being investigated for possible sexual abuse have been found to have genital warts, and sexual abuse was implicated in 42% of those presenting with anogenital warts (mean figure from reported surveys). However, HPV types 1 and 2 (the most common type in cutaneous warts) may cause anogenital warts suggesting possible non-sexual acquisition, including auto-inoculation (although abuse, e.g. by fondling, must be considered).

Syphilis

Introduction

The origins of syphilis are unclear, but it became an epidemic in Europe in the late fifteenth century (although skeletal evidence suggests earlier endemic infection). The name originates from a poem about the infected shepherd Syphilis written by Fracastoro in 1530.

Aetiology: *Treponema pallidum*

Delicate spiralled spirochaete, 6–20μm long by 0.1–0.18μm in diameter. Consists of a cylindrical nucleus and cytoplasm contained within a cell wall and outer envelope with flagella in the periplasmic space. Microaerophilic and can only be grown on tissue culture. Limited viability outside its host (obligate human parasite), so is usually transmitted sexually to and from mucosal skin through tiny abrasions.

Epidemiology and transmission

Currently high rates in Eastern Europe. In UK disproportionately high rates of infection in ♂ who have sex with ♂, especially as outbreaks through anonymous sex in saunas and 'cruising sites' by orogenital sex and in association with HIV infection. Circumcised ♂ are at lower risk.
- Sexual (only from early syphilis): ~30–50% of contacts are infected.
- Accidental infection by inoculation (e.g. healthcare professionals).
- Blood-borne—needle sharing, blood transfusion (very rare as blood is screened and organisms die after 96–120 hours at 4°C).
- Transplacental (from 9th week of pregnancy). More common in early syphilis (80–90% risk); rare after 4 years.

Natural history

Acquired

Early (infectious) syphilis
- 1°: 9–90 days after infection (average 3 weeks) resolving within 3–8 weeks (occasionally with small pale scar).
- 2°: 6 weeks–6 months after infection, associated with a persisting 1° lesion in 33%. Lesions may relapse (in 25% if untreated) and regress over a period of 2 years. Permanent depigmentation of the skin of the neck (leucoderma colli) rarely occurs.
- Early latent: within first 2 years of infection (1 year in USA).

Late syphilis
- Late latent—after 2 years of infection (1 year in USA). Also separate category in USA of latent infection of unknown duration. End result in two-thirds of those who are not treated (data from pre-antibiotic area)
- Gummatous ('benign'): can appear within 2 years, usually 10–15 years.
  - Musculoskeletal (10%), visceral and mucosal (15%).
- Cardiovascular (10%)—after ~10–30 years.
- Neurological (10%):

- Meningovascular: after ~2–7 years; general paresis, after ~10–20 years; tabes dorsalis, after ~15–25 years.

Congenital
- Early, first 2 years of life.
- Late, lesions usually from 2–3 years of age.

Frequently asked questions

Can I catch syphilis from oral sex?
Yes, unprotected oral sex is a risk factor.

Is it true that you can go 'mad' with syphilis?
Neurosyphilis may lead to general paralysis with dulling of the intellect, judgement, and insight, memory loss, antisocial behaviour, grandiose delusions, depression, and dementia. It takes 20–25 years to develop but is prevented by earlier treatment. It is extremely rare nowadays.

When I've been treated, am I immune?
No, it is possible to catch syphilis again after reinfection. Having been infected once with syphilis does not give any lasting immunity.

Do I have to have an injection for treatment? Can I have tablets instead?
The first-line recommended treatment is with long-acting penicillin injections. For those who are allergic to penicillin, oral doxycycline is recommended. The dosage and duration of treatment depends on the stage of infection.

My blood tests are still positive after treatment. Does this mean I still have syphilis?
No. Many of the blood tests used for detecting syphilis measure anti-treponemal antibodies, which are usually produced for life even after successful treatment. They do not provide protection against future infection. It is important to measure their nadir after treatment as reinfection will produce a rise in their levels.

Does my partner need treating?
If you have been diagnosed with:
- 1° syphilis—your current partner needs to be seen to be tested for syphilis, and any other partners seen within the previous 3 months
- 2° syphilis—all sexual contacts within the previous 2 years need to be seen with serological review for 3 months from the last sexual risk.

Partners will only be treated if they test positive for syphilis. If surveillance is not possible, epidemiological treatment may be considered.

If you have been diagnosed with late latent syphilis you are not sexually infectious. However, we need to work out when infection was most likely acquired and partners from within 2 years of this time should be notified for testing.

Clinical features: early syphilis

Primary syphilis: lesion(s) at site(s) of infection

Classical presentation

Initial painless papule at inoculation site which expands and ulcerates, producing a round or oval painless chancre 1–2cm in diameter with an indurated margin and clear moist base exuding serum without blood on pressure (Plate 2). Typically solitary, although multiple lesions may occur. Moderate, usually bilateral, painless enlargement of regional inguinal lymph nodes if chancre is within the area of drainage.

Contemporary presentation

it has become more common to find multiple painful ulcers with little induration mimicking genital herpes, especially in ♂ homosexual outbreaks (Plate 3). Orogenital sex is a major vehicle for transmission, with oral ulceration seen more frequently.

Sites

- Genitals: may appear anywhere but more likely on mucosal surfaces, i.e. sub-preputial sac, glans penis, labia, fourchette, and cervix (the latter without inguinal adenopathy and usually asymptomatic). Rarely an intra-urethral chancre presenting as urethritis may occur in ♂. Rare reports of balanitis (including balanitis of Follmann).
- Extra-genital: oral (lips, mouth, tongue, tonsils, and pharynx—the last two may be painful), anal margin (often resembling a fissure with local tenderness), rectum (unusual), and rarely other sites (including finger, hand, arm, supraclavicular, nipple, eyelid).

Secondary syphilis—from haematogenous dissemination

- Constitutional: malaise, fever, headache, anorexia, myalgia.
- Skin lesions (syphilides), often polymorphic (~80%), pruritus in ~40%:
  - Macular: pink, 1cm diameter, mostly on trunk, often overlooked.
  - Papular (dull red with shiny surface) and papulosquamous (with surface scaling). Extensive, typically affecting flexor surfaces and involving palms (Plate 4) and soles (firm non-prominent papules, scaling common). May form condylomata lata, hypertrophied wart-like lesions on moist areas, especially around vulva and anus (Plate 5). Brittle nails.
  - Other: pustular (especially with debility), hyper- or hypopigmented (leucoderma) lesions.
- Lymphadenopathy: 75% inguinal, 60% generalized; also splenomegaly.
- Mucous membrane lesions in 30%: 'mucous patch'—ulcer with white/grey border (may coalesce with others forming 'snail track ulcers'). Found in the oral cavity and larynx (sore throat, hoarseness), nasal mucosa (discharge), genitalia, anus, and rectum (diffuse, distal proctitis).
- Alopecia: specific—'moth-eaten'; non-specific—telogen effluvium (diffuse).
- Musculoskeletal: periostitis—bone pain (25% prior to antibiotic era), especially tibia; bursitis; arthralgia (6%).

- Hepatitis: usually subclinical, raised enzymes, mainly alkaline phosphatase, in 20%.
- Renal: rarely glomerulonephritis; nephrotic syndrome (both mild and self-limiting).
- Neurological: meningism in 1–2%; transitory cerebrospinal fluid (CSF) white cell and protein ↑ in 5–40%; very rarely meningitis/meningovasculitis; perceptive nerve deafness; peripheral neuritis.
- Eyes: iritis (<1%); anterior uveitis (more common in HIV infection); choroidoretinitis, including optic atrophy (usually asymptomatic).

Early latent

No signs or symptoms, positive serology, within 2 years of acquisition.

Differential diagnosis of 2° syphilis

Macular rash

- Pityriasis rosea—initial herald patch
- Tinea (pityriasis) versicolor—hypo- or hyperpigmented scaly macular rash, mostly over trunk. Culture scales for *Malassezia furfur*
- Measles—oral Koplik spots
- Rubella—posterior cervical lymph node enlargement
- Infectious mononucleosis—may be associated with biological false-positive VDRL/RPR test result
- Drug reaction—associated with drug intake and pruritus

Papular lesions

- Psoriasis—extensor surfaces, knees and elbows, scalp, nail pitting
- Lichen planus—oral lesions, Wickham's striae

Clinical features: late syphilis

Late latent

No signs or symptoms, positive serology, >2 years after acquisition. Proportionately, more common now as active late syphilis has declined with the widespread use of antibiotics for other purposes.

Gummatous (late benign) syphilis

Gumma formation (syphilitic granulation tissue) is due to reactivation of residual treponemes in sensitized host. Gummata are nodules or nodulo-ulcers, indurated and indolent, single or few in number. They commonly heal with central scarring while peripherally still active. Ulcers are described as 'punched out' with a basal 'wash leather' appearance due to slough. They are not contagious.

Sites

- Skin: especially below knee, buttocks, thighs, shoulders, scalp, face.
- Bones: gummatous periostitis (bony proliferation) e.g. sabre tibia; gummatous osteitis (bone destruction).
- Mouth and throat: palatal perforation; gumma of tongue or superficial glossitis (associated with leucoplakia and malignancy); epiglottis destruction and laryngeal infiltration (hoarseness).
- Other organs: gummata of liver, testis, oesophagus, stomach, intestine, cerebrum, spinal cord, aortic wall, myocardium. Also reported in bronchi and lungs, kidney, bladder adrenal glands, and breast.

Cardiovascular syphilis

- Conduction defects: if gummatous involvement (e.g. Stokes–Adams syndrome).
- Aortitis leading to:
  - Aortic aneurysm: proximal ascending aorta, fusiform or saccular, without dissection. Presents as chest pain or signs of compression of adjacent structures (e.g. hoarseness, dysphagia).
  - Aortic regurgitation (30% of those with cardiovascular syphilis)—insidious so well compensated. Typical early diastolic murmur on forced expiration with patient inclined forward.
  - Coronary ostial stenosis leading to angina and heart failure.

Neurosyphilis

- Asymptomatic: just abnormal CSF findings. Found in up to 30% of 1° and 2° syphilis and in most does not become clinically relevant. In the pre-antibiotic era 23–87% of cases progressed to clinical neurosyphilis.
- Meningovascular: focal arteritis causing infarction and meningeal inflammation. Now the most common neurosyphilitic presentation. Consider if cerebrovascular accident in a young adult. Often sudden onset preceded by prodromal headache, insomnia, emotional lability, and mental deterioration. Hemiplegia/paresis, aphasia, seizures typical features but ocular palsy and trigeminal neuralgia may occur. Pupillary abnormalities are frequent with a full Argyll Robertson pupil (constriction on accommodation, not to light) in 10%.

- General paralysis: cortical neuronal loss. Insidious, dulling of intellect, judgement, and insight. Memory loss, antisocial behaviour, grandiose delusions (now rare), hand and facial tremor, depression, and dementia. Seizures and paresis (spastic) are late complications. Full Argyll Robertson pupil in 25%.
- Tabes dorsalis: selective inflammation and degeneration of the spinal dorsal columns and nerve roots. Lightning pains, paraesthesia, visceral crises (smooth muscle spasm), sensory ataxia with stamping gait, and positive Romberg sign. Diminished or absent reflexes, deep pain, vibration, and position sense. Trophic changes lead to neuropathic joints (Charcot) and painless perforating plantar ulcers. Optic atrophy and bilateral ptosis are common. Argyll Robertson pupil seen most commonly in tabes dorsalis, with at least 80% developing pupil abnormalities.

Pregnancy and congenital infection

Syphilis in pregnancy

All pregnant ♀ should be screened for syphilis at the initial booking visit. Syphilis can be transmitted at any stage of pregnancy, with fetal infection reported from 9th week of gestation. However, it is most likely to arise after the 18th week. It may result in polyhydramnios, preterm labour, hydrops, congenital syphilis, miscarriage, and stillbirth, with spontaneous abortion most commonly occurring in 2nd and early 3rd trimester. Outcome in untreated infection varies with stage.

- 1° or 2° syphilis: up to 50% prematurity/perinatal death and 50% congenital infection.
- Early latent syphilis: up to 40% prematurity/perinatal death and 20% congenital infection.
- Late latent syphilis: up to 20% prematurity/perinatal death and 10% congenital infection.

(Normal control: 9% prematurity/perinatal death).

▶ Despite treatment in early syphilis up to 14% may result in fetal death or congenital infection.

If untreated syphilis is detected, consideration should be given to testing children from earlier pregnancies.

Early congenital syphilis (within first 2 years of life)

Clinical manifestations do not normally appear until 2–12 weeks after birth. Features include:

- failure to thrive
- mucosal lesions—with pharyngeal and nasal involvement (snuffles), progressing to local destruction and perforation
- skin lesions:
  - rashes similar to 2° syphilis but prominent around the mouth and body orifices leading to scarring (rhagades)
  - blistering bullous eruption of palms and soles (syphilitic pemphigus)
  - condylomata lata around anus and genitalia
  - sparse hair and brittle, atrophic nails
- hepatosplenomegaly and moderate generalized lymphadenopathy
- osteochondritis and later periostitis especially of the long bones (may present as pseudoparalysis)
- others (meningitis, nephrotic syndrome, choroidoretinitis, anaemia, thrombocytopenia).

Late congenital syphilis (after 2 years of age)

No clinical features in about 60% (diagnosed on serology). Otherwise many features are similar to accelerated late-stage acquired syphilis (though the cardiovascular system is usually spared) and usually appear near puberty.

Inflammation

- Interstitial keratitis (most common late feature, 20–50%).
- Deafness (2° to otolabyrinthitis).
- Clutton's joints (bilateral painless effusion of the knee joints).
- Gummata of nasal septum, palate and throat; skin and bone (as acquired syphilis).
- Neurosyphilis (seizures, mental deficiency, juvenile tabes dorsalis and general paralysis).
- Paroxysmal cold haemoglobinuria.

Malformations

- Craniofacial: frontal bossing; 'bulldog' appearance—hypoplastic maxilla, high arched palate, and prominent mandible; 'saddle-nose'; circumoral rhagades.
- Dental:
  - Hutchinson's incisors (usually upper central)—conical, tapered towards the apex and notched. Hutchinson's triad ≈ Hutchinson's incisors, interstitial keratitis, and nerve deafness.
  - Moon's (Mulberry) molars—1st lower molars dome-shaped with hypoplastic cusps.
- Skeletal: bony sclerosis (generalized) or nodules (localized). Long bones primarily affected especially the tibia with anterior bowing ('sabre tibia').

Frequently asked questions

I am pregnant, is syphilis harmful to my baby?

Syphilis in pregnancy is associated with a high risk of spontaneous abortion, premature delivery, perinatal death, and congenital syphilis. Risks are greater in 1° and 2° syphilis. Despite treatment in early syphilis during pregnancy, up to 14% will have a fetal death or a baby with congenital syphilis.

Can I have passed it on to my children?

There is a high risk of congenital syphilis in offspring of ♀ with early syphilis during pregnancy, and may even occur when the syphilis is treated during pregnancy. Early congenital syphilis occurs within the first 2 years of life, late congenital manifestations occur after 2 years of age.

Diagnosis and investigations

Regular

Dark ground microscopy (📖 Slide preparation for obtaining specimen p. 69)
Material

- 1° syphilis: serum from chancres (79–86% sensitivity)—less reliable for non-genital lesions, especially oral, because of other treponemes.
- Aspiration of a regional lymph node (especially if the chancre is secondarily infected).
- 2° and early congenital syphilis: serum from mucous patches, ulcers, and condylomata lata.

Examination

- Treponemes are very slender with tight spirals moving forwards and backwards, rotating about longitudinal axis and angulating to ~90°.
- If negative and clinical suspicion repeat daily for 3 days.
- If 2° infection saline lavage or consider antibiotics inactive against *T.pallidum* to clear contaminants (e.g. co-trimoxazole, quinolones).

Serological tests (all stages—see Table 6.1)
Positive serology usually found ~4 weeks after infection but may take up to 3 months to develop. Therefore it is essential to repeat then when single high-risk exposure. Negative in up to 15% of those with chancre. Similar response with endemic treponematoses (📖 Chapter 18, Endemic syphilis p. 245). Positive results should always be confirmed by testing a second sample.

Non-specific
Cardiolipin antigen tests (reagin): e.g. Venereal Disease Research Laboratory (VDRL) slide test, rapid plasma reagin (RPR) test. Inexpensive, readily quantifiable (useful in assessing serial titres), biological false positives (Box 6.1), poor sensitivity in late syphilis. Usually positive 4 weeks after infection. Prozone phenomenon (false-negative results from strongly positive samples due to blocking antibodies) is excluded by specimen dilution.

Specific for anti-treponemal antibodies

- Agglutination: *T.pallidum* (TP) particle assay (TPPA) is now recommended in preference to the TP haemagglutination assay (TPHA) or microhaemagglutination assay for TP (MHA-TP) as it is more sensitive in 1° infection. TPPA titre does not correlate with disease activity or treatment response. Its use is only to distinguish weak from strong reactivity (BASHH 0408).
- Enzyme immunoassay (EIA): simple, can be automated, widely used for screening and confirmation. EIAs that detect both IgG (4–5 weeks post-infection) and IgM (2–3 weeks post-infection) recommended as more sensitive for 1° syphilis.
- Specific antitreponemal immunoglobulin M (IgM) detection. EIA or FTA abs): usually first serological response. May remain reactive for 1–2 years. Important in diagnosing early congenital syphilis.
- Immunoblot test (also known as Western blot): antibody detection by response to recombinant antigens. Used in cases with discrepant isolated EIA and TPPA results.

- Fluorescent treponemal antibody absorbed (FTA abs) test:
  (if available): useful in cases of discrepant EIA and TPPA results but
  largely replaced by immunoblotting and not recommended as a
  standard confirmatory test.

Rapid point of care tests
Rapid POCTs are available but use is generally confined to outreach
projects or field conditions in developing countries.

Serological diagnosis
- EIA or TPPA alone recommended for routine screening. If ↑ syphilis
  risk (e.g. contact, suspicious oro-anogenital ulceration) include EIA IgM.
- Quantitative TPPA should be used to confirm +ve EIA.
- EIA should be used to conform +ve TPPA.
- If discrepant results, test with immunoblot (or FTA abs).
- Quantitive VDRL/RPR testing and EIA IgM should be performed if
  screening test(s) +ve prior to treatment.

In patients previously treated for syphilis a 4-fold VDRL titre ↑ and/or
confirmed change in EIA IgM to +ve suggests reinfection or relapse.

Table 6.1 Syphilis—serological response. Repeat to confirm

Stage	VDRL	TPPA/TPHA	EIA	IgM
Primary	Positive (60–90%)	Positive (90–100%)	Positive (90%)	Positive
	Usual titre Neat—1:16	Usual titre; 80–320		
Secondary	Positive	Positive	Positive	Positive
	Usual titre 1:32–1:256	High titres (about 5120)		
Early latent	Positive	Positive	Positive	Usually positive
	Usual titre 1:16–1:64	Titres still usually high		
Late syphilis	Positive (50–65%)	Positive	Positive	Usually negative
	Usual titre Neat—1:16 but often high if active	Low titres (80–640) unless active syphilis		
Old treated syphilis†	Usually negative or very low titre	Usually positive	Usually positive	Negative (unless recently treated early syphilis)
Congenital syphilis	The demonstration of IgM is important as it does not cross the placenta and usually represents active infection. May take up to 3 months to appear.			

Box 6.1 Biological false-positive reactions (VDRL/RPR tests) occur in <1% of the normal population

- Acute (disappear within 6 months)—usually <30 years of age:
  - acute febrile illnesses (e.g. infectious mononucleosis, viral hepatitis).
  - vaccination
  - pregnancy.
- Chronic (persist beyond 6 months)—usually >30 years of age:
  - chronic infections (e.g. leprosy)
  - autoimmune conditions (e.g. lupus erythematosus)
  - drug addiction.

Additional investigations

Other direct diagnostic tests which may be available in early syphilis
- Direct fluorescent antibody stain (of acetone fixed smears).
- Polymerase chain reaction (95% sensitive, 99% specific for 1° syphilis and 80% sensitive, 99% specific for 2° syphilis): especially useful if infectious oral lesions suspected as *T.denticola* in the mouth does not cross-react. If combined (multiplex) PCR test is used, high herpes simplex viral loads could lead to a false-negative PCR for *T.pallidum*.

Cerebrospinal fluid (CSF): suspected or increased risk of neurosyphilis (acquired and congenital)
CSF examination is required if neurological or ophthalmic symptoms or signs or treatment failure. In latent syphilis a negative VDRL is 100% sensitive in excluding CSF abnormalities compatible with neurosyphilis. Arrange head CT scan if clinical evidence of ↑ intracranial pressure prior to lumbar puncture.
- ↑ white cell count $>5 \times 10^6$/L
- ↑ protein >0.4g/L
- Positive VDRL/RPR, providing no blood contamination (~50% sensitive, 90% if symptomatic).
- Negative treponemal antibody test excludes neurosyphilis but +ve test lacks specificity; if TPHA titre <320 or TPPA titre <640 neurosyphilis is unlikely.
- TPHA index >70 (not readily available).
TPHA index ≈ CSF TPHA titre ÷ albumin quotient (CSF albumin × 10^3 ÷ serum albumin)

Biopsy and histology
For gummata—important to exclude malignancy in oral lesions.

X-ray

- Cardiovascular: aortic dilatation with linear 'egg-shell' calcification.
- Tabes dorsalis: neuropathic joints (bone destruction and osteophyte formation).
- Bone gummata: osteomyelitic lesions sometimes hidden by reactive osteosclerosis; periosteal thickening.
- Early congenital: periostitis (new bone formation), metaphyseal calcification, dactylitis (spindle-shaped finger swelling).

CT angiography

Cardiovascular syphilis (level of ventricular reflux).

Ophthalmic slit lamp examination

If eye pathology suspected.

Neurological imaging

Consider if neurological clinical features and certainly before lumbar puncture if risk of ↑ intracranial pressure.

Ultrasonography

For intra-uterine congenital syphilis:

- hepatomegaly
- splenomegaly
- placentomegaly
- scalp oedema
- polyhydramnios.

Infants born to women with syphilis and congenital infection

All infants born to mothers with syphilis require thorough clinical assessment with following investigations.

- Dark ground microscopy—e.g. from suspicious lesions, nasal discharge
- Infant serology (NB: not cord blood), in parallel with maternal serum if +ve (IgG type +ve tests may be passive transfer of maternal antibodies):
  - Positive IgM EIA test ± sustained VDRL/RPR or TPPA titres >4 times maternal level diagnostic of congenital infection (confirmed on repeat testing). Further investigations include full blood count, electrolytes, liver function tests, long-bone X-rays, and ophthalmic assessment.
  - If IgM EIA –ve, TPPA titre <4 times maternal level, and no signs of congenital syphilis, repeat reactive tests at 3, 6, and 12 months or until all tests become –ve. Repeat IgM at 3 months.
  - If neonatal serology –ve and no signs of congenital infection, no further testing required.

Syphilis management: early and late

Treatment principles

Optimal treponemal antibody sensitivity occurs during bacterial division (every 33 hours). Penicillin (1st line treatment) levels must be >0.018mg/L for 7–10 days (early syphilis) and 14–21 days (late syphilis). Desensitization should be considered as an option in those with penicillin allergy. Antibiotic free time or suboptimal levels should not exceed 24–30 hours. To reduce the pain associated with benzathine benzylpenicillin injections the use of 1% lidocaine (lignocaine) as a diluent is recommended. (Reconstitute vial with 8mL of 1% lidocaine hydrochloride solution, divide resultant solution into two equal volumes, and administer by deep IM injection into two different sites).

Early syphilis

- Benzathine benzylpenicillin G 2.4 mega-units (MU), single dose.
- IM procaine benzylpenicillin G 600mg (600,000units) daily for 10 days.

Alternatives (e.g. penicillin allergy/refusing parenteral treatment)

- Oral doxycycline 100mg twice daily for 14 days.
- IM ceftriaxone 500mg daily for 10 days (if no penicillin anaphylaxis).
- Oral erythromycin 500mg 4 times a day for 14 days (but less CSF and placental penetration than other treatments).
- Oral amoxicillin 500mg with oral probenecid 500mg each 4 times a day for 14 days.
- Oral azithromycin 2g single dose or 500mg daily for 10 days.
  ▶Resistant cases have been reported from the USA and Ireland and congenital syphilis following use in pregnancy.

▶If ophthalmic involvement treat as for neurosyphilis.

Late latent, cardiovascular, and gummatous syphilis

- IM benzathine benzylpenicillin G 2.4MU weekly for 3 doses (over 2 weeks).
- IM procaine benzylpenicillin G 600mg (600,000units) daily for 17 days.

Alternatives

- Oral doxycycline 100mg twice daily for 28 days.
- Oral amoxicillin 2g 3 times a day plus probenecid 500mg 4 times a day for 17 days.

Neurosyphilis

- IM procaine benzylpenicillin G 1.8–2.4g daily with oral probenecid 500mg 4 times a day for 17 days (Box 6.2).
- IV benzylpenicillin 18–24MU daily, given as 3–4MU every 4 hours for 17 days.

Alternatives

- Oral doxycycline 200mg twice daily for 28 days.
- Oral amoxicillin 2g 3 times a day with oral probenecid 500mg 4 times a day each for 28 days.
- IV ceftriaxone 2g (diluted with water) or IM ceftriaxone 2g (diluted with lidocaine) daily for 10–14 days (if no penicillin anaphylaxis).

Box 6.2 Procaine benzylpenicillin G: directions for administering 1.8MU for treating neurosyphilis

UK availability limited but may be imported (Farmapriona)— 1.2MU/vial. To produce standard dose of 1.8MU

- Obtain two 1.2MU vials
- Reconstitute the powder in each vial with the solvent provided (5mL). The resultant solution will be ~6mL, containing 1.2MU procaine benzylpenicillin G.
- Inject 4.5mL (900,000U) in each buttock, totalling 1.8MU.

Steroids and Jarisch–Herxheimer reaction

To protect against the series effects of a Jarisch-Herxheimer reaction (Box 6.3) steroid cover should be considered in the following situations.

- Interstitial keratitis—0.1% betamethasone eye drops, starting prior to antibiotics.

Oral prednisolone: 10–20mg 3 times a day for 3 days starting 1 day prior to antibiotics for:

- neurological involvement, e.g. optic atrophy, optic neuritis, 8th nerve deafness
- cardiological disease, e.g. involvement of coronary ostia.
- pregnancy with fetal involvement
- laryngeal involvement, e.g. gumma.

Box 6.3 Jarisch–Herxheimer reaction

Non-specific acute febrile illness associated with the start of antibiotic treatment, especially 2° (about 75%) and 1° (about 50%) syphilis, developing in 4 hours and resolving within 24 hours. Rare in late syphilis but potentially life threatening if strategic sites involved (e.g. coronary ostia, larynx, nervous system).

Features
Myalgia, rigors/chills, flush/fever/hypotension/deterioration of clinical lesions (therapeutic paradox), then resolution.

Management
Warn and reassure, bed rest, aspirin/paracetamol.

Special care required
Involvement of coronary ostia, larynx, optic neuritis, uveitis, nerve deafness (severe deterioration) and pregnancy, especially if fetal infection (see steroids).

Pregnancy

- Early—procaine benzylpenicillin G 750mg IM daily for 10 days or benzathine benzylpenicillin, single dose in 1st and 2nd trimester with a second dose if treated during 3rd trimester after 1 week (physiological changes in pregnancy may ↓ penicillin concentrations). Second-line treatments include amoxicillin plus probenecid, ceftriaxone (limited data), and macrolides (erythromycin and azithromycin) for 10 days as detailed. However, there are case reports of congenital infection with macrolides, so if used neonatal treatment is required after delivery.
- Late—as for non-pregnant patients but excluding doxycycline.
- Previously treated syphilis—consider retreatment if doubt about initial treatment, high reinfection risk, 4-fold drop in VDRL/RPR not achieved, serofast VDRL/RPR >1:8.

Consider penicillin desensitization if allergic.

Refer to fetal medicine if diagnosed after 26 weeks gestation for evaluation of fetal involvement and assessment of fetal distress during the first 24 hours (more likely if the fetus has stigmata of congenital syphilis). In early syphilis, Jarisch–Herxheimer reaction may cause uterine contractions, fetal distress, and preterm labour, especially if the fetus is infected, and steroids should be considered. Serological review of the mother after treatment should include repeat tests in the 3rd trimester and at term.

Neonates and congenital infection

Treatment for congenital syphilis should be provided if:
- mother has untreated syphilis
- suspected congenital syphilis and mother treated <4 weeks prior to delivery
- mother treated with non-penicillin regimens
- serological evidence of congenital syphilis

Special care required if maternal serology remains serofast, especially if reinfection risk

Paediatric treatment regimens

- IV benzyl penicillin 60–90mg (100,000–150,000U) per kg body weight daily in divided doses of 30mg (50,000U) 12 hourly for first 7 days, then 8 hourly for 10 days.
- IM procaine benzylpenicillin G 50mg (50,000U) per kg body weight daily for 10–14 days.
- If penicillin allergy, consider desensitization.

Serology should be repeated every 2–3 months to ensure a satisfactory response to treatment (4-fold ↓ in VDRL/RPR titre).

HIV co-infection

There is a paucity of evidence on the treatment of syphilis in those also infected by HIV. UK and USA guidelines recommend treatment for the stage of infection as in HIV-negative individuals. However, some specialists advocate treating as for neurosyphilis, especially if CD4 count very low and/or VDRL/RPR titres very high.

Management of anaphylactic shock
(Penicillin is one of the most common causes)

- IM epinephrine (adrenaline) 1:1000, 0.5mL
- followed by IM/IV antihistamine (e.g. chlorphenamine, 10mg) and IM/IV hydrocortisone, 100mg, if necessary.

Syphilis: review and contacts

Review

- Early syphilis: serological review monthly for 3 months, then at 6 months and 1 year until VDRL/RPR –ve or serofast.
- Late syphilis: serological review 3 monthly until VDRL/RPR –ve or serofast.

Treponemal antibody tests (except IgM) often remain +ve for life. It is important to communicate this to patients (as they may be tested elsewhere) and ensure that latest results and titres are clearly documented.

- Neurosyphilis: 6 monthly CSF cell count until normal.
- HIV co-infection: maintain annual serological review for life extending to every 3 months (coinciding with HIV review visits) in outbreak areas.

Consider reinfection or relapse if VDRL/RPR antibody titres ↑ 4-fold (or greater), ideally compared with previous samples run in parallel, or clinical evidence of infection. If reinfection cannot be confirmed CSF examination is required to exclude neurosyphilis and should also be considered for those whose VDRL/RPR fails to ↓ 4-fold within 6–12 months of treatment when initially high (>1:32). If CSF, is normal recommended first-line re-treatment is IM benzathine benzylpenicillin 2.4MU weekly for three doses.

Partner notification and contact management

Early syphilis

- 1°: all sexual partners within previous 3 months.
- 2° and early latent: consider all sexual contacts within previous 2 years.

Maintain under serological review for 3 months from last sexual risk. 46-60% of contactable partners are infected.

Epidemiological treatment (and for incubating infection)
Consider in contacts of early syphilis if full surveillance is impossible.

- IM benzathine benzylpenicillin 2.4MU, single dose.
- Oral doxycycline 100mg twice daily for 14 days.
- Oral azithromycin 1g single dose.

Late syphilis

As index case is not sexually infectious at diagnosis an estimate of when the infection was acquired should be made (e.g. from previous negative serology) and contacts from within 2 years of this time notified. However, vertical infection, although most common in early syphilis, can occur for at least 10 years after infection. Therefore more extensive screening may be required for children of infected ♀.

Co-infection with HIV

- Temporary ↓ of CD4 count and ↑ viral load and shedding with new syphilis infection.
- ↑ risk of HIV acquisition with infectious syphilis from 3–5-fold.
- Maternal co-infection with HIV may ↑ transmission risk of syphilis.
- In early syphilis incidence of symptomatic neurosyphilis in HIV-infected people 2.1% compared with 0.6% for those who are HIV negative.
- More rapid progression to gummatous syphilis.
- Syphilis serological response is usually normal, but rarely atypical reactions arise with a tendency for VDRL/RPR titres to be lower in 1° syphilis and higher in 2° syphilis.
- Prozone phenomenon is more likely.

Gonorrhoea

Introduction

Gonorrhoea—literally 'flow of seed' as named by Galen, Greek physician, in the 2nd century AD—has probably been known to be sexually transmitted for several millennia as shown by references in the Old Testament (Leviticus 15) and attribution of 'strangury' to 'pleasures of Venus' by Hippocrates.

Aetiology: *Neisseria gonorrhoeae*

Gram-negative kidney-shaped coccus about 1μm in diameter; appear in pairs (diplococci) with concave aspects facing each other, typically inside polymorphonuclear leucocytes (PMNLs). Fastidious growth requirements: temperature 35–37°C, pH 6.5–7.5, atmosphere containing 5–7% carbon dioxide, and selective and enriched culture media (e.g. Thayer–Martin or Modified New York City) supplemented with iron, essential amino acids, glucose, and antimicrobials to inhibit other organisms

Humans are the only natural host. Primarily infects the columnar epithelium of lower genital tract, rectum, pharynx, and conjunctiva with transluminal spread to epididymis and prostate in ♂ and endometrium and pelvic organs in ♀ with occasional haematogenous dissemination.

Epidemiology and transmission

WHO estimates 62 million cases annually worldwide. In the UK the incidence peaked in the late 1960s and early 1970s. This was followed by a marked fall between 1985 and 1995 coinciding with the AIDS awareness campaign. However, since 1997 there has been a steady upward trend.

Highest incidence in the following: young people, urban dwellers, socioeconomically deprived persons, migrants, and certain ethnic minorities. Rates of gonorrhoea are regarded as surrogate markers of unsafe sexual behaviour. An episode of gonorrhoea does not confer immunity as outer membrane proteins vary. Reinfection is common.

Closely associated with other STIs, especially *Chlamydia trachomatis* (up to 40% of ♀ and 25% of ♂ with gonorrhoea).

Sexual and non-sexual transmission

Anogenital and pharyngeal infections

Almost exclusively sexually transmitted. Although recoverable from laboratory, suspensions left on surfaces, such as toilet seats for up to 24 hours; loses viability on drying and evidence of transmission from toilet seats is contentious. Fomite transmission is very unusual but anecdotal cases have been reported following the shared use of a portable male urinal and inflatable sex doll.

Adult conjunctivitis

Often associated with anogenital infection due to autoinoculation but non-sexual transmission is possible as reported in sporadic epidemics and isolated cases attributed to poor hygiene, accidental inoculation, or irrigation with urine (folk remedy). Flies have been implicated as vectors responsible for an outbreak in Australia.

Neonatal infection

Vertical transmission due to exposure in birth canal following rupture of membranes.

Infectivity

- ♂ to ♀ infection after one episode of sex: 60–80%. Risk reduced by about 40% by use of condom.
- ♀ to ♂ infection after one episode of sex: 20%. Risk reduced by up to 75% by use of condom.
- Pharynx to urethra: 26% of partners.
- Vertical transmission: up to 30%.

Spontaneous clearance

- Pharyngeal infection: almost 100% in 12 weeks.
- Anogenital and conjunctival infections: no data available.

Clinical features

Sites of infection
Commonly identifiable at several different sites (Table 7.1).

Table 7.1 Sites of infection

	Heterosexual ♂ (%)	MSM* (%)	♀ (%)
Urethra	>90	60–70	65–75
Cervix	–	–	80–90
Pharynx ± other site(s)	3–10	10–30	5–15
Pharynx only	<5	10–15	<5
Rectum ± other site(s)	–	25–50	25–40
Rectum only	–	20–40	5

*MSM = ♂ who have sex with ♂

Male genital infection
Symptoms
- Incubation period: 5–8 days, range 1–14.
- Urethral discharge in 80% (typically profuse and yellow/green/white) and/or dysuria in 50%. May be scanty and mucoid initially but becomes profuse and purulent within 24 hours. Asymptomatic in 5–10%.

Signs
- Mucopurulent or purulent urethral discharge, typically profuse but if scanty can be elicited by urethral massage.
- Erythema of the urethral meatus sometimes with oedema.
- Urine 'threads'—plugs of pus from urethral (Littré's) glands in first passed 20mL urine indicating anterior urethritis.

Female genital infection
Symptoms
- Asymptomatic in 50–70% (>50% are usually seen as contacts).
- Symptoms, when present, appear within 10 days of infection.
- ↑ vaginal discharge in up to 50% (often related to co-infection).
- Lower abdominal pain in up to 25%.
- Dysuria without frequency ~12%.
- Intermenstrual bleeding or menorrhagia (unusual).

Signs
- Commonly no abnormal findings.
- Cervix: mucopurulent discharge and easily induced bleeding (<50%).
- Pelvic/lower abdominal tenderness (<5%).

Extragenital infections in ♂ and ♀

Rectal infection
In MSM
In the UK ↓ between 1985 and 1995 (following AIDS awareness campaign) but has since ↑. Usually asymptomatic (~90%) but may cause anal discharge, pain, discomfort, or pruritus, and less frequently rectal bleeding, tenesmus, and constipation. Proctoscopy may show mucoid or purulent discharge, erythema, oedema, and friability.

In ♀
An estimated 10% (possibly more) may be due to anal sexual intercourse. The positive correlation with duration of cervical infection suggests tracking of infected material into the anal canal as the main cause. Usually asymptomatic but symptoms and signs as in ♂.

Pharyngeal infection
Asymptomatic in >90%. Occasional mild pharyngitis and/or cervical lymphadenopathy. Almost 100% spontaneous clearance within 12 weeks but significant association with disseminated gonococcal infection.

Conjunctival infection
Adult infection, which is uncommon, presents with purulent discharge and inflammation affecting one or both eyes. If untreated, complications such as keratitis and pan-ophthalmitis, can lead to blindness.

Prepubertal children
In girls the vulval and vaginal epithelium are vulnerable to infection. Although theoretically infection may be acquired accidentally from infected secretions, especially with poor sanitation and hygiene, gonorrhoea is a strong indicator of sexual abuse. It usually presents as a purulent oedematous vulvovaginitis.

Gonococcal urethritis in boys, or pharyngeal and rectal infection in both sexes, is almost always the result of sexual abuse.

Complications

In ♂
- Infection of the median raphe: linear erythematous swelling.
- Tysonitis: painful swelling of parafrenal gland.
- Meatal para-urethral gland abscess.
- Peri-urethral cellulitis and abscess: inflammation of Littré's glands with duct obstruction produces small cysts and abscesses causing tender swelling in fossa navicularis or bulb. Urine flow may be restricted. Painful erections ± ventral angulation if corpus spongiosum is affected.
- Urethral strictures and fistulae: sequelae of peri-urethral abscess in untreated infection.
- Cowperitis and abscess: Cowper's (bulbo-urethral) glands at the base of the prostate are affected, causing fever, pain in perineum, particularly on defecation, and urinary frequency or retention. Abscesses usually point to one side of the perineum or are palpable rectally.
- Prostatitis and seminal vesiculitis: acute features include: fever, malaise, perineal discomfort, tenesmus, suprapubic pain, urgency of micturition or retention, haematuria, and painful erections. A tender swollen prostate on rectal examination. Chronic prostatitis may develop.
- Epididymitis (<1%): 📖 Chapter 12, Aetiology p. 186.

In ♀
- Inflammation of para-urethral (Skene's) glands.
- Bartholinitis ± Bartholin's abscess: single or bilateral. Vulval pain and erythema with tender cystic swelling of the posterior half of the labium majora. Pus may be seen or expressed from the duct orifice.
- Pelvic inflammatory disease (PID) may occur in 10–20% of untreated infections (📖 Chapter 10, Aetiology p. 168).

Systemic

Perihepatitis (Fitz-Hugh–Curtis syndrome)
Usually found in ♀ with associated PID, suggesting intra-abdominal spread, but also rarely reported in ♂ implicating lymphatic or haematogenous dissemination (📖 Chapter 10, Complications/perihepatitis p. 170).

Disseminated gonococcal infection (DGI)
Occurs in <1% with mucosal infection.
- Host factors:
  - 4-fold ↑ in ♀ (especially during or just after menstruation or in pregnancy particularly with pharyngeal infection)
  - complement deficiency predisposing to recurrent episodes in <10% with DGI.
- Bacterial factors:
  - serogroup IA-1(WI)
  - auxotype AHU⁻ (arginine, hypoxanthine, and uracil dependent)
  - complement resistance.
  - penicillin sensitivity and vancomycin susceptibility but these vary over time and penicillin-resistant strains now play a significant role.

Clinical features

The preceding mucosal infection tends to be asymptomatic. Usual presentation: mild fever, skin rash, and arthralgia ± arthritis.

- Skin (gonococcal dermatitis) in 67%: initial macules develop into papules, vesicles with petechiae, and then typical necrotic pustules surrounded by erythema. Usually at extremities (especially hands).
- Skeletal: tenosynovitis (in ~33%) producing migratory arthralgia mostly in wrists, fingers, toes, and ankles. Arthritis (single joint), in ~50%, with effusion typically involving the knee, wrist, or metacarpo-phalangeal joints.
- Other sites (rare):
  - heart: endocarditis in 1–3% leading to aortic incompetence and cardiac failure; also pericarditis and myocarditis.
  - hepatitis
  - meningitis, similar to meningococcal (very rare).

Pregnancy and the neonate

In pregnancy the proportion of pharyngeal infection is ↑ by 15–35%, presumably due to ↑ in oral sex. Genital infection is less likely to be complicated by PID (because of thickening of cervical mucus) but cases of salpingitis have been reported in the 1st trimester.

Adverse pregnancy outcomes

- Infection of chorio-amnion can cause septic abortion but there is no consistent evidence for ↑ risk.
- Preterm delivery and low birth weight ↑ 3- to 6-fold.
- Premature rupture of membrane (PROM) is more frequent.
- Postpartum/intrapartum or postabortal endometritis and pyrexia illness are ↑ (3-fold) and occur in ~42% with gonorrhoea.
- Some studies suggest that risk of DGI is ↑, reflecting ↑ pharyngeal infection.

Screening in pregnancy advisable in PROM, septic abortion, intra/postpartum fever, or those considered to be at risk.

Neonatal gonococcal infection

Occurs because of exposure in birth canal during labour.

Gonococcal ophthalmia neonatorum

A notifiable disease in the UK, defined as conjunctivitis with a purulent discharge in an infant arising within 21 days of birth. Occurs in 30–40% of those exposed with ↑ risk if PROM or preterm delivery. Typically develops within 2–5 days of delivery and presents with oedema of the conjunctiva and eyelids with profuse discharge. Without treatment infection may extend to sub-conjunctival connective tissue and the cornea leading to ulceration. If ulcers perforate, anterior synechiae formation or panophthalmitis may follow, which can result in blindness.

The rate of infection in at-risk infants is ↓ to 2–5% by prophylaxis (1% silver nitrate solution ('Crede prophylaxis'), 1% tetracycline, or 0.5% erythromycin ointment) applied to the eyes soon after birth.

Gonococcal arthritis

Associated with vulvovaginitis, proctitis, or ophthalmia neonatorum. Usually polyarticular, presenting as pseudoparalysis. Rarely progressive. Skin lesions not usual.

Scalp abscess

Follows trauma to scalp, e.g. with intra-uterine fetal monitoring.

Other neonatal gonococcal infection

- Pharyngeal infection in ~33% with ophthalmia neonatorum. Rhinitis may be associated.
- Vaginitis, urethritis, and anorectal infection.
- Neonatal sepsis without arthritis particularly in preterm infants. *N.gonorrhoeae* is recoverable from nasogastric aspirate or blood. Rarely complicated by meningitis.

Frequently asked questions

How long can I have had gonorrhoea for?

In ♂ urethral symptoms usually appear within 10 days of exposure to gonorrhoea, although 5–10% are asymptomatic when diagnosed. Symptoms are much less common with rectal and throat infection. Up to 70% of ♀ diagnosed with gonorrhoea are asymptomatic. Therefore, although most people are probably diagnosed shortly after being infected, it is possible that it may have been present for weeks or months.

Can it be cured?

Yes, gonorrhoea can be cured by antibiotics. When swabs are taken for gonorrhoea culture, the laboratory also tests for antibiotic sensitivities, so that the appropriate antibiotic is identified. It is recommended that, while awaiting these results, an antibiotic be used to which >95% of the local stains of *N.gonorrhoeae* are sensitive.

Will it have done any damage?

- In ♀: PID may occur in 10–20% of untreated cases of gonorrhoea. Infertility may occur as a result of PID.
- In ♂: urethral strictures and fistulae are sequelae of periurethral abscesses in untreated gonorrhoea and it may also cause epididymitis.

Do I need a test of cure?

No. Although this was a recommended practice, audit studies have shown that it is unnecessary provided that the isolate is fully sensitive to the antibiotic administered, and the patient has taken all of their medication correctly and has not been re-exposed to the infection.

Can I have caught this from a toilet seat?

Not normally. However, in prepubertal girls the vulvovaginal skin is vulnerable to *N.gonorrhoeae* and a report has alleged acquisition of gonorrhoea from a dirty toilet seat in an aeroplane by an 8-year-old girl.

I'm pregnant. Can it harm my baby?

There is a risk of neonatal infection due to exposure in the birth canal during labour. Gonococcal ophthalmia neonatorum is acquired by 30–40% of infants exposed to *N.gonorrhoeae*.

Without treatment there are ↑ risks of preterm delivery, low birth weight, premature rupture of membranes, and postpartum/post-abortion endometritis.

Diagnosis

Screening

- Genital: ♂ urethra, ♀ cervix and urethra. Vaginal or vulval if sensitive nucleic acid amplification test (NAAT) is used.
- Pharynx: all MSM and heterosexuals with symptoms of gonorrhoea elsewhere or history of contact.
- Rectum: all MSM (advised as ~20% with rectal infection deny receptive anal intercourse) and ♀ with symptoms, gonorrhoea elsewhere, or history of contact

▶ Sensitivity of cervical culture alone is 75–85%. A single set of tests from the urethra, cervix, rectum, and pharynx ↑ this to >95%.

- Conjunctivitis: include potential 1° infection sites.
- DGI:
  - from potential 1° infection sites
  - material from skin lesions and joint aspirate
  - blood culture.

Culture of joint fluid and skin lesions is insensitive; therefore NAAT is recommended.

Microscopy

Microscopy (1000×) of Gram-stained genital specimens shows *N.gonorrhoeae* as Gram-negative diplococci within PMNLs (Plate 6). Smear sensitivity (compared with culture):

- in ♂—urethra 90–95% (symptomatic) and 50–75% (asymptomatic)
- in ♀—cervix 23–65% and urethra 20%
- rectum—blind swab 40%, using proctoscope 70–80%.

Microscopy is not appropriate for pharyngeal specimens as other neisserial commensals are commonly seen. Conjunctival specimens are suitable for Gram staining and microscopy.

Laboratory detection of *N.gonorrhoeae*

Culture—isolation and identification of *N.gonorrhoeae*

Dependent on good specimen collection and efficient transport to the laboratory. ▶ Caution with lubricants during examination, as they may inhibit the growth of *N.gonorrhoeae*.

Specimens for culture may be:

- directly inoculated onto culture medium and incubated
- transported in a non-nutrient medium (e.g. Amies, Stuart) or a CO_2-producing culture medium.

Transport media should be kept at ≤4°C after inoculation (check product information or with local laboratory). Provided that the material in the transport medium is processed within 48 hours, there is only ~5% loss in sensitivity compared with direct inoculation.

The culture medium is examined for growth at 24 and 48 hours. Presumptive identification is by positive cytochrome oxidase reaction and microscopy. Definitive identification by a combination of further tests, e.g. carbohydrate utilization (*N.gonorrhoeae* utilizes glucose only), monoclonal antibody test (e.g. Phadebact), and enzyme substrate degradation.

Molecular detection

NAATs are ~100% sensitive for genital, rectal, and pharyngeal specimens compared directly with culture (75–85% endocervix, <60% rectum, <50% pharynx) but cannot identify antibiotic sensitivities. They are suitable for urine, vaginal (including self-collected), and vulval samples. They are un-licensed for rectal and pharyngeal specimens, although there are some data showing >90% sensitivity with NAAT (culture <60%). Transcription-mediated amplification and Strand displacement assay methods are more sensitive than polymerase chain reaction in women. False-positive reactions may ↓ positive predictive value to <90% with some reagents in low prevalence populations. Confirmation of NAAT reactivity by culture is recommended and allows antimicrobial sensitivity assay.

Typing

Serotyping, auxotyping, opa-typing, and plasmid analysis are not applicable to routine clinical practice but are useful in monitoring the epidemiology of the infection and the identification of transmission chains.

Antibiotic sensitivity

Identifies appropriate treatment. Sensitivity predicts success in >95% with intermediate sensitivity suggesting failure in 5–15% although ↑ dosage may be effective. Resistance may be due to plasmids (circular DNA fragments independent of chromosome) or chromosomal mutations.

Management

▶Advise avoidance of sexual intercourse until the patient and partner(s) have completed treatment and resolution has been established. Screen for *C.trachomatis* using a sensitive assay (NAAT) or provide epidemiological treatment. Treatment before antibiotic sensitivity is known should be with an antibiotic to which >95% of local strains are sensitive.

Uncomplicated genital and rectal infections (all single doses)
Recommended:
- Ceftriaxone 250mg IM
- Cefixime 400mg oral
- Spectinomycin 2g IM.

Alternative (if regional prevalence of resistance <5%):
- Ciprofloxacin 500mg oral
- Ofloxacin 400mg oral
- Ampicillin 2g or 3g plus probenecid 1g oral.

Complicated genital infection (📖 Chapter 10, Management p. 174, Chapter 12, Management p. 192)

Pharyngeal infection (all single doses)
- Ceftriaxone 250mg IM
- Ciprofloxacin 500mg oral
- Ofloxacin 400mg oral

Pregnancy and breastfeeding (all single doses)
Quinolone and tetracycline antimicrobials are contraindicated.
- Ceftriaxone 250mg IM
- Cefotaxime 500mg IM
- Ampicillin 2g or 3g plus probenecid 1g oral (provided that local prevalence of penicillin-resistant *N.gonorrhoeae* <5%)
- Spectinomycin 2g IM

Adult gonococcal conjunctivitis
Ceftriaxone 1g IM as a single dose (limited evidence base).

Disseminated gonococcal infection
Hospital admission is recommended. Assess for endocarditis/meningitis.
- A parenteral antibiotic is necessary initially, e.g.
  - ceftriaxone or cefotaxime or ceftizoxime 1g IM 8 hourly
  - ciprofloxacin or ofloxacin 400mg IV 12 hourly
  - spectinomycin 2g IM 12 hourly.
- The parenteral antibiotic should be continued for 24–48 hours until improvement, and then replaced with oral cefixime 400mg, ciprofloxacin 500mg, or ofloxacin 400mg twice daily for 7 days.

Other situations

- Gonococcal meningitis and endocarditis: IV antibiotic for at least
  2 weeks and 4 weeks, respectively.
- Ophthalmia neonatorum: single dose of ceftriaxone 25–50mg/kg up to
  a maximum of 125mg.
- Neonatal sepsis, scalp abscess, meningitis, and arthritis: ceftriaxone
  25–50mg/kg daily IV or IM for 7–14 days.
- Neonatal prophylaxis: if mother is not treated before delivery a single
  dose of ceftriaxone 25–50mg/kg to a maximum of 125mg.
- Prepubertal infection:
  - weight >45kg—adult regimens.
  - weight <45kg—ceftriaxone 125mg IM (single dose).

Partner notification

Partner notification is essential. Contact tracing period:

- ♂ symptomatic urethral infection—2 weeks prior to onset of
  symptoms or until last sexual partner, if longer.
- Other—3 months prior to diagnosis or until the last sexual partner.

Epidemiological treatment and, ideally, screening should be offered to
sexual partners. Similar principles should apply to the mother of a neonate
with gonococcal infection and her sex partner(s).

Follow-up

Tests of cure are unnecessary provided that the isolate is sensitive to the
antibiotic prescribed and the patient has adhered fully to the treatment
and advice provided. If required, culture should be delayed for at least
72 hours and NAAT for at least 2 weeks after treatment.

HIV infection

Gonorrhoea facilitates HIV transmission, producing ↑ in detectable virus
in genital secretions. This is reversed following antibiotic treatment.

Chlamydia trachomatis infections

Introduction

Although recognized since antiquity (e.g. description of trachoma in Egyptian papyri), the discovery of *Chlamydia trachomatis* as a cause of genital tract and ocular infections was only made in the early part of the 20th century.

Aetiology

C.trachomatis is a bacterial species within the genus *Chlamydia* (Table 8.1). It is divided into four biovars—lymphogranuloma venereum (LGV), trachoma, murine, and swine—which are subdivided into several serovars based on the major outer membrane protein (MOMP) antigens. Serovars D to K of the trachoma biovar are sexually transmissible and 'chlamydial infection' commonly refers to infection with this group. Genotyping based on MOMP genes increasingly refines classification of the species and is a useful research tool.

C.trachomatis is an obligate intracellular pathogen depending entirely on host cell adenosine triphosphate for its energy. Two distinct structures appear during its life cycle of 48–72 hours.

- Elementary body (0.35μm). Infectious form, attaches to and enters host cells (columnar and pseudostratified columnar), transforming after 6–9 hours into:
- Reticulate body (1μm). Non-infective replicative phase within intracellular vacuoles (endosomes). These fuse into an inclusion where reticulate bodies multiply for 24–48 hours. Maturation back into elementary bodies is followed by their release.

Epidemiology and transmission

The WHO estimated the annual worldwide incidence of new infections to be 92 million in 1999. Genital chlamydial infection is the most common STI in the UK with the highest incidence amongst ♀ aged 16–19 and ♂ aged 20–24. Factors associated with ↑ prevalence of chlamydial infection include being unmarried, ↑ number of sexual partners, ethnic minority status, inconsistent or no use of barrier methods of contraception, and use of oral contraceptive pill. Prevalence of the infection in various settings is shown in Table 8.2.

- Transmissibility of the infection after a single act of unprotected penetrative sexual intercourse is estimated to be ~10% for both sexes. Correct use of condoms reduces the risk by ~40%.
- Spontaneous bacterial clearance is estimated to occur in ~20–28% within 3 months and 50% by 15 months. Persistence for up to 6 years has been reported and is believed to be longer in ♀ than ♂.

Table 8.1 *C.trachomatis* and related species

Species	Biovar	Serovar	Natural host	Human disease
C.pecorum	–	Multiple	Sheep, cattle, swine	None
C psittaci	–	Multiple	Birds, lower mammals	Psittacosis
C pneumoniae	–	TWAR	Human	Respiratory disease
C.trachomatis	LGV	L1, L2, L3	Human (infects macrophages)	Lymphogranuloma venereum
	Trachoma	A, B, Ba, C	Human	Hyperendemic trachoma
		D–K	Human (infects squamocolumnar cells)	Conjunctivitis, non-gonococcal urethritis, cervicitis, salpingitis, proctitis, epidydimitis, pneumonia of newborn
	Murine	–	Mouse	None
	Swine	–	Swine	None

Table 8.2 Mean prevalence of chlamydial infection in 5 in different settings*

Survey population	Prevalence (%)				
	Overall	<20 years	20–24 years	25–29 years	>30 years
General population	1.6	3.8	2.7	2.2	0.9
General practice	7.1	8.6	5.9	2.9	1.1
Family planning	8.1	10	7.4	3.8	1.5
Antenatal clinic	8.5	13.5	6.5	7.2	0.1
Termination service	8.5	13.5	9.7	2	1.2
Youth clinic	12.2	12.3	10	–	–
GUM clinic	12.7	17.3	12.4	4.9	5.1

* UK data based on a meta-analysis published in 2004.
Source: E J Adams, A Charlett, W J Edmunds, and G Hughes (2004).
Chlamydia trachomatis in the United Kingdom: a systematic review and analysis of prevalence studies. *Sex Transm Infect.* 80: 354–62, Table 4. Reproduced with permission from the BMJ Publishing Group.

Clinical features

Sites of infection

- ♂: Urethra (35–50% of non-gonococcal urethritis (NGU)); epididymis; prostate (inconclusive evidence).
- ♀: Cervix (75–85%); urethra (50–60% overall, 15–20% urethra only); Bartholin's gland; endometrium; fallopian tubes; vagina if prepubertal.
- ♂ and ♀: conjunctiva; rectum (8–10% in homosexual ♂); pharynx (1–2%); hepatic capsule; synovium; rarely endocardium and meninges.

Male genital infection

Symptoms

- Incubation period: 7–21 days.
- Urethral discharge and/or dysuria in ~50%. Remainder asymptomatic.

Signs

About 60% of ♂ have signs.

- Usually mild to moderate opaque or clear urethral discharge.
- Sometimes oedema and erythema of the urethral meatus.
- Often urine 'threads'—plugs of pus from urethral (Littré's) glands in first passed 20mL urine indicating anterior urethritis.

Female genital infection

Symptoms

- Asymptomatic in up to 80%.
- Symptoms include:
  - increased vaginal discharge
  - dysuria without frequency
  - intermenstrual bleeding and/or menorrhagia
  - post-coital bleeding
  - low abdominal pain.

Signs

- Usually no abnormal findings.
- Cervix: mucopurulent cervicitis (MPC)—mucopurulent discharge and/or oedema, congestion, and friability (easily induced bleeding) present in about a third including those who are asymptomatic.
- Incidental finding on colposcopy of 'cobblestone' appearance of the cervix due to raised lymphoid follicles.
- Cervical ectopy is positively correlated with chlamydial infection.

Extragenital infections in ♂ and ♀

Rectal infection

In homosexual ♂

- Attending GUM clinics:
  - up to 15% of those with proctitis; also consider LGV (📖 Chapter 17, Lymphogranuloma venereum p. 238)
  - up to 10% on routine screening (67% without urethral infection).

- Usually asymptomatic (>60%) but may cause anal discharge, pain, discomfort, or pruritus, and less frequently rectal bleeding, severe anal pain, tenesmus, and constipation with overt proctitis.
- Occasionally external anal erythema or discharge. Proctoscopy may show mucoid or purulent discharge, erythema, oedema, or friability in those who are symptomatic.
- 'Cobblestone' appearance if magnified with a colposcope.

In ♀
- Attending GUM clinics—up to 5% (may occur without urogenital infection).
- Usually asymptomatic but symptoms and signs as with ♂.

Pharyngeal infection
- Limited data: ♂ (including homosexual) <1% and ♀ <3%.
- Usually asymptomatic but mild pharyngeal symptoms may be reported.

Conjunctival infection
- Concomitant anogenital infection in 60–70%.
- Partners: ~50% ♀ and ~80% ♂ have chlamydial or non-specific genital infection.

Unilateral or bilateral follicular conjunctivitis presenting 1–2 weeks after exposure with conjunctival irritation, discharge ± photophobia/periorbital pain. Signs include conjunctival injection ± chemosis and ulceration (Herber's pits) in severe cases and hyperaemia with follicles 0.5–1mm in diameter ± palpebral conjunctival oedema. May result in conjunctival scarring. Epithelial keratitis (unusual) does not lead to corneal scarring.

Prepubertal children
In girls the vulval and vaginal epithelium are vulnerable to infection. Urethral, pharyngeal, and rectal infections may also occur. Prepubertal infection is a strong indicator of sexual abuse. ►However, perinatal *C.trachomatis* infection may persist for at least 3 years following delivery.

Complications

Local

In ♂
- Prostatitis and seminal vesiculitis: the role of chlamydial infection is not well established.
- Epididymitis (📖 Chapter 12, Aetiology p. 186).

In ♀
- Bartholinitis ± Bartholin's abscess—one or both sides. Pain in vulva with tender cystic swelling of the posterior half of labia majora with erythema; pus may exude or be expressed from the duct orifice.
- Endometritis: may cause irregular vaginal bleeding.
- Pelvic inflammatory disease (PID) and sequelae: may occur in about 10–30% of untreated infections.
- Cervical neoplasia: epidemiological studies show a correlation with previous chlamydial infection.

Systemic
- Perihepatitis (Fitz-Hugh–Curtis syndrome): usually found in ♀ with associated PID suggesting intra-abdominal spread, but also rarely reported in ♂ implicating lymphatic or haematogenous dissemination.
- Sexually acquired reactive arthritis (SARA) or Reiter's syndrome: polyarthritis affecting mostly weight-bearing joints usually preceded by urethritis and conjunctivitis in <1% of chlamydial infections.

Pregnancy and the neonate

The infection rate in pregnancy varies from 2% to 30%. Genital infection is less likely to be complicated by PID (because of thick cervical mucus), but cases of salpingitis have been reported in the 1st trimester.

Adverse pregnancy outcomes of untreated chlamydial infection
- Chlamydial infection in pregnancy may be associated with preterm delivery and low birth weight.
- Premature rupture of membrane (PROM) more frequent.
- *C.trachomatis* has been isolated from amniotic fluid.
- Intrapartum pyrexia and late postpartum endometritis ↑ by 20–25%.
- Post-abortal PID.

Neonatal chlamydial infection
Occurs because of exposure in birth canal during labour.
- Chlamydial ophthalmia neonatorum
  - 30–50% of exposed infants acquire chlamydial conjunctivitis, ↓ to 1–2% if mother treated before delivery.
  - Incubation period 5–14 days (from delivery or PROM) but can be up to 2 months.
  - Conjunctivitis—mild (scant mucoid discharge) to severe (profuse discharge). Bilateral involvement in 67%. Corneal scarring is rare.

- Respiratory tract infection
  - The nasopharynx is the most frequent site of neonatal infection (70–80% of infected infants) where it is usually asymptomatic.
  - 30% with nasopharyngeal infection develop apyrexial pneumonia at 4–12 weeks of age with cough, tachypnoea, and crepitations on auscultation. Apnoeic episodes may occur. Long-term outcome includes impaired lung function and obstructive pulmonary disease.
  - Investigations show hyperinflation on radiography, peripheral eosinophilia, and ↑ serum immunoglobulins.
- Others
  - Otitis media complicating nasopharyngeal infection may become chronic if not treated early.
  - Vaginal and rectal infection in 10–15% of exposed infants. Usually asymptomatic and may persist for at least 3 years.

Frequently asked questions

How long could I have had chlamydia for?
Up to 80% of ♀ and 50% of ♂ infected with chlamydia are asymptomatic. Therefore it is possible to be infected for months and in some cases years before it is diagnosed.

Could I have caught if from a toilet seat?
No. There is no evidence for this.

Does my partner need to be seen?
Yes. There is a very high chance of infection. Screening for STIs is recommended and treatment to cover chlamydial infection should be taken.

Although my partner has not been treated, since I finished my treatment we have been using condoms. This is OK, isn't it?
No. Condoms only reduce the risk of infection, not eliminate it. Your partner needs treatment and you need to be retreated.

How have I caught chlamydia when my only ever partner has tested negative?
Although tests for chlamydia are now very reliable, they are not 100% sensitive and therefore infection may be missed, especially if EIAs are used. In addition, your partner may have received antibiotics for something else or the infection may have cleared spontaneously. Despite conflicting results in a partnership we recommend treatment for both.

Will it have affected my fertility?
Chlamydial infection is extremely common and does not appear to impair fertility in most people who are treated properly. Untreated chlamydia can lead to either symptomatic PID or silent episodes which are associated with infertility.

Can you test my fertility?
Fertility is not assessed at a GUM clinic. 90% of couples will conceive within 12 months of trying with regular intercourse. Couples who do not conceive within 12 months may undergo infertility investigations. If a ♀ has a history of chlamydia and/or PID, she may be offered investigations to check her fallopian tubes.

Diagnosis

Investigations

1° analysis—initial investigations in the clinic
Anogenital specimens

Light microscopy (1000×) of Gram-stained smears does not show *C.trachomatis* but can demonstrate PMNLs which may indicate chlamydial infection in the appropriate clinical context.

- Urethral in ♂: ≥5 PMNL/high power field (HPF) in the absence of Gram-negative intracellular diplococci = NGU.
- Cervical: ≥30 PMNL/HPF suggests cervicitis.
- Rectal: ≥1 PMNL/HPF suggests proctitis.

Urine

- ≥10 PMNL/HPF in threads from the first voided urine (FVU) in ♂.
- Sterile pyuria may be due to *C.trachomatis* infection.

Laboratory detection of *C.trachomatis*

DNA assays—nucleic acid amplification tests (NAATs) and DNA probe—are recommended as they are more accurate than cell culture or antigen detection.

Cell culture

100% specificity and therefore still essential for medico-legal cases. Sensitivity ~70%. Vulnerable to invalidation by toxins in specimens. Suitable for genital and extra-genital swabs but not urine. Should be maintained at 4°C and received by the laboratory within 24 hours.

Enzyme-linked immunosorbent assay (EIA)

Several commercial assays are available. High specificity (>95%) when combined with confirmatory test, e.g. blocking antibody. Sensitivity (variable between assays) 15–94% on urine sample (less for ♀) and 60–85% for other specimens. Inexpensive—automation permits mass testing. Unsuitable for rectal swabs (interference by normal flora). Should be received by the laboratory in 3–5 days and preferably maintained at 4°C.

Direct fluorescent antibody (DFA)

Specificity 82–99% (observer dependent), sensitivity 68–100%. Unsuitable for large numbers (labour intensive). Suitable for all specimen sites. Swab rolled onto a slide and fixed. No special transport conditions.

Nucleic acid amplification tests (NAAT)

Amplification of:

- plasmid DNA, MOMP1, or ribosomal RNA genes—polymerase chain reaction (PCR).
- plasmid DNA + probe—ligase chain reaction (LCR). No longer available.
- RNA and hybridization with a labelled DNA probe—transcription mediated amplification (TMA).
- plasmid DNA—strand displacement amplification (SDA).
- MOMP1 RNA—nucleic acid sequence based amplification assay (NASBA).

High specificity (98–100%) and sensitivity, e.g. LCR, PCR, and TMA with urine >95%, >85%, and 92%; cervical swabs >88%, >95%, and >92%, respectively. Other NAATs have similar sensitivities. Suitable for any site including self-collected vulval and tampon samples. Not yet acceptable for medico-legal diagnosis. Currently unlicensed and non-validated for ano-rectal and oropharyngeal specimens. If delays >24 hours are anticipated, storage at 4°C is recommended to avoid sample degradation. Manufacturer's instructions should be followed.

DNA probe
- Probe Assay Chemiluminescence Enhanced (PACE®).
- Hybrid Capture II.

Similar to cell culture in sensitivity and rarely used.

Chlamydial antibody in serum
While complicated infections (PID, epidydimitis) elicit strong antibody responses, most mucosal infections do not. Microimmunofluorescent assay necessary to identify species-specific antibody. Only useful in retrospective diagnosis. IgG titre >1:64 may indicate a recent episode but does not exclude past infection. IgA may indicate active infection. IgM is useful in the diagnosis of neonatal pneumonia.

Frequently asked questions
I'm pregnant can it harm my baby?
Chlamydia in pregnancy is associated with ↑ risk of preterm delivery and low birth weight. Premature rupture of membranes is more frequent, as is intrapartum pyrexia, postpartum endometritis, and post-abortal PID.

Neonatal chlamydia infection is due to exposure in the birth canal during labour. 30–50% of exposed infants will develop chlamydia ophthalmia neonatorum. Treatment of the mother for chlamydia prior to delivery is associated with a decrease in incidence to 1–2%. There is a risk of respiratory tract infection in the neonate after birth canal exposure.

Do I need a test of cure?
Routine test of cure is not necessary following standard 1st line treatment, e.g. doxycycline 100mg twice daily for 7 days or azithromycin 1g single dose. If a ♀ has been treated with erythromycin (usually in pregnancy when doxycycline is contraindicated), a test of cure isrecommended 3 weeks after completion of therapy.

Management

▶Advise avoidance of sexual intercourse including with condoms until the patient and partner(s) have completed treatment and symptoms have resolved.

Uncomplicated genital and rectal infections

Recommended treatment regimens

- Doxycycline 100mg twice daily for 7 days
- Azithromycin 1g as a single dose

Alternative regimens

- Tetracyclines:
  - tetracycline 500mg 4 times a day for 7 days (compliance problem)
  - minocycline 100mg once daily for 7 days.
- Macrolides:
  - erythromycin 500mg twice daily for 14 days or 500mg 4 times a day for 7 days (↑ side-effects with the latter)
  - clarithromycin 400mg twice daily for 7 days.
- Fluoroquinolones:
  - ofloxacin 200mg twice daily or 400mg once daily for 7 days
  - levofloxacin 500mg once daily for 7 days.
- Penicillins
  - amoxicillin—used in pregnancy (📖 Pregnancy and breastfeeding)
  - pivampicillin 700mg twice daily for 7 days (limited evidence).
- Other antibiotics (limited efficacy or applicability)
  - co-trimoxazole two tablets (trimethoprim 160mg + sulfamethoxazole 800mg) twice daily for 7 days (limited evidence)
  - rifampicin 600mg once daily for 6 days.

Complicated genital infection (📖 Chapter 10, Management p. 174; Chapter 12, Management p. 192).

Pregnancy and breastfeeding

- Erythromycin 500mg daily for 14 days or 500mg 4 times a day for 7 days.
- Amoxicillin 500mg three times day for 7 days (better tolerated than erythromycin).
- Azithromycin 1g as a single dose—restricted licence in pregnancy but available data indicate no teratogenicity or adverse pregnancy outcomes.

❶ Tetracyclines, fluroquinolones, and co-trimoxazole are contraindicated in pregnancy.

Other situations

- Adult chlamydial conjunctivitis: treatment as for genital infection, i.e. systemic treatment required.
- Ophthalmia neonatorum and infant pneumonia:
  - erythromycin 50mg/kg/day oral divided into 4 doses daily for 14 days.

- Neonatal prophylaxis: silver nitrate drops and erythromycin and tetracycline ointments are ineffective, and infants born of mothers with untreated chlamydial infection should be monitored carefully for signs of conjunctivitis. Swabs should be taken for *C.trachomatis* from everted eyelids 5–10 days after birth.
- Prepubertal infection:
  - erythromycin 50mg/kg/day (up to 1g) divided into 4 doses for 14 days
  - Alternative treatments: age ≥8 years—doxycycline 100mg twice daily for 7 days; weight >45kg—azithromycin 1g as a single dose.

Partner notification

Partner notification is essential. Contact tracing period:
- symptomatic ♂—4 weeks prior to onset of symptoms or until last sexual partner.
- asymptomatic ♂—6 months prior to presentation or until the last sexual partner.

Similar principles should apply to the mother of a neonate with chlamydial infection and her sex partner/s.

Follow-up

Need not necessarily be through re-attendance at the clinic. The objectives of follow-up are to assess management compliance, resolution of any symptoms, and partner notification. A test of cure is only recommended if not treated with doxycycline or azithromycin or symptoms persist. Repeat treatment if risk of reinfection with untreated partner.

NAAT testing, if required, should be delayed until at least 3 weeks after the end of the treatment.

HIV infection

Chlamydial infection facilitates HIV transmission, producing ↑ in detectable virus in urethral/cervical secretions when infection is present. This is reversed following antibiotic treatment.

Non-chlamydial non-specific genital infection

Introduction

Non-specific genital infection (NSGI) refers to ♂ urethritis in the absence of gonorrhoea, non-gonococcal or non-specific urethritis (NGU or NSU), and the equivalent but less well-defined condition in ♀, mucopurulent cervicitis (MPC). *Chlamydia trachomatis* is the cause in 30–50% of NGU and 25–45% of MPC. Non-chlamydial NSGI has been attributed to several causes supported by variable evidence.

Aetiology

Non-chlamydial NGU

Microorganisms

- *Mycoplasma genitalium*—up to 20% of NGU (Box 9.1).
- *Ureaplasma urealyticum*—association with non-chlamydial NGU in up to 52% (similar prevalence in the absence of NGU). Serovar 4 more likely to play a role in NGU.
- Bacterial vaginosis (BV)—30% of ♂ with NGU have ♀ partners with BV which may be implicated in an undetermined proportion.
- Bacteria causing urinary tract infections (UTIs)—up to 6% of NGU seen in GUM clinic is due to UTI. Coliform bacteria may be associated with NGU in ♂ practising insertive anal sex.
- *Trichomonas vaginalis*—up to 15% of NGU in high-prevalence areas.
- Herpes simplex virus (HSV)—up to 2% of NGU without external genital ulcers. 30% of primary genital HSV episodes in ♂ include NGU.
- Adenovirus—types 8, 19, and 37 (subgenus D) isolated from 0.4% of ♂ attending GUM clinics. 75% of isolates associated with NGU, often with conjunctivitis, pharyngitis, and constitutional symptoms. Transmission probably by oral sex.

The following organisms show a possible or occasional causal role:
- *Neisseria meningitidis*
- *Candida* species (rarely): if present usually associated with balanitis (possible reaction to partner's candidal infection)
- *Haemophilus influenzae and parainfluenzae*
- *Staphylococcus saprophyticus*
- *Corynebacterium genitalium*
- *Bacteroides urealyticus*
- *Mycobacterium tuberculosis*.

Non-microbial

- Congenital anomalies, e.g. urethral stricture
- Physical irritation—trauma related to sex, manipulation, or foreign body (e.g. urinary catheter)
- Chemical irritation
- Reactive urethritis (e.g. reactive arthritis, allergens)
- Stevens–Johnson syndrome.

Non-gonococcal non-chlamydial MPC

- *M.genitalium* implicated in up to 10%
- HSV infection
- Possibly other as yet unidentified causes

Box 9.1 *Mycoplasma genitalium*

- A bacterium:
  - discovered in 1980 in the urethra of 2 ♂ with NGU
  - classified as belonging to the family Mycoplasmateles
  - 1 of 14 mycoplasmas of human origin
  - long flask shape with a narrow terminal rod binding to eukaryotic cells
  - fastidious and slow growing (difficult to isolate)
  - forms fried-egg-like colonies within agar medium incubated in nitrogen and 5% carbon dioxide
  - genome—580 kilobase, smallest of any self-replicating bacterium.
- Urogenital tract—preferred site of colonization where it may invade epithelial cells.
- Sexual transmission—causal role in NGU/MPC and possibly pelvic inflammatory disease (PID)/epididymitis. Identified in:
  - 18–45% of non-chlamydial NGU (odds ratio 7.1)
  - up to 10% of MPC
  - 16% of endometritis
  - 15% of PID.
  - ~7% of tubal factor infertility (by serology) (odds ratio 4.5)
- Sensitive to tetracyclines (except when the *tetM* gene is present), macrolides, ketolides, and fluoroquinolones, and resistant to penicillins, sulphonamides, and rifampicin. Antibiotics only suppress growth and a competent immune system is necessary for eradication.

Clinical features

Male—NGU

Symptoms	Signs
• Urethral discharge • Dysuria • Penile irritation • None (asymptomatic)	• Urethral discharge—varyingamounts, clear to yellow, spontaneous, or expressed • None (subclinical)

Up to 20% of ♂ with observable discharge have no symptoms. NGU without symptoms and signs (in ~25%) is less likely to be due to *C.trachomatis* or *M.genitalium*.

Female—MPC

Usually asymptomatic, but if severe may cause vaginal discharge and vulval irritation. Dysuria unusual.

Cervix appears inflamed, oedematous, and friable with an overlying mucopurulent discharge.

Complications

Epididymo-orchitis (☐ Chapter 12)
Sexually acquired reactive arthritis (☐ Chapter 13).
Pelvic inflammatory disease (☐ Chapter 10).

Diagnosis

NGU

Urethral specimen using a 5mm plastic loop or cotton-tipped swab (better quality if bladder not emptied in preceding 3 hours). If no urethral material check first voided urine (FVU).

Urethritis diagnosed by high-power (1000×) microscopy of Gram-stained material:

- ≥5PMNL)/field of urethral smear
- ≥10PMNL/field of threads or deposits from FVU.

Symptomatic ♂ without evidence of urethritis may be re-assessed after retaining urine overnight (or for at least 3 hours).

MPC

No clear microscopic criteria for diagnosis as the number of cervical polymorphonuclear leucocytes (PMNLs) varies physiologically. Diagnosis based on the cervical appearance possibly supported by microscopy (>30PMNLs/high-power field).

Other investigations

- *N.gonorrhoeae* and *C.trachomatis*—as routine.
- Midstream sample of urine (MSSU)—positive dipstick for leucocyte esterase, nitrites, and blood suggests UTI. Confirm with microscopy and culture.
- *M.genitalium*—culture difficult and not readily available. Polymerase chain reaction ↑ sensitivity but not yet available for routine use.

Management

▶ Advise avoidance of sexual intercourse, including with condoms, until the patient and partner(s) have completed treatment and symptoms have resolved. Discourage repeated self-examination and advise that other factors (e.g. spicy food) may aggravate or prolong symptoms. Standard anti-chlamydial regimens are generally effective against non-chlamydial NSGI (except if 2° to UTI/coliforms).

Recommended treatment regimens

- Doxycycline 100mg twice daily for 7 days.
- Azithromycin 1g—single dose. 87% effective in *M.genitalium* infection with failures likely to be associated with resistance due to mutation in region V of 23S rRNA. Azithromycin 500mg followed by 250mg daily for 4–6 days is 97% effective and less likely to induce the mutation.

Alternative regimens

Tetracyclines
- Tetracycline 500mg 4 times a day for 7 days
- Minocycline 100mg once daily for 7 days

Macrolides
- Erythromycin 500mg twice daily for 14 days
- Clarithromycin 400mg twice daily for 7 days

Fluoroquinolones
- Ofloxacin 200mg twice daily or 400mg once daily for 7 days.
- Moxifloxacin 400mg daily for 10 days if resistant *M.genitalium* and no response to other treatments because of risk of serious side-effects.
  - ⚠ ↑ risk of life-threatening liver reactions, cardiac arrhythmias with QTc prolongation, rhabdomyolysis, and tendon rupture.

Complicated genital infection (📖 Chapter 10. Management p. 174; Chapter 12, Management p. 192).

Epidemiological treatment regimens

As for uncomplicated infection.

Partner notification

Assessment of sexual partners may reveal possible causes (e.g. trichomoniasis) which could affect overall management. Epidemiological treatment of sexual partners of ♂ with chlamydia-negative NGU may ↓ recurrence and possibly↓ ♀ morbidity. Suggested 'look-back' periods: 4 weeks for symptomatic ♂; up to 6 months for asymptomatic ♂.

Similarly, sexual partners of ♀ with MPC should be offered epidemiological treatment and routine screening for STIs.

Follow-up

May be by telephone to ensure management compliance, resolution of symptoms, and partner notification. If symptoms or signs persist/recur, repeat urethral smear/FVU specimen. Repeat treatment if risk of reinfection.

Persistent, relapsing, and chronic NGU

- Persistent NGU—continuing despite treatment of initial episode
- Relapsing NGU—recurrence following resolution of initial episode
- Chronic NGU—persistent or relapsing NGU ≥30 days post-treatment

All without a risk of re-infection.

Persistent or relapsing NGU occurs in 20–60% of ♂ treated for acute NGU and half of these may become chronic with *U.urealyticum* and *M.genitalium* of possible importance. A continuing inflammatory response following eradication of active chlamydial infection has also been suggested. In this situation there is no ↑ risk of PID in ♀ partners.

Recommended treatment regimen

- Azithromycin 500mg stat followed by 250mg daily for 4 days plus metronidazole 400mg twice a day for 5 days.
- Erythromycin 500mg 4 times a day for 3 weeks *plus* metronidazole 400mg twice a day for 5 days.
- Repeat epidemiological treatment of partner using erythromycin if doxycycline used initially.
- Moxifloxacin 400mg daily if resistant *M.genitalium* for 10 days.
  - ⚠ ↑ risk of life-threatening liver reactions and other serious risks. Use only if no alternative suitable.

Continuing symptoms

Microscopic urethritis with no signs or symptoms after two courses of treatment is of little clinical significance. Further re-treatment of sexual partners is not beneficial. Limited evidence on how best to manage patients who either remain symptomatic or have frequent relapses following a 2nd course of treatment. Consider:

- urological investigations—usually normal unless the patient has urinary flow problems
- chronic abacterial prostatitis
- psychosexual causes.

HIV infection

M.genitalium may enhance transmission of HIV. Impaired immune function hampers its eradication (detection rate in urethra—56% with AIDS compared with 12% without AIDS).

Pelvic inflammatory disease

Introduction

Pelvic inflammatory disease (PID) refers to inflammation of the upper female genital tract (endometrium, fallopian tubes, and ovaries) and supporting structures (parametrium and pelvic peritoneum). It is usually a result of infection:

- ascending from the endocervix
- less commonly spread from other abdominal organs (e.g. appendicitis) or disseminated by blood.

Endometritis and endosalpingitis produce a purulent exudate that may escape into the rectovaginal pouch resulting in a pelvic abscess. Inflammation may spread to the ovaries (oophoritis), parametrium, and pelvic peritoneum (peritonitis).

Aetiology

Sexually transmitted infections

- *Neisseria gonorrhoeae* in 5–75%: produces complement-mediated necrosis of ciliated epithelial cells.
- *Chlamydia trachomatis* in 5–45%: induces Th-2 type immune response damaging tubal epithelium.

Worldwide data—wide ranges relate to variable infection rates and availability of reliable tests.

PID in 10–30% of untreated cervical chlamydial and gonococcal infections.

Other micro-organisms

- Bacterial vaginosis (BV) associated organisms: anaerobic bacilli (e.g. *Prevotella* and *Bacteroides* spp), anaerobic cocci (e.g. *Peptosreptococcus* spp, *Gardenerella vaginalis*, *Mycoplasma hominis*, α and non-haemolytic streptococci). Recovered from fallopian tubes in up to 20% of ♀ with PID and 80% of endometrial samples in plasma cell endometritis (accompanying PID in ascending infection). Statistically significant association between BV and PID. Sialidase activity of *Prevotella* and *Bacteroides* spp, weakening cervical mucous barrier, possibly promotes ascending infection.
- Other organisms have also been recovered from the fallopian tubes: viridans group streptococci, group A–D streptococci, *Escherichia coli*, *Bacteroides fragilis*, and coagulase –ve staphylococci).
- *Mycoplasma genitalium*: cervical infection in ~15% ♀ with PID. Experimental evidence for PID in chimpanzees.
- *Actinomyces israelii* and related species: occasionally cause a chronic pelvic abscess (<1 in 3000 cases of PID and 3% of all human actinomyces infections) usually in association with plastic intra-uterine devices (IUDs) and anaerobic co-infection.
- *Mycobacterium tuberculosis*: haematogenously disseminated; an important cause in areas of high prevalence.
- *Salmonella* spp: rarely as a result of abdominal spread from an intestinal focus of infection in typhoid and paratyphoid.

Factors facilitating ascending infection

Physiological

- Uterine contractions: ↑ in the follicular phase until ovulation.
- Loss of cervical mucus plug (formed in the luteal phase) and retrograde flow during menstruation.
- Possible carriage of bacteria by spermatozoa.

Iatrogenic

- Uterine instrumentation.

Epidemiology

Estimated annual incidence in industrialized countries ~1 in 1000 in ♀ aged 15–34 years (1.5–2/1000 if 15–24) with wide geographical and temporal variations. Sexual transmission is the major aetiological factor.

Factors increasing risk

- Young age: peak incidence in age group 15–24 years
- Multiple partners
- New partner within previous 3 months
- Frequency of sexual intercourse
- Past history of STI (patient or partner)
- Past history of PID
- Uterine instrumentation:
  - termination of pregnancy
  - insertion of IUD within the previous 6 weeks—not a high risk alone (overall incidence of PID only 0.15%) but concomitant cervical chlamydial/gonococcal infection ↑ risk to 3–5%
  - hysterosalpingography/hysteroscopy
  - endometrial biopsy, curettage, and ablation
  - *in vitro* fertilization procedure
- Postpartum endometritis
- Vaginal douching
- Cigarette smoking

Factors reducing risk

- Hormonal contraception especially progesterone-only preparations (production of a 'luteal-type' cervical mucus plug and reduction in the tubal inflammatory response)
- Consistent use of condom or diaphragm
- Spermicide
- Pregnancy: PID is uncommon because of thickened cervical mucus plug and is limited to the 1st trimester (protection afforded by the amniotic sac filling the uterine cavity is absent)

Clinical features

Acute PID (symptoms for <3 weeks)
Onset within 7 days of the 1st day of menstruation correlates with gono-coccal/chlamydial infection. Symptoms and signs tend to be more acute/intense in gonococcal than chlamydial PID.

Symptoms
- Lower abdominal pain; usually subacute if mild and acute if severe
- Deep dyspareunia, common
- Menstrual irregularity in ~40%
- Abnormal bleeding
- Dysmenorrhoea
- Vaginal discharge
- Nausea ± vomiting if severe

Signs
- Lower abdominal tenderness with guarding; rebound if severe
- Adnexal and cervical motion (excitation) tenderness
- Fever (>38°C) in ~50%; more likely in severe or gonococcal PID
- Adnexal mass in 50% of ♀ with gonococcal PID
- Abdominal distension due to paralytic ileus if very severe (~1%)

Chronic PID ('silent PID')
May be asymptomatic and discovered only on investigation of infertility. Symptoms include constant or intermittent pain/discomfort in lower ab-domen, groin or back, dyspareunia, malaise, and frequent/heavy menstrual periods. Usually no appreciable signs, but thickening of tubes and/or fixed retroverted uterus may be palpable.

Complications and sequelae

Tubo-ovarian and pelvic abscess
Late complication, likely to be associated with anaerobic bacteria.

Peri-appendicitis
Direct spread of infection from the right fallopian tube to the appendiceal serosa may produce external inflammation (serositis) without mucosal in-volvement. Tubo-appendiceal mass develops. 2–10% of acute appendicitis in ♀ may be due to peri-appendicitis, 25–50% of which may be linked to tubal inflammation.

Infertility
Occurs in 8%, 20%, and 40% after 1, 2, and 3 episodes of PID, respectively. Due to tubal occlusion and peritubal adhesions. The more severe the episode the higher the incidence of infertility. Conflicting evidence on risk ↓ with treatment of PID.

Ectopic gestation

Sevenfold ↑ in risk of ectopic gestation (9% compared with 1.3% in the absence of PID). Risk ↑ directly with PID severity and number of episodes.

Chronic pelvic pain

Incidence 12%, 33%, and 66% after 1, 2, and 3 episodes of PID, respectively. Due to pelvic adhesions that form after the initial or recurrent episodes. Affects psychosocial functioning and quality of life.

Perihepatitis (Fitz-Hugh–Curtis syndrome)

Inflammation of the hepatic capsule with 'violin string' adhesions between anterior surface of liver and abdominal wall. Results from peritoneal or lymphatic spread of pelvic gonococcal/chlamydial infection. Occurs in 10–20% with PID.

▶ Haematogenous spread possible (case reports in ♂ with gonorrhoea).

Symptoms and signs of PID are not always present but a past history of PID or lower genital infection may be obtained. Typical presentation is acute, often severe, with right upper quadrant pain radiating to the back and shoulder tip, made worse by deep inspiration and movement. Examination demonstrates tenderness and guarding in the right upper abdominal quadrant with Murphy's sign (↑ pain on deep inspiration, examining hand just below the right costal margin). Hepatic rub may be heard on auscultation. Pyrexia in ~50%.

Differential diagnosis: acute cholecystitis, biliary colic, pleurisy, pneumonia, or pulmonary embolism.

Investigations

Routine

- Swabs for *N.gonorrhoeae* and *C.trachomatis*.
- Gram-stained smear of cervical material: may provide presumptive diagnosis of gonorrhoea. Polymorphonuclear leucocytes (PMNLs) are non-specific (positive predictive value only 17%) but useful for exclusion of PID (negative predictive value 95%).
- Peripheral blood white blood cell (WBC) count: ↑ in ~50%.
- Erythrocyte sedimentation rate (ESR)—↑ in ~75%.
- C-reactive protein (CRP): ↑ in ~75%, level reflects severity.
- Chlamydial antibody: only provides retrospective or inconclusive evidence, hence of limited value in acute PID. However, in ♀ investigated for infertility antibody, especially at high level, correlates closely with frequency and severity of tubal damage and adverse pregnancy outcome. Therefore useful as a screening test to determine the likelihood of tubal damage and need for early laparoscopy.
- ▶ Pregnancy test (urine or plasma β-hCG): essential for acute pelvic pain in all ♀ of childbearing age.
- Urine analysis ± MSU if urinary tract infection is suspected.

Specialized

Endometrial histology/microbiology

- Sensitivity ~70%, specificity ~90%.

Pelvic imaging

Abdominal ultrasound useful for detection of pelvic abscess. Transvaginal ultrasonography reported to have ~80% sensitivity and specificity (compared with laparoscopy/endometrial biopsy). May be necessary for differential diagnosis, particularly ectopic gestation.

Laparoscopy

- Regarded as the gold standard but not routinely performed (time/cost/complication risk). Allows:
- diagnosis of acute PID by identifying
  - pronounced hyperaemia of tubal surface
  - oedema of tubal wall
  - sticky exudate from fimbriae
- collection of laboratory specimens from affected sites
- identification of other causes (e.g. ectopic gestation, appendicitis, endometriosis) or complications (e.g. abscess, pelvic adhesions, 'violin string adhesions' of perihepatitis).

May fail to identify endosalpingitis/endometritis in early/mild infection.

Diagnosis

The presence of all main criteria plus one of the additional criteria is widely used for clinical diagnosis (Table 10.1). Positive predictive value of 65–90% compared with laporoscopy. In routine clinical practice a lower threshold is often applied for prompt antibiotic treatment.

Table 10.1 Diagnostic criteria

Main	Additional
Low abdominal or pelvic pain	Temperature >38°C
Abdominal ± rebound tenderness/ adnexal tenderness	↑ CRP/ESR WBC >10 x 10⁹
Cervical motion (excitation) Tenderness	Adnexal mass PMNLs in cervical/vaginal Gram-stained smears

Differential diagnosis of PID

Acute/subacute

- Ectopic pregnancy: in ruptured ectopic pregnancy sudden onset of iliac fossa or hypogastric pain often associated with syncope. Vaginal spotting in early stages. Shoulder tip pain if blood tracked into abdominal cavity. Shock with intra-abdominal haemorrhage.
- Acute appendicitis: initial peri-umbilical pain later localizing to right iliac fossa with pronounced nausea and vomiting.
- Ruptured ovarian or endometriotic cyst: sudden onset of perimenstrual lower abdominal pain, usually afebrile.
- Complications of ovarian neoplasms.
- Acute pyelonephritis: pyrexia of sudden onset, rigors, loin/iliac fossa pain, urinary symptoms.
- Mesenteric lymphadenitis, inflammatory bowel disease.
- Adnexal torsion.
- Other abdominal emergencies.

Chronic/recurrent

- Endometriosis.
- Pelvic congestion syndrome.
- Ovarian cysts.
- Ovarian and uterine neoplasms.
- Interstitial cystitis.
- Urethral syndrome.
- Irritable bowel syndrome.
- Inflammatory bowel disease.
- Previous surgery, leading to pelvic adhesions or nerve entrapment.
- Myofascial pain syndrome.
- Psychosocial causes: depression, previous physical and sexual abuse/ trauma, leading to somatization disorder.

Management

General principles

To minimize sequelae commence treatment promptly (even before definitive diagnosis). Hospital admission if:

- systemic disturbance is severe
- surgical/gynaecological emergency cannot be excluded
- patient is pregnant or immunocompromised
- tubo-ovarian or pelvic abscess is detected or suspected.

Rest and adequate analgesia. IUD removal is indicated only if severe PID, no improvement after 72 hours of treatment, actinomyces-like organisms present, or patient requests. Offer emergency contraception on removal if pregnancy risk within preceding 7 days. ▶ Advise avoidance of sexual intercourse until the patient and partner(s) have completed treatment.

Treatment regimens

When choosing antibiotic regimen consider:

- severity and systemic disturbance—may need parenteral treatment
- local prevalence of *N.gonorrhoeae* and antibiotic sensitivity
- patient preference and likelihood of adherence.

Initial regimens (may need to be altered when antibiotic sensitivities are available)

Out-patient

- Ceftriaxone 250mg IM single dose followed by doxycycline 100mg oral twice daily for 14 days plus metronidazole 400mg twice daily for 7–14 days (90–95% clinical cure rate).
- Ofloxacin 400mg twice daily for 14 days plus metronidazole 400mg twice daily for 7–14 days (95% clinical cure rate).
- Doxycycline 100mg twice daily for 14 days plus metronidazole 400mg twice daily for 7–14 days (70–81% clinical cure rate). Does not cover *N. gonorrhoeae*, viridans streptococci and coliforms.
- Moxifloxacin 400 mg daily for 14 days (no metronidazole) but because of serious side-effects should only be used if no other treatment is suitable. ⚠ ↑ risk of life-threatening liver reactions, cardiac arrhythmias with QTc prolongation, rhabdomyolysis and tendon rupture.

In-patient

- Cefoxitin 2g IV 4 times a day plus doxycycline 100mg orally (or IV if vomiting makes oral treatment intolerable) twice daily. Add metronidazole 500mg IV if pelvic or tubo-ovarian abscess develops.
- Clindamycin IV 900mg 3 times a day plus gentamicin 2mg/kg IV or IM loading dose followed by 1.5mg/kg 3 times a day.
- Ofloxacin 400mg IV infusion twice daily plus metronidazole 500mg IV 3 times a day.
- Ampicillin/sulbactam IV infusion 3g 3 times a day plus doxycycline oral or IV 100mg twice daily.

Parenteral regimen is replaced after clinical improvement by one of the oral regimens and continued for a total of 14 days.

Treatment in pregnancy
Parenteral treatment advisable. Replace doxycycline with erythromycin (50mg/kg daily by continuous IV infusion).

Treatment of actinomycosis
Remove IUD. Benzylpenicillin 18–24MU (10.8–14.4g) IV daily as infusion (or 4 hourly injections) and metronidazole 500mg IV 8 hourly. Doxycycline, erythromycin, and clindamycin are alternatives to benzylpenicillin. Change to oral regimen after clinical improvement and continue for at least 4–6 weeks. Drainage of abscess relieves bowel or urinary tract compression. Salpingo-oophorectomy and hysterectomy may be necessary.

Partner notification

Sexual partner/s within a 6 month period of onset of symptoms should be contacted and offered screening for STIs and epidemiological treatment for chlamydia ± gonorrhoea taking into consideration the proven or probable aetiology.

Follow-up

Review diagnosis and management after 72 hours if acute symptoms and signs do not improve. Reassess after 2–4 weeks.

HIV infection

- ↓ production of interferon-γ may ↑ susceptibility to PID
- Tubo-ovarian abscess formation more likely if immunocompromised
- Symptoms may be more severe but respond well to parenteral antibiotic therapy

Prostatitis/chronic pelvic pain syndrome

Introduction

Prostatitis affects up to 50% of ♂ at some time in their lives, with a prevalence of 10–16% of all ages and ethnic origins. The National Institutes of Health produced a classification following two consensus conferences in 1995 and 1998, detailed below and now widely used:

I   Acute bacterial prostatitis
II Chronic bacterial prostatitis
III Chronic prostatitis/chronic pelvic pain syndrome
    A. Inflammatory
    B. Non-inflammatory (previously prostatodynia)
IV Asymptomatic inflammatory prostatitis

The majority of cases are chronic, and probably 90–95% of these are abacterial. Diagnosis is largely based on symptoms, as signs and objective clinical data may be inconclusive or lacking. Symptoms which may be attributed to prostate dysfunction include the following.

Pain
- Perineum
- Low abdomen/suprapubic
- Penis (especially tip)
- Testes
- Rectum
- Retropubis and upper thighs
- Low back/coccyx

Urinary dysfunction
- Frequency/nocturia
- Urgency
- Incomplete voiding
- Abnormal flow
- Urethral discharge
- Double voiding

Ejaculatory disturbance
- Pain with/after ejaculation
- Discoloration of or blood in semen

Acute bacterial prostatitis (ABP)

Uncommon but clearly identifiable and easiest to diagnose and treat effectively. Should be considered as a complication of acute urinary tract infection (UTI), caused by urinary pathogens especially *Escherichia coli*. Less common organisms include *Klebsiella pneumoniae*, *Proteus mirabilis*, *Pseudomonas aeruginosa*, *Enterobacter* spp, and other urinary tract pathogens. There may be an underlying structural abnormality of the urinary tract which should be investigated after resolution of the acute episode. In the pre-antibiotic era gonorrhoea was a frequent cause of a prostatic abscess.

Symptoms
- Prostatitis—perineal prostatic pain
- UTI—dysuria, frequency, urgency, incomplete bladder emptying
- Bacteraemia—pyrexia, rigors, myalgia, arthralgia
- Abscess (rare complication)—intense pain and acute urinary retention

Diagnosis

- Gentle digital rectal examination—prostate enlarged, tender, warm, and/or boggy. ⚠ Prostatic massage contraindicated in ABP as it may precipitate bacteraemia.
- Midstream sample of urine (MSSU).
- Blood cultures.
- Transrectal ultrasound (also useful to exclude prostatic abscess).
- Residual bladder ultrasound to check for urinary retention.

Management

- Mild to moderate: oral fluoroquinolone (e.g. ciprofloxacin 500mg twice daily or ofloxacin 200mg twice daily). Trimethoprim 200mg twice daily (if fluoroquinolone intolerant or allergic). All for 28 days.
- Severe: initial parenteral broad-spectrum cephalosporin (e.g. cefuroxime) plus gentamicin then switch to oral regimen during convalescence. Intravenous fluids and urinary drainage (if retention) may also be required. If abscess present which fails to respond to antibiotics—transurethral resection with drainage.

Causes of haematospermia

- Trauma (most common cause in young ♂). Generally mild, often isolated episodes. Usually self-limiting.
- Inflammation: prostatitis, seminal vesiculitis, urethritis, epididymitis.
- Obstruction/dilatation of urogenital ducts: prostatic cysts, urethral strictures, ejaculatory duct cysts, and strictures.
- Vascular abnormalities: arteriovenous malformations, venous malformations, haemangiomata.
- Systemic disorders:
  - severe hypertension
  - haematological disorders—coagulation disorders, leukaemia
  - cirrhosis.
- Drugs: e.g. warfarin.
- Tumours:
  - benign—polyps, warts, benign prostatic hyperplasia
  - malignant—carcinoma of genital tract.

Chronic bacterial prostatitis (CBP)

Unusual, accounting for ~2–5% of prostatitis cases. Chronic or persistent prostate infection usually due to *E.coli* (~80%). Patients experience recurrent UTIs with the prostate gland as the infection source, warranting urological referral. In addition, there may be obstructive urinary symptoms, perineal prostatic pain, and possibly sexual dysfunction but, unlike ABP, no systemic symptoms.

Diagnosis

- Consider if recurrent UTIs.
- Digital rectal examination: normal, hypertrophied, and/or tender prostate.
- Evidence of prostatic infection: bacterial colony count in expressed prostatic secretions or post-prostate-massage urine specimen (Box 11.1) at least 10× greater than first voided urine or midstream sample.

Management

Antibiotics for 4–8 weeks according to antimicrobial sensitivity, prefer-ably a fluoroquinolone (high relative concentration in prostate tissue, 2–3× serum levels), e.g. ciprofloxacin 500mg, ofloxacin 200mg, norfloxacin 400mg all twice daily. Trimethoprim, 200mg twice daily, which also has good prostate penetration, can be considered as second-line treatment.

Chronic prostatitis/chronic pelvic pain syndrome (CPPS)

The most common form of prostatitis (>90% of all cases). Understanding of the causes of this syndrome is limited and other organs, including pelvic floor, bladder, and seminal vesicles, may be involved. ↑ genital-tract post-inflammatory cytokines possibly suggest autoimmunity, post-infective triggers, or neurogenic inflammation. Genital or pelvic pain is required in its diagnosis, and exclusion criteria include urethritis, uro-genital cancer, urinary tract disease, functionally relevant urethral stricture, or bladder neurological disease. Undiagnosed depression or anxiety states may be important factors in ♂ with severe refractory CPPS.

Subclassified as inflammatory if polymorphonuclear leucocytes found in expressed prostatic secretions (EPS) (Box 11.1), semen, or post-prostate-massage urine. Patients with the non-inflammatory subtype have no evidence of inflammation. In practical terms this differentiation is of little value as the clinical presentation and response to treatment are almost identical.

CPPS may present as chronic unilateral testicular pain, which may be provoked by coitus. This is usually idiopathic but may follow acute epididymitis, vasectomy, previous trauma, or be associated with a varicocele, hydrocele, or sexual dysfunction.

Box 11.1 Prostatic assessment for inflammation and infection

Prostatic massage
Patient should not have:
  • taken antibiotics within previous 4 weeks
  • ejaculated within previous 48 hours
  • evidence of urethritis or UTI (exclude prior to prostatic massage).
• Place patient in left lateral position and ensure that he is breathing easily through his mouth (to avoid Valsalva manoeuvre).
• With lubricated forefinger in rectum gently press on right and left lateral aspects of prostate gland in turn and move finger to the midline. Repeat 3–4 times.
• Press on superior aspect of prostate gland in midline and move finger to its lower pole. Repeat 2–3 times.
• Prostatic fluid should appear at the urethral meatus although sometimes gentle milking of the urethra is required.
If this fails, the process can be repeated. However, a dry massage is fairly common.

Expressed prostatic secretions (EPS)
• pH≥8 suggestive but not diagnostic of prostatitis.
• Bacterial colony count in the EPS and post-prostate massage urine sample must be at least 10× greater than first voided urine and pre-massage midstream sample of urine to diagnose chronic bacterial prostatitis.
• ≥10 PMNL/high power field (×400) is considered diagnostic of inflammation. If dry massage, PMNLs 10/HPF greater in post-massage urine than first voided urine and MSU. ⚠: EPS PMNLs may be absent in cases of inflammation with infection and ≥10/HPF found in up to 6% of healthy controls Therefore unreliable in subclassifying CPPS into inflammatory and non-inflammatory categories.

Symptoms

- Pain (essential feature): perineum, suprapubic, coccygeal, rectal, urethral, testicular/scrotal, penile (especially the tip).
- Urinary obstruction: poor stream, incomplete emptying, double voiding, frequency, urgency, dysuria.
- Sexual dysfunction: erectile dysfunction, premature/painful ejaculation.

Quantitative assessment of severity of prostatitis useful in temporal review or in gauging therapeutic response using Chronic Prostatitis Symptom Index (Box 11.2).

Diagnosis

- By exclusion of other causes including bladder or prostate infection, urinary obstruction, testicular cancer, genitourinary tract calculi, hernias, radiculopathies, other chronic pain syndromes.
- The prostate gland usually feels normal on digital examination with variable degrees of tenderness (local, diffuse) or none.

Management

In view of lack of understanding and imprecision in diagnosis it is difficult to evaluate treatments properly. No therapy has been demonstrated to be absolutely effective.

- Antibiotics: although CBP regimens are prescribed, because of an assumed bacterial association there is no clear evidence in support.
- Alpha-blocking drugs (e.g. terazosin and alfuzosin): relax the bladder neck and prostate gland but limited and inconsistent evidence of benefit. May have a useful role in treatment of severely symptomatic naive patients if administered for at least 3 months.
- Allopurinol: inadequate data but improvement in patient-reported symptoms and investigator-graded prostate pain reported.
- Quercetin: a naturally occurring bioflavonoid with reported benefit in two-thirds of ♂ in one small study. Available from herbalists.
- Non-steroidal anti-inflammatory drugs: helpful for pain relief.
- Tricyclic antidepressants (e.g. amitriptyline) or anticonvulsant, gabapentin): anecdotal reports of benefit due to pain modulation as with other chronic pain conditions.
- Serotonin specific reuptake inhibitor (sertraline) has been shown in one small study to improve prostatic symptoms although cannot exclude a placebo effect.
- Frequent ejaculation (≥2× a week) reduces prostatic congestion and may ameliorate symptoms.
- Prostatic hyperthermia (by microwave): data limited but benefit has been demonstrated, meriting further investigation.
- Psychological treatment: assessment required if depressed or distressed. Behavioural therapy or pain clinic referral are options.
- Chronic testicular pain may respond to doxycycline (anti-chlamydia), anti-inflammatory agents, amitriptyline, gabapentin, local anaesthetic spermatic cord infiltration followed by cord denervation (if successful), transcutaneous electrical nerve stimulation, and even orchidectomy if severely intractable.

Box 11.2 Chronic Prostatitis Symptom Index (from National Institutes of Health)

Pain or discomfort in the last week

1. Have you experienced any pain or discomfort in the following areas?
    (a) Perineum (i.e. from rectum to testicles)—Yes(1)/No(0)
    (b) Testicles—Yes (1)/No (0)
    (c) Penile tip (unrelated to urination)—Yes(1)/No(0)
    (d) Below waist (pubic/bladder area)—Yes(1)/No(0)
2. Have you experienced?
    (a) Pain/burning during micturition—Yes(1)/No(0)
    (b) Pain/discomfort during/after ejaculation—Yes(1)/No(0)
3. How often have you had pain or discomfort in any of these areas?
Never(0)/Rarely(1)/Sometimes(2)/Often(3)/Usually(4)/Always(5)
4. Which number describes your **average** pain/discomfort on the days you had it on a 0–10 point scale?
'No pain' (0) to 'Pain as bad as you can imagine' (10)

Urination over the last week

5. How often have you sensed incomplete bladder emptying?
Never(0)/<1 in 5(1)/<half(2)/about half(3)/>half(4)/almost always(5).
6. How often have you had to repeat urination within <2 hours?
Never(0)/<1in5(1)/<half(2)/about half(3)/>half(4)/almost always(5)

Impact of symptoms over the last week

7. How much have the symptoms restricted you from doing things?
None(0)/only a little(1)/some(2)/a lot(3)
8. How much have you thought about your symptoms?
None(0)/only a little(1)/some(2)/a lot(3)

Quality of life based on your symptoms over the past week:

9. How would you feel if they persisted for the rest of your life?
Delighted(0)/Pleased(1)/Mostly satisfied(2)/Mixed(3)/
Mostly dissatisfied(4)/Unhappy(5)/Terrible(6)

Scoring

- Calculate and report 3 separate scores: pain (1–4), urinary symptoms (5 and 6), and impact of symptoms/quality of life (7–9).
- Calculate and report a pain and urinary score (range 0–31) referred to as the 'symptom scale score':
    - Mild = 0–9
    - Moderate = 10–18
    - Severe = 19–31

Calculate and report total score (range 0–43), referred to as the 'total score'. Assess at baseline and follow over time (and treatment) using each patient as his control. Can also be used to compare with established and published 'norms'.

Asymptomatic inflammatory prostatitis

Usually an incidental finding arising during the investigation of the genito-urinary tract for other reasons (e.g. prostate biopsy for possible prostate cancer because of an elevated serum prostate specific antigen test or infertility investigations). The patient has no symptoms but excess leucocytes in the seminal fluid are common findings. No treatment is required.

Other rare causes of prostatitis

- *Mycobacterium tuberculosis* and other atypical mycobacteria—granulomatous prostatitis
- Parasites—e.g. *Trichomonas vaginalis, Schistosoma haematobium*.
- Viruses—e.g. herpes simplex virus and cytomegalovirus in immunocompromised patients. May also present acutely.
- Mycoses—e.g. coccidioidomycosis, blastomycosis, cryptococcosis, histoplasmosis, candidiasis. More common in the immunosuppressed causing a granulomatous reaction.

Sexually transmitted infections

Chlamydia trachomatis, Ureaplasma urealyticum, Mycoplasma genitalium, and *Mycoplasma hominis* have been implicated in chronic prostatitis. Their nucleotide sequences have been reported in up to 10% of cases from prostatic secretions or semen without associated demonstrable urethral infection. However, there is no clear consistent evidence to support a causative role.

Prostatitis and HIV infection

↑ risk of prostatic abscess in those immunosuppressed with acute prostatitis.

Epididymitis, orchitis, epididymo-orchitis

Aetiology

Inflammation of the epididymis (epididymitis), the testicle (orchitis), or both (epididymo-orchitis) may be caused by spread of infection, or less commonly other agents, from:
- the urethra or bladder through the ejaculatory duct, seminal vesicle, and vas deferens
- distant sites through the lymphatic or blood vessels.

Genital infection
- *Chlamydia trachomatis* and/or *Neisseria gonorrhoeae* cause ~70% of acute epididymitis in sexually active ♂ aged <35 years and 5–30% in older ♂. Up to 30% of untreated urethral infections may lead to acute epididymitis, usually unilateral.
- Coliform enteric bacteria (acquired through insertive anal sex) in up to 65% of ♂ who have sex with ♂ (MSM) with non-gonococcal non-chlamydial epididymitis.
- *Treponema pallidum* is a rare cause of diffuse chronic interstitial inflammation of the testis in late benign syphilis which may lead to a gumma (or atrophy).

Urinary tract infection (UTI)
- Coliform bacteria (*Escherichia coli*, *Klebsiella* spp, and *Proteus* spp) and *Pseudomonas aeroginosa* cause up to 80% of acute epididymitis in ♂ aged ≥35. May be associated with an underlying urological abnormality e.g. obstruction, calculus, chronic bacterial prostatitis. Urethral instrumentation (e.g. catheterization) is a predisposing factor.
- *Mycobacterium tuberculosis* associated with renal, prostatic, or seminal vesicle infection is an uncommon cause with usually insidious, occasionally acute, onset. 75% of ♂ with renal tuberculosis have associated epididymitis, 65% of which is bilateral.

Other micro-organisms
- *Mycobacterium leprae* commonly involves the testes ± the epididymes causing atrophy.
- Mumps: epididymo-orchitis in 20% of cases in adult ♂, 16% bilateral.
- *Brucella* spp (*Br.melitensis* 5× more than *Br.abortus*) may cause orchitis in 5–18% of cases (epididymitis less evident).
- Coxsackie virus B infections may include orchitis in up to a third of cases.
- Systemic fungal and yeast infections (e.g. cryptococcosis, histoplasmosis, coccidioidomycosis, and blastomycosis) may produce orchitis.
- Filarial organisms, *Wuchereria bancrofti* and *Wuchereria pacifica*, and less commonly *Brugia malayi*. If present in inguinal lymph nodes may cause chronic allergic lymphangitis of the spermatic cord and testis. This produces chronic epididymitis and orchitis with profuse effusion within the tunica vaginalis leading to scrotal oedema and elephantiasis.
- *Streptococcus pneumoniae*, *Nocardia* spp, *Haemophilus parainfluenzae*, group B *Salmonella* spp, *Neisseria meningitidis*, *Schistosoma haematobium*, and cytomegalovirus have been reported as probable causes.

Non-infective causes

- Spermatic granuloma: extravasation of spermatozoa into adjacent tissue inducing autoimmune granulomatous epididymitis (a cellular reaction) leading to fibrosis.
- Granulomatous orchitis: idiopathic or ♂ to systemic granulomatous disorders.
- Behçet's disease: epididymo-orchitis in up to 20% of ♂.
- Amiodarone: side-effects in up to 11% of ♂. Causes lymphocytic infiltration and fibrosis, usually bilateral.
- Sarcoidosis: may rarely cause non-caseating granulomatous epididymo-orchitis.
- Idiopathic lymphocytic orchitis.

Clinical features

Acute

- Typically unilateral scrotal pain and swelling.
- Pyrexia may be present.
- If sexually acquired probable urethritis, often asymptomatic.
- Scrotal erythema.
- Tenderness and palpable swelling of the epididymis.
- Development of oedema and formation of a hydrocele may lead to a grossly enlarged scrotum.
- Haematospermia (rarely).
- In mumps orchitis the onset is usually within a week of parotid enlargement but sometimes follows resolution of parotitis.

Chronic

Symptoms are of >3 months duration. Pain is of variable intensity. Epididymial and testicular swelling is gradual and depends on the underlying cause.

Complications

- Hydrocele in ~10% (usually resolves with antibiotics).
- Abscess in up to 3% of cases.
- Infarction of the testicle in <1% (due to compression of the swollen spermatic cord at the external inguinal ring).
- Recurrence due to lack of adequate treatment, reinfection, or chronic inflammation. High recurrence rates in MSM (coliform infection).
- Chronic epididymitis follows ~15% of acute episodes.
- Infertility due to:
  - occlusion of vasa deferentia (following bilateral epididymitis)
  - impaired spermatogenesis (following bilateral orchitis).
  Possibility of infertility after unilateral epididymitis ± orchitis due to sperm agglutinins (suggested but unproven).
- Chronic prostatitis (unusual).

Investigations

Gram stain of urethral smear

May show urethritis, i.e. ≥5PMNL/HPF ± Gram-negative intracellular diplococci.

Tests for *N.gonorrhoeae* and *C.trachomatis*

Urine examination
- First-voided urine (FVU): for threads containing ≥10 PMNL/HPF (if no urethral material).
- Midstream specimen of urine (MSSU): dipstick test for leucocyte esterase, nitrites, and blood. Send to laboratory for microscopy and culture.
- Early morning urine ×3: microscopy and culture for *M.tuberculosis* if suspected.

Screening for other STIs

If sexually transmitted, epididymo-orchitis is likely.

Ultrasonography

Doppler ultrasonography (stethoscope or colour-coded duplex): useful in the differential diagnosis of acute scrotal pain and swelling. Acute epididymitis/orchitis ↑ blood flow. Radionuclide scanning may provide similar information.

Real-time ultrasonography: of great value in the differential diagnosis of scrotal swellings, particularly when malignancy or complications of acute epididymitis, requiring surgical intervention, are suspected.

Additional investigations
- Epididymal aspiration for microbiological specimens (usually during surgical exploration).
- Magnetic resonance imaging when diagnosis is unclear despite ultrasonography.
- Further urological investigations (e.g. urethrocystoscopy and excretion urogram) if an underlying urological abnormality is likely.

Diagnosis

Age, clinical features including sexual history, urethral Gram stain, and urine examination are important in establishing a diagnosis, supported by specialized investigations if indicated (Boxes 12.1 and 12.2). It is essential to exclude testicular torsion in acute presentation (requires emergency surgical intervention).

In the differential diagnosis of non-acute scrotal pain and swelling (Table 12.1) clinical assessment should attempt to identify if the lesion is within the body of the testis (malignancy more likely).

Table 12.1 Main differential diagnosis

	Testicular torsion	Epididymitis	Testicular cancer
Age range (years)	Most common 12–18 Less common 18–30	Most common 19–40 Less common <18 and >40	Peak incidence 25–35. 74% in 20–49
Pain	Sudden onset. 50% report previous short episodes of pain resolving spontaneously	Onset over 24–48 hours	Typically painless but diffuse pain or dragging sensation/ache in 730%; 5–15% present with acute pain
Urinary symptoms	90% normal urinalysis 4% ↑ frequency	Dysuria, frequency or urgency. Urethritis (smear/ FVU) or pyuria	No association
GI symptoms	~33% nausea and vomiting. 20–30% abdominal pain	Nausea and vomiting if acute orchitis develops	May be due to metastases
Pyrexia	Usually absent	May be low grade. >40°C in acute orchitis	Usually absent
Inspection and palpation	Oedema and erythema of affected side Enlarged and exquisitely tender testis, high in scrotum Transverse lie and anterior epididymis on unaffected side	Oedema and erythema of affected side. Epididymis distinguishable from tests unless very advanced or scrotum grossly enlarged	Testicle enlarged, 15% with inflammation Solid lump not separated from testis
Cremastric reflex	Absent	Present	Present
Ultrasonography	↑ blood flow	↓ blood flow	Hypo-echoic mass within the testis

Box 12.1 Causes of scrotal mass/pain

- Trauma
- Hydrocele
- Epididymo-orchitis
- Testicular torsion
- Torsion of testicular appendix (in 6–12 year old children)
- Spermatocele
- Epididymal cyst
- Varicocele
- Hernia
- Testicular tumour:
  - germ cell tumours—seminoma and malignant teratoma
  - lymphoma and other malignancies
- Epididymal and non-testicular neoplasms
- Fournier's gangrene
- Vasculitis: Henoch–Schönlein purpura and Kawasaki disease
  (<15 years), Bürger's disease (adults)

Box 12.2 Three clues to diagnosis of scrotal mass

Clinical assessment should aim to answer three important questions in
diagnosing the cause of scrotal mass.
- Is the mass intrascrotal ('get above the swelling')?Hernia extends
  above the scrotum.
- Is the mass cystic?Cystic mass (e.g. hydrocele) is usually
  transilluminable.
- Is the mass an integral part of the testis?

Solid testicular mass should be regarded as malignant until proven otherwise, and urgent investigations should be arranged.

Management

General
- Scrotal elevation/support and analgesics (non-steroidal anti-inflammatory) are recommended.
- Avoid sexual intercourse until both patient and partner are treated and follow-up is complete.

Treatment
- Empirical therapy should be commenced immediately, taking into consideration the likely cause and local antibiotic sensitivities, andaltered if necessary when laboratory results are available.

Treatment regimens
- Chlamydia/gonorrhoea (suspected/confirmed):
  - doxycycline 100mg oral twice daily for 10–14 days *plus* ceftriaxone 250mg single IM dose if gonorrhoea diagnosed or probable
  - ofloxacin 200mg oral twice daily for 14 days
- Coliform (suspected/confirmed):
  - ofloxacin 200mg oral twice daily for 14 days
  - ciprofloxacin 500mg oral twice daily for 10 days

Partner notification
If the cause is or likely to be sexually transmitted, sexual contacts should be offered screening and epidemiological treatment. If chlamydia is found in index case or aetiology is undetermined, provide anti-chlamydia treatment (as for uncomplicated infection). If gonorrhoea found/probable, add treatment for gonorrhoea (as for uncomplicated infection).

Follow-up
If no improvement after 3 days review diagnosis and management. Reassess if swelling and tenderness persist after antimicrobial therapy is completed (swelling may take several weeks to resolve).

HIV infection

- Case reports of poor response to standard treatment in HIV infection
- Unusual causes (cytomegalovirus, *M.tuberculosis*, *H.influenzae*, *Nocardia asterioides*, *Candida* spp, and *Cryptococcus neoformans*) more common

Sexually acquired reactive arthritis

Introduction

Reactive (or post-infectious) arthritis (ReA) is a seronegative sterile inflammation of the synovial membrane initiated by an external stimulant, usually an enteric or sexually transmitted infection (STI). Estimated prevalence is 30–40/100,000 adults).

When ReA is associated with both urethritis and conjunctivitis (minority of cases), it is commonly referred to as Reiter's syndrome (after Hans Reiter who described a case preceded by dysentery in 1916).

As Reiter's syndrome may be incomplete and other clinical features may be present, the term sexually acquired ReA (SARA) is commonly used when the main component, arthritis, follows an STI. The manifestations of post-enteric ReA are similar.

Aetiology

Although an infective urethritis or enteritis commonly triggers ReA its multisystem involvement and potential for relapse/remission (similar to other seronegative spondylo-arthropathies) imply an underlying reactive aetiology. However, the detection of bacterial antigen or sensitized CD4 cells in inflamed synovial material from organisms which may provoke SARA suggests a more direct relationship. Other infections and conditions may be associated with ReA (e.g. rheumatic fever) but have different clinical features. In ~25% of cases no trigger can be identified.

Sexually acquired infection

SARA typically presents in ♂ 2–4 weeks after urethritis, usually non-gonococcal (NGU). Although found in ♀ it is much less common and more likely to be unrecognized as it is associated with cervicitis, usually latent. Therefore certain organisms associated with urethritis/cervicitis are linked to SARA. Their role is unclear and SARA may arise without any demonstrable infection.

NGU (and cervicitis)
<0.8% of those with NGU develop SARA.
- *Chlamydia trachomatis*: the only urogenital pathogen consistently implicated in sporadic SARA. Chlamydia-like particles, seen by electron microscopy, and chlamydial DNA, using nucleic acid amplification tests (NAATs), have been identified from synovial fluid of some patients with SARA. Associated urogenital infection has been found by non-NAATs in 30–70% (no data using NAATs).
- *Ureaplasma urealyticum*: ↑ urogenital detection rate in some with SARA without evidence of chlamydial or enteric infection. *U.ureaplasma* DNA from synovial fluid has been reported in those with SARA (using NAAT).
- *Mycoplasma genitalium*: DNA found in synovial fluid (using NAAT).

Gonorrhoea

Neisseria gonorrhoeae has been implicated in up to 14–16% cases of SARA, distinct from its more common association with septic arthritis.

Enteric infection (frequency of ReA 1–4%)

- *Shigella* spp
- *Salmonella* spp
- *Campylobacter* spp
- *Yersinia enterocolitica* and *Yersinia pseudotuberculosis*
- *Clostridium difficile*

Other factors

Urethral or bowel trauma (e.g. catheterization, surgery). Unusual but may precipitate recurrence.

Associations

- Gender
  - SARA ~98% in ♂ (falsely high as under-diagnosed in ♀)
  - Enteric ReA ~90% in ♂.
- Age: usually young adults.
- Geography: urethritis appears to precede ReA more commonly in the UK and USA, whereas an initial dysenteric illness has been reported more frequently in studies from continental Europe.
- Human leucocyte antigen B27 (HLA-B27) positivity. However, an association has only been established with the following infections: *Chlamydia, Campylobacter, Clostridium, Salmonella, Shigella* and *Yersinia.*
- Diagnostic relevance dubious although may be associated with ↑ risk of chronicity and recurrence:
  - 30–90% of those with SARA
  - 50–80% with ReA following enteric infection.

  Controls
  - Native Americans, Lapps, northern Scandinavians: 26–50%
  - Most Europeans: 7–10%
  - Blacks: <2%.
- Genetic predisposition: May be family history of
  - SARA
  - other seronegative spondylo-arthropathy (e.g. associated with ankylosing spondylitis, inflammatory bowel disease, psoriasis)
  - iritis.

Clinical features

Usually starts within 4 weeks of 1° urogenital or enteric infection. Malaise, fever, and fatigue are common but ~10% do not have a preceding symptomatic infection.

Urogenital

Men

- Urethritis (usually NGU): discharge/dysuria in ~80% with SARA, NGU in:
  - ~70% of ♂ with post-enteric ReA
  - ~60% of cases of recurrent SARA which may be associated with a new infection or may arise spontaneously (a new infection does not necessarily trigger a recurrence).
- Chronic prostatitis in 95% of cases of SARA.

Women

- Urethritis (dysuria/discharge) uncommon (short urethra).
- Cervicitis usually asymptomatic but may be visible on examination
- Salpingo-oophoritis (rarely).

Bladder and upper urinary tract

Mild sterile (by conventional culture) cystitis found in 20% although severe haemorrhagic manifestations have been reported. Glomerulo-nephritis and IgA nephropathy rarely associated.

Musculoskeletal

- Arthritis: asymmetrical polyarthritis (>95%) predominantly affecting the lower limbs starting ~14 days after genital symptoms. Low back pain common (~50%) with sacroiliitis in 10%. Joints not involved simultaneously, but overall severity peaks ~14 days after the onset of the arthritis. Rapid muscle wasting in relation to joints involved is common.
- Enthesitis (inflammation at insertion point of ligaments, tendons, and capsules) and tenosynovitis:
  - plantar fasciitis in ~20%, may be associated with calcaneal enthesitis
  - Achilles tendonitis in 10–15%.
  Contributes to painful feet and difficulty walking. Enthesitis may also be found at insertion points around the pelvis and ribs.

Ophthalmic

- Conjunctivitis: usually bilateral. Found in 20–50% of cases of SARA. Generally mild and self-limiting. Typically develops after the appearance of symptoms from the provoking infection and the onset of arthritis.
- Iritis (acute anterior uveitis): late manifestation of an initial episode or recurrence in 2–11%. Usually unilateral, presenting as a painful eye with blurred vision and inflammation at the margins of the cornea. Associated with sacroiliitis.
- Episcleritis: keratitis and corneal ulceration have also been reported.

Dermatological (skin manifestations commonly occur together)

- Keratoderma blennorrhagica (KB): identical to pustular psoriasis and found in up to 33%, although may be greater as often asymptomatic. Most commonly found on the soles of the feet (often the only site involved), although other sites may be affected (e.g. penis, especially if circumcised, palms, toes, scalp, scrotum, and sometimes a generalized rash). The lesions, which may exhibit the Koebner phenomenon, typically appear as hard parakeratotic nodules or soft limpet-like patches, usually brown in colour and becoming pustular.
- Erythema nodosum: rarely reported with *Yersinia* infection.
- Nails: ~10% of patients develop thickening and ridging of the nails which may progress to subungual abscess formation with shedding. Pitting is not a feature.
- Genital lesions: balanitis (often asymptomatic) is found in 20–40% and is an early finding. If circumcised the psoriatic lesions are elevated, dry, and scaly (as KB). In the uncircumcised erythematous confluent patches appear circumscribed by a well-defined pale margin creating a geographical appearance and referred to as circinate balanitis. May be found in ♂ presenting with urethritis and no other clinical features. Circinate vulvitis has also been reported in ♀. Lesions usually resolve spontaneously within 4 weeks.
- Oral lesions: found in 10–16% (although under-diagnosed as asymptomatic). The palate, buccal mucosa, gingiva, and tongue may show erythematous or circinate lesions and ulceration. Patchy loss of papillae can appear over the tongue (geographical tongue).

Other manifestations

- Constitutional symptoms: malaise and fever in ~10%.
- Cardiovascular system:
  - thrombophlebitis (deep leg veins) in ~3% (symptoms may resemble a ruptured knee joint capsule, a rare complication of arthritis)
  - myocarditis—1° heart block in up to 14%
  - pericarditis—rare
  - aortitis with aortic incompetence—very rare.
- Respiratory system: pleurisy in up to 8%.
- Nervous system: <2%—meningoencephalitis, peripheral neuropathies, amyotrophic lateral sclerosis.
- Enteric: non-specific mucous enterocolitis may occasionally appear at onset of symptoms.
- Amyloidosis: very rare.

Natural history

Most initial episodes resolve within 2–6 months, although they may extend to >1 year in ~35%. 15–30% may develop progressive chronic arthritis, sacroiliitis, and dactylitis ('sausage digits'). Recurrences occur in ~50% with an annual risk of ~15%. Chronic development and recurrences more common if HLA-B27 +ve.

Without treatment urethritis and conjunctivitis usually resolve in up to 4 weeks. The dermatological manifestations also generally settle within 4 weeks, although KB may persist for 2–3 months or longer.

Iritis is liable to recur, especially if associated with sacroiliitis.

Diagnosis

▶Clinical: there is no simple diagnostic test for SARA and Reiter's syndrome. Diagnosis is made on clinical grounds, although it may be supported by the following investigations.
- Screen for STIs (including rectal gonorrhoea and chlamydial infection if indicated by the sexual history).
- Stool cultures and *Yersinia* spp serology if enteric infection suspected.
- Full blood count:
  - normochromic normocytic anaemia in severe cases
  - polymorphonuclear leucocytosis in up to 30%.
- Erythrocyte sedimentation rate/C-reactive protein: elevated in >90% with SARA. Level gives an indication of disease activity.
- Urinalysis: proteinuria, microscopic haematuria, pyuria in up to 50%.
- Radiology: early SARA—no findings. In progressive disease:
  - periostitis (tibia, fibula, hands, and feet)
  - articular erosions with joint narrowing (hands, feet, posterior aspect of calcaneous)
  - periosteal reaction at sites of tendon insertion producing 'spurs', especially calcaneum (>50% of chronic cases)
  - sacroiliitis in 50% with severe chronic disease.
- Slit-lamp examination: suspected iritis.
- Electrocardiography (variable degrees of heart block) and echocardiography if suspected cardiac involvement.
- Synovial fluid: polymorphs in acute disease followed by lymphocytes. Sterile culture and no crystals.
- Synovial biopsy: polymorph infiltrate as with other rheumatic disease.
- HLA-B27 test: debatable value. It has low diagnostic predictive value but may be of value in determining management and prognosis.
- Negative/normal findings:
  - antistreptolysin O titre
  - rheumatoid factor (although 4% positivity rate in normal population)
  - antinuclear antibody test
  - uric acid levels.

The most common differential diagnosis (Box 13.1) is gonococcal arthritis, especially if SARA presents as a monoarthritis (3–7% of cases). Culture of synovial fluid is usually negative but gonorrhoea may also trigger SARA. If in doubt treatment should be given to cover disseminated gonococcal infection which, unlike SARA, should show rapid improvement.

Box 13.1 Other causes of acute painful swollen joint(s)

Direct infection
- Acute septic arthritis (~80% due to Gram-positive aerobes)
- Tuberculosis
- Fungal infections—unusual (e.g. blastomycosis, candida species)

Direct infection and/or reactive arthritis
- Gonococcal arthritis (usually monoarthritis)
- Meningococcal arthritis
- Reaction to streptococcal infection (e.g. rheumatic fever)
- Bacterial endocarditis
- Syphilis
- Viral infections (including HIV, hepatitis B, herpes simplex virus, and parvovirus)
- Lyme disease
- Cat-scratch disease (atypical presentation)
- Brucellosis
- Leptospirosis

Others
- Trauma and foreign body reaction (also exacerbation of osteo-arthritis)
- Seronegative HLA-B27 associated spondylo-arthropathies
- Rheumatoid arthritis and other seropositive connective tissue diseases
- Still's disease (juvenile rheumatoid arthritis, seronegative)
- Erythema multiforme and Stevens–Johnson syndrome
- Reaction to drugs and vaccines
- Behçet's disease
- Gout/pseudogout
- Haemachromatosis
- Sarcoidosis
- Haemophilia and other clotting deficiencies
- Acute leukaemia

Management

General

Full information on SARA and its clinical course should be provided with advice on the avoidance of future potential triggers. Partner notification (with epidemiological treatment) may be required depending on the initial provoking infection.

▶ Liaise with or refer to the appropriate specialty for extra-genital manifestations, especially if severe.

Antibiotics

SARA

The provoking infection in acute SARA (usually NGU) should be treated as for an uncomplicated infection (📖 Chapter 9, Management p. 164). Treatment of the triggering infection does not appear to affect the course of any established skeletal, skin, or ophthalmic manifestations. Otherwise, short-term antibiotics are not advised unless the triggering infection is still active. Although long-term (3 months) treatment does not alter the course of the disease during the 1st year, there is conflicting evidence that it may have a long-term benefit in the prognosis of those HLA-B27 +ve.

Early treatment of urogenital infection may ↓ risk of relapsing arthritis in those with a history of ReA.

Enteric

Short-term antibiotics for the underlying enteric infection do not appear to alter the course of ReA or Reiter's syndrome. Any associated urethritis should be treated as above.

Prolonged treatment for 4–6 weeks may be of benefit for arthritis triggered by *Yersinia enterocolitica*.

Ophthalmic

- Conjunctivitis: usually no treatment required
- Iritis: mydriatics and topical steroids

Arthritis and enthesitis

- Rest, avoidance of weight-bearing, passive muscle exercises to limit wasting.
- Non-steroidal anti-inflammatory drugs (NSAIDs) with dosage at night to reduce morning stiffness. If at high risk of upper gastrointestinal (GI) complications (e.g. GI bleeding) consider:
  - a cyclo-oxygenase 2 (COX-2) selective NSAID
  - or the addition of gastroprotective agents (e.g. misoprostol, histamine-2 blockers and a proton pump inhibitor).

In view of possible long-term increased cardiovascular risks, treatment duration should be kept as brief as possible.

- Corticosteroids:
  - systemic prednisolone only rarely indicated if severe polyarthritis with other systemic symptoms
  - local injection at tendon insertion or into a severely swollen knee joint following aspiration may be of value.
- Options for chronic disabling arthritis (persistence for ≥3 months or erosive joint damage) include:
  - sulfasalazine
  - methotrexate
  - azathioprine
  - gold salts.
  - Tumour necrosis factor alpha (TNF-α) blocking agents are highly effective in treatment of other spondylo-arthropathies. Data are largely anecdotal and still undergoing evaluation, but the initial impression is of short-term effectiveness in ReA, although drugs may re-activate the infective trigger.

Skin

Manifestations are self-limiting and, unless unusually severe, treatment is not required. However, topical corticosteroids may be indicated for severe circinate balanitis and KB with the options of topical calcipotriol, systemic methotrexate, and retinoid for intractable cases.

Pregnancy

- Antibiotics: for sexually transmitted infections as indicated (see relevant chapter).
- NSAIDs: may produce sub-fertility in women, and if used regularly in pregnancy may produce premature closure of the fetal ductus arteriosus, oligohydramnios, and delayed onset and ↑ duration of labour.
- Corticosteroids: low risk but may cause growth restriction and fetal adrenal suppression.
- Sulfasalazine: small theoretical risk so use with caution.
- Azathioprine: appears to be safe.
- Methotrexate, gold salts, and TNF-α blockers should be avoided.

HIV infection

Rising incidence in association with HIV in sub-Saharan Africa (up to 11%) but not in Caucasian populations. Musculoskeletal features are similar to those in non-HIV patients, but cutaneous manifestations and urethritis are common and more severe. White patients are usually HLA-B27 +ve whereas non-whites are generally −ve.

Frequency of spondylo-arthropathies is unchanged with anti-retroviral treatment, although cutaneous lesions are less severe. Otherwise, management is similar to non-HIV-infected cases, with sulfasalazine beneficial in long-standing cases.

Bacterial vaginosis and anaerobic balanitis

Introduction

First described as 'non-specific vaginitis' in 1955 by Gardner and Dukes with the term 'bacterial vaginosis' (BV) formally introduced in 1984.

Characterized by bacteriological imbalance of vaginal flora with overgrowth of characteristic commensal bacteria (*Gardnerella vaginalis*, anaerobic bacteria, and mycoplasmas), replacing normally predominant *Lactobacillus* spp and producing an altered vaginal discharge. Most common cause of acute vaginitis/osis, accounting for 15–50% of cases and experienced by 10% of ♀ over a lifetime.

Aetiology

Vaginal hydrogen peroxide (H_2O_2) producing lactobacilli, ~60% of vaginal lactobacilli strains (especially *Lactobacillus crispatus* and *Lactobacillus jensenii*), appear to be protective as the prevalence of BV is only 4% compared with 32% in those with non-H_2O_2-producing organisms. A mean of 13 different bacterial phylotypes has been demonstrated by molecular analysis in ♀ with BV compared with three without BV.

Organisms

- *G.vaginalis*: facultative anaerobic small Gram-negative bacillus (often stains Gram positive). Found in high concentrations (>100× normal) in up to 95% of BV but can be isolated in up to 58% of those with normal discharge. In virginal ♀ vaginal carriage is associated with oral sex and hand-to-genital non-penetrative contact.
- Anaerobic bacteria in high concentrations:
  - *Mobiluncus* spp—sickle-shaped rods displaying vigorous motility, including corkscrew motion, in vaginal wet mounts. Cultured in 14–96% ♀ with BV (<6% without) and seen on microscopy in up to 77%. *Mobiluncus mulieris*—long, Gram negative. *Mobiluncus curtisii*—short, Gram variable but usually stain positive.
  - *Prevotella* spp (e.g. *P. bivia*).
  - *Prophyromonas* spp.
  - Peptostreptococci (e.g. *Streptococcus intermedius*).
  - *Fusobacterium* spp.
  - *Bacteroides* spp.
- Aerobic bacteria, e.g. α-haemolytic streptococci, coliforms.
- *Mycoplasma hominis*: found in 24–75% ♀ with BV (13–22% without BV).
- Recently described bacteria:
  - *Atopobium vaginae*—a metronidazole-resistant Gram-positive anaerobe. Frequently demonstrated in BV and may be responsible for metronidazole treatment failure.
  - *Leptotrichia/Sneathia*, *Eggerthella*-like bacterium, *Megasphaera* spp—three novel bacteria (BV-associated bacteria 1-3) in the order *Clostridiales*. BV diagnostic sensitivity is 99%, specificity 89% (compared with Amsel criteria) if *Megasphaera* spp or one of the *Clostridiales* bacteria is detected.

Factors

- Non-white ethnicity.
- Hormonal contraception: combined oestrogen/progesterone associated with a ↓ risk probably related to oestradiol levels but shift to anaerobic predominance aided by progesterone injection.
- Intra-uterine device (IUD): variable data but no consistent evidence of ↑ risk
- Vaginal douching: although only apparently associated with BV if flora already imbalanced
- Diet: BV has been shown to be associated with ↑ consumption of fat and severe vaginosis associated with both saturated and mono-unsaturated fat. ↑ intakes of folate, vitamin E, and calcium inversely related to the risk of severe vaginosis.
- Cigarette smoking: ↑ risk of BV possibly due to anti-oestrogenic effect.
- Sexual: not considered to be sexually transmitted although following features suggest a sexual link.
  - Lower mean age of coitarche.
  - New sex partner within previous 30 days, multiple sex partners, unprotected heterosexual intercourse with associated anal sex.
  - Associated with *Neisseria gonorrhoeae* and *Chlamydia trachomatis*.
  - BV discharge (but not *G.vaginalis* in pure culture) inoculated into healthy vagina can induce BV in recipient
  - Lesbians—2.5-fold ↑ rate compared with heterosexual ♀. Prevalence up to 25–52% with 20-fold ↑ if ♀ partner has BV. Apparent relationship with recent partner change, multiple partners, and receptive cunnilingus (receiving oral sex), but no other practices including the shared use of dildos and anal penetration with fingers.
- Against sexual transmission (heterosexual);
  - comparative study—BV found in similar proportion of virginal and sexually active adolescents (12% and 15%, respectively).
  - Although *G.vaginalis* is isolated from the urethra in up to 80% of ♂ sex partners of ♀ with BV, their concurrent treatment does not ↓ ♀ recurrence rate.

There is conflicting information regarding the circumcision status of ♂ partners.

Clinical features

- Asymptomatic: ~50%.
- Vaginal discharge: symptom in 49% (20% without BV), sign in 69% (3% without BV).
  - Volume—usually moderate (varies from scanty to profuse).
  - Colour—grey in 65–85%, white in 7–30% (remainder yellowish).
  - Nature—homogeneous vaginal discharge adhering to vaginal walls as a thin film). Frothy in 27–80% (1–18% normal ♀).
- Malodorous—fishy ammoniacal smell reported in 20–49% but probably higher as may not be volunteered because of embarrassment (reported in 20% without BV). Smell enhanced when vaginal pH ↑ (e.g. during menstruation and following contact with alkaline prostatic fluid after intercourse) releasing volatile amines.
- Irritation—a non-inflammatory process so absent in most cases.

Associations

- *N.gonorrhoeae* and *C.trachomatis*:
  - 3.8-fold risk of *N.gonorrhoeae* or *C.trachomatis* in ♀ with symptomatic BV
  - ↑ in ♀ with BV if ♂ partners have urethritis.
- Cervicitis (with risk factors distinct from gonococcal and chlamydial infections). May be related to absence of H_2O_2-producing lactobacilli.
- Non-specific urethritis (NSU) in ♂ partner.
- Trichomoniasis: bacterial overgrowth as BV but purulent discharge.
- HSV-2 infection and viral shedding.
- Cytomegalovirus infection and replication (multiple strains).

Complications

- Persistence (11–29%) and recurrence (72% by 7 months).
- Post-hysterectomy vaginal cuff cellulitis.
- Post-abortion pelvic inflammatory disease (PID).
- Possibly contributes to spontaneous PID.
- ↓ probability of successful *in vitro* fertilization.
- In pregnancy increased bacterial production of cytokines and prostaglandins and amniotic fluid/chorioamniotic infection leading to:
  - chorioamnionitis
  - low birth weight
  - preterm birth (relative risk 1.5–2.3) from preterm labour and premature rupture of membranes
  - 2nd trimester miscarriage (up to 3–6-fold risk)
  - endometritis (pre/post-delivery including Caesarean section).

History of previous premature delivery increases risk of further preterm birth 7-fold with BV.

Frequently asked questions

What is bacterial vaginosis?

It is a condition caused by the overgrowth of normal vaginal bacteria causing an imbalance and an altered vaginal discharge.

Is it sexually transmitted?

It is not thought to be sexually transmitted, and so partners of ♀ with BV are not treated. Lesbian partners of ♀ with BV also have a higher incidence of BV although the reason is not clear.

Is it like thrush?

Thrush (candidiasis) is caused by a yeast, usually *Candida albicans* (90%). Bacterial vaginosis is due to an imbalance of normal vaginal flora, with a loss or reduction in lactobacilli and an overgrowth of largely anaerobic bacteria, especially *Gardnerella vaginalis*.

Thrush usually causes a thick white vaginal discharge, itching, and soreness. BV is usually associated with a thin white/grey discharge and an offensive fishy smell.

Both thrush and BV are prone to recur.

Is it treated with anti-thrush preparations?

No. Thrush is treated with topical azoles (pessaries/creams) or oral azoles. BV is treated with metronidazole or clindamycin either topically or orally.

Can my partner catch it from me?

It is not sexually transmitted. ♂ may occasionally develop balanitis with bacteria similar to those found with BV but it does not appear to be related to intercourse with a partner who has BV. However, the increased incidence of BV in lesbian couples suggests a sexual link.

Does my partner who has no symptoms need treatment?

No. Treating an asymptomatic partner does not make any difference to recurrence rate.

Will I ever get rid of it?

Overall cure rate is 95%. Recurrence rate is about 15–30% with the majority recurring within 7 months of treatment.

Diagnosis

The sensitivity and specificity of the following diagnostic tests are shown in Table 14.1.

Gram stain

Simple, fast, and accurate way to diagnose BV. Typical appearance is substantial reduction or absence of lactobacilli (Gram-positive rods) replaced by small Gram-variable bacilli (*G.vaginalis*) adhering to shed epithelial ('clue') cells without polymorphs (Plate 7). Other small Gram-negative bacilli (e.g. *Bacteroides* spp), Gram-positive cocci (e.g. peptostreptococci), Gram-variable sickle-shaped rods (*Mobiluncus* spp) may be found. The last of these are seen more easily as motile organisms on a wet mount which may also show long thin pointed rods (fusiform bacilli).

Hay–Ison Gram-stain method

Simple qualitative method grading smears as follows:
- grade 0: epithelial cells/no bacteria
- grade I (normal): lactobacilli only
- grade II (intermediate): reduced lactobacilli/mixed bacteria—not found in BV as diagnosed by Amsel's criteria
- grade III (consistent with BV as diagnosed by Amsel's criteria)—mixed bacteria with few or absent lactobacilli
- grade IV—epithelial cells covered with Gram +ve cocci only.

Nugent Gram-stain method

Although sensitive, this method is too complex and time-consuming for routine clinical use. It is based on the quantitative scoring of *Lactobacillus*, *G.vaginalis*, and *Bacteroides* morphotypes, and *Mobiluncus* spp on a Gram-stained vaginal smear. High scores (>6) equate to BV, medium scores (4–6) intermediate, and 0–3 normal.

Amsel's criteria (regarded as 'gold standard' for research)

Three of four criteria to be fulfilled:
- characteristic discharge
- positive amine ('sniff' or 'whiff') test—drop of 10% potassium hydroxide on vaginal fluid releases 'fishy' smelling amines (avoid semen which may give false-positive result). ⚠ No longer recommended for safety reasons.
- pH >4.5 (avoiding cervical mucus (pH 7.0), blood, and seminal fluid)
- vaginal 'clue' cells on wet-mount microscopy
- detection of amines in vaginal fluid by chromatography, biochemical assays, or electronically (the 'electronic nose')—not generally available for routine clinical use.

▶Detection of *G.vaginalis* by culture cannot be used to diagnose BV as it can be isolated in >50% of normal ♀.

Table 14.1 Diagnostic methods

	Sensitivity (%)	Specificity (%)
Amsel criteria		
Atypical discharge	52–69	78–97
pH >4.5*	97	53
Amine test*	43–80	99
Clue cells	80–90	94
Nugent Gram-stain method†	86–89	83–96
Hay–Ison Gram-stain method†	94	93
Detection of amines in vaginal fluid†	79–87	76–95

*Provided that sample is not contaminated with blood or seminal fluid.

† Compared with Amsel criteria (on premise that they are most accurate method for diagnosing BV).

Frequently asked questions

Can I prevent it from coming back?

♀ who suffer from recurrent BV can be treated with episodic, anticipatory, or cyclical metronidazole or clindamycin. As BV is associated with a high vaginal pH it is advisable to try to keep it low to prevent recurrences. This can be done by decreasing menstruation, e.g. with Depo-Provera® or using acetic acid vaginal jelly. If a ♀ has an IUD and suffers from recurrent or persistent BV it may be advisable to remove the IUD and try another method of contraception.

Is it the cause of my abdominal pain?

Usually not on its own. However, BV is associated with PID especially when there is an IUD *in situ*. BV is also associated with post-abortion PID and post-hysterectomy vaginal cuff cellulitis.

Is it harmful in pregnancy?

BV is associated with an increased risk of preterm delivery. Therefore it is recommended that ♀ with a history of a preterm delivery are screened for BV during pregnancy and treated if positive. It is not recommended that all pregnant ♀ are screened for BV. However, if a pregnant ♀ is found to have BV during routine testing (e.g. for a symptomatic discharge), she should be treated. Meta-analysis has shown that metronidazole is safe in pregnancy at all trimesters, although large doses are best avoided.

Management

Variations in vaginal bacterial flora are common and BV-type features are often transient and self-limiting. Treatment is recommended for those with symptoms, those with clear signs of BV (who may report improvement after treatment), and those undergoing certain surgical procedures, but otherwise not for asymptomatic BV or *G.vaginalis* colonization.

- Metronidazole:
  - oral—400–500mg twice daily for 5–7 days (single-dose treatment not advised as failure rate of 50% has been reported)
  - intravaginal—0.75% gel 5g once daily for 5 days.
- Clindamycin:
  - oral—300mg twice daily for 7 days
  - intravaginal—2% cream 5g once daily for 7 days (can weaken condoms), 2% extended-release clindamycin cream (single application).
- tinidazole (oral)—1g daily for 5 days, 2g daily for 2 days, or 2g as a single dose.

Studies show that 7 days of oral metronidazole are as effective as 5 days of vaginal gel (symptomatic and microbiological cure rates of about 80% and 70%, respectively, at 1 month) and similar to clindamycin cream.

Alcohol produces disulfiram-like reaction with metronidazole and possibly tinidazole, and should be avoided. No data are available on intravaginal preparations but alcohol ingestion is not recommended.

Partners

No evidence of ↓ relapse rate if male partners are treated epidemiologically, but male condom may reduce the BV recurrence rate up to 5-fold. No data are available on the value of treating female partners concurrently.

Pregnancy

Caution is advised in the use of metronidazole during pregnancy and breastfeeding with high-dose regimens avoided. However, meta-analyses have shown no evidence linking birth defects to the use of metronidazole in early pregnancy. Antibiotic treatment can eradicate BV in pregnancy and it is advised for those with symptoms. Conventional screening and treatment of asymptomatic ♀ for BV occurs in the 2nd and 3rd trimester (there are insufficient data on 1st trimester interventions, which may be more effective). Based on current data there is little evidence that screening and treating all pregnant ♀ with asymptomatic BV will prevent preterm birth and its consequences, although there is some suggestion that treatment before 20 weeks' gestation may ↓ risk of preterm birth. ♀ with recurrent or persistent bacterial vaginosis may be at highest risk of associated adverse outcomes but, from studies to date, there is a lack of information about the impact of these interventions on the health of the baby. Therefore currently there is no evidence to support the introduction of screening (and treating) pregnant ♀ in the 2nd and 3rd trimester even if high risk.

Breastfeeding—as both systemic metronidazole (especially in high dosage) and clindamycin enter the breast milk, intravaginal treatment should be considered.

Termination of pregnancy (TOP)

- Based on three independent studies, screening for and treating BV with metronidazole or clindamycin cream prior to TOP is recommended to ↓ the incidence of subsequent endometritis and PID.

Persisting or recurrent BV

Eliminate possible factors that may influence the microbiological flora (e.g. douching, shampoos, spermicides, etc.). Lack of evidence but consider the following.

- Persistent:
  - change treatment (metronidazole to clindamycin or vice versa)
  - consider removing IUD if *in situ*
  - oral co-amoxiclav (amoxicillin 250mg + clavulanic acid 125mg) 375mg 3 times a day for 7 days, as possibility of resistance or metronidazole de-activation by other vaginal bacteria. May also be considered initially if metronidazole and clindamycin cannot be used.
- Recurrent: following initial treatment mildly abnormal microscopy or elevated pH may be found suggesting relapse rather than a new episode. If relevant, consider providing a contraceptive method which reduces or stops menstrual flow (e.g. progesterone-only preparation) to maintain low pH. Ten days of induction therapy with vaginal metronidazole followed by twice weekly gel for 16 weeks can establish clinical cure of 75% at 16 weeks and 50% at 28 weeks. Other strategies include episodic, anticipatory, pulse, suppressive (e.g. twice weekly for 4–6 months using metronidazole gel 0.75% or clindamycin cream), or cyclical treatment (e.g. oral metronidazole 400mg bd for 3 days at the start and end of menstruation).
- Other approaches:
  - 3% hydrogen peroxide single vaginal wash
  - probiotics—oral/vaginal lactobacillus replacement (e.g. with *L.acidophilus*, *L.rhamnosus* GR-1, *L.fermentum* RC-14) or live yoghurt (limited data but no conclusive evidence of benefit)
  - agents lowering vaginal pH (e.g. lactic or acetic acid gel)—suggested in those with normal microscopy but ↑ vaginal pH, in those with recurrent BV as maintenance treatment, or in situations which raise pH such as seminal fluid or menstrual blood in the vagina (e.g. for 3 days post-menstruation).

Anaerobic and *G.vaginalis*-associated balanitis/balanoposthitis

♂ partners of ♀ with BV are usually asymptomatic and unlikely to develop balanitis/balanoposthitis.

G.vaginalis can be found in 31% of those with a non-candidal balanoposthitis. Usually mild but may be foul smelling in association with anaerobes, especially *Bacteroides* spp (commonly *B.melaninogenicus*). Normally found in those with underlying phimosis and poor hygiene. An offensive sub-preputial discharge may occur with 2° erosions and preputial oedema. Usually resolves with advice on hygiene and the use of saline lavage, although oral metronidazole is sometimes required. Clindamycin cream 2% twice daily or oral co-amoxiclav 375mg 3× a day for 1 week may also be used.

HIV infection

- Acquisition and transmission ↑ with BV 2–5-fold.
- The acquisition of H_2O_2-producing lactobacilli significantly ↓ cervico-vaginal HIV RNA while their loss ↑ these levels compared with stable colonization.

Trichomoniasis

Introduction

Trichomonas vaginalis was first described by Donné in 1836.

Aetiology

Flagellated protozoan of the order Trichomonadida which is parasitic to the human genitourinary tract (Fig. 15.1 and Plate 8). *T.vaginalis* (TV) is usually oval and measures up to 15µm in length *in vivo* (the size of a leucocyte). It is propelled by four anterior flagella arising from an anterior kinetosomal complex. An additional 5th flagellum is attached to an undulating membrane that extends halfway down the organism and an axostyle projects from the end of the body. Trichomonads lack mitochondria but contain hydrogenosomes, large cytoplasmic granules involved in catabolism. It grows in a moist environment at 35–37°C and pH 4.9–7.5 (similar to bacterial vaginosis). Multiplication is by mitosis occurring optimally every 8–12 hours and cysts are not produced.

Trichomonads infected by double-stranded RNA viruses have been identified, and are termed type II in contrast with virus-negative organisms designated type I. In a small comparative study type II isolates were found proportionately more commonly in ♀, especially older ♀.

Epidemiology and transmission

Common worldwide but steady decline in developed countries over the past 20 years. Reason is unclear but may relate to standard cervical cytology screening which can also detect TV. Almost exclusively sexually transmitted from infected genital secretions.

The parasite can be found:
- ♀: vagina, cervix, urethra, bladder, and the ducts of Bartholin's and Skene's (per-iutheral) glands.
- ♂: anterior urethra, sub-preputial sac, glans penis, prostate, epididymis, and semen.

Sexual transmission
- Most commonly found in ♀ during the most sexually active years (16–35 years) and in those more sexually active (change in partner, intercourse twice weekly or more, ≥3 partners in past month).
- Recognized association with other STIs (e.g. gonorrhoea).
- High rate of reinfection unless ♂ partners are treated (up to 70% carry the parasite).

Detection rates in ♂ contacts of infected ♀:
  - sex within previous 48 hours—70%, previous 5 days—40%, after 14 days—33%, after 21 days—12%.
Detection rates in ♀ contacts of infected ♂: 67–100%.
♀ to ♀ sexual transmission is well recognized and may relate to the shared use of sex toys.

Non-sexual transmission

Protozoa may survive up to 45min on toilet seats and for several hours in moist clothes, although transmission is unlikely.

- Direct ♀ to ♀ transmission related to poor hygiene has been suggested but lacks evidence.
- Neonatal vulvovaginitis arising from infection acquired at delivery may arise but is rare (5% of those born to mothers with TV). Commonly asymptomatic and usually spontaneously clears in 3–6 weeks as maternal oestrogen level falls.

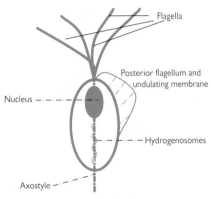

Fig. 15.1 *Trichomomas vaginalis*

Frequently asked questions

Is it always sexually transmitted?

Generally yes, although it has been suggested that transmission could occur through moist flannels which are shared.

How long has it been present?

Symptoms usually develop within a month of acquiring infection although up to 50% of ♀ are diagnosed without symptoms.

Does my boyfriend require treatment?

Yes. ♂ commonly carry *T.vaginalis* without any symptoms. Unless he is treated there is a high rate of reinfection.

Clinical features

Women

Incubation period (before symptoms develop): 4–28 days.

Symptoms
- 20–50% asymptomatic (depending on criteria)
- Vaginal discharge: 56%
- Dysuria: 18%
- Low abdominal pain (probably related to vaginitis): up to 12%
- Vulval discomfort
- Vaginal malodour: ~50%, associated with anaerobic bacterial overgrowth (similar to bacterial vaginosis)

Signs
- Altered vaginal discharge in up to 70%, frothy yellow in 10–30%, otherwise thin/thick, scanty/profuse
- Vulvovaginitis
- 'Strawberry cervix' (colpitis macularis): small punctate cervical haemorrhages with ulceration found in 2–5%
- Urethritis: ~25%
- No signs: 5–15%
- Isolated case reports of detection from fallopian tubes (in salpingitis) and peritoneal fluid.

Complications
- Independent association in pregnancy with premature rupture of the membranes, preterm delivery, and low birth weight. Although treatment of symptomatic ♀ is advocated, the risk of preterm birth is not ↓ with metronidazole treatment. One study of asymptomatic ♀ treated with metronidazole was stopped as there was an association with ↑ risk of preterm birth; hence routine screening in pregnancy is not advised.
- Association with cervical carcinoma reported but uncontrolled for other genital pathogens (e.g. human papilloma virus); therefore no proven causal relationship.

Spontaneous resolution occurs in 20–25%.

Men
- ~50% asymptomatic.
- Most common feature: small to moderate urethral discharge—non-gonococcal urethritis (NGU). Trichomonal infection may be the cause in up to 15% of cases in high-prevalence areas.
- Balanoposthitis: 4–11% (rarely with 2° ulceration).
- Prostatitis, epididymitis, cystitis alleged but probably due to other associated infection.
- Isolated case reports associated with penile ulceration and median raphe suppuration.

Diagnosis

Direct microscopy

Vaginal discharge examined as an isotonic saline suspension by dark ground or phase contrast microscopy. Readily recognizable motile protozoa propelled by flagella and undulating membrane but must be examined immediately otherwise 20% failure within 10min (Fig. 15.1 and Plate 8). ♂ urethral discharge and sub-preputial material can be examined in a similar fashion. Alternatively, dried smears can be stained with acridine orange and viewed using fluorescent microscopy. This is more sensitive than using wet preparations.

Compared with culture the overall sensitivity of microscopy in ♀ is 40–80%, but in ♂ it is only ~30% although the specificity is high.

Gram-stained vaginal smears typically show polymorphonuclear leucocytes, reduced or absent lactobacilli, and a mixed bacterial flora as seen with bacterial vaginosis. However, there is considerable variability.

Culture

As well as vaginal, urethral, and sub-preputial samples, a centrifuged deposit of first morning urine can also be tested by culture (especially useful for ♂). Ideally specimens should be placed in culture medium (e.g. Feinberg–Whittington). Otherwise forward in transport medium (e.g. Amies or Stuart) and inoculate in growth medium within 24 hours. Culture under partial or complete anaerobic conditions.

Prior to the introduction of PCR testing, the sensitivity of culture for urethral and urine samples was ~95% for ♀ and 60–80% for ♂.

Latex agglutination

Eluate prepared by agitating vaginal swab in phosphate-buffered saline. One drop of material is mixed with a drop of test latex on a black slide and rocked for 2min. Agglutination of test, but not control, latex indicates TV antigen. Sensitivity 95–98.8%, specificity 92–99% (compared with culture).

Papanicolaou-stained cervical smears

TV is sometimes reported on cervical cytology. Compared with culture, this is reasonably sensitive (60–80%) but specificity varies and may be only ~70% although liquid-based cytology has been shown to enhance specificity up to 99%. Despite this, positive cases should be confirmed by microscopy ± culture.

Polymerase chain reaction (PCR)

PCR tests are not available for routine use in the UK although they have been widely reported. Although detection of TV by culture remains the 'gold standard' its sensitivity compared with PCR is poor, ranging from 34% to 59%, although its specificity is high at ~100%. However, the specificity of PCR testing ranges from 83% to 98% so there are concerns about false-positive results.

Management

- ▶Sexual partners should be treated simultaneously and sexual intercourse avoided until treatment has been completed.
- If ♂ contacts present with NGU, it is reasonable to treat initially as TV infection and review after treatment.
- Screening for other STIs for patients and their contacts is advised.
- Treatment should be systemic in view of the high rates of urethral and periurethral gland involvement.

Treatment

Oral metronidazole: 400–500mg twice daily for 5–7 days or 2g in a single dose. The only effective agents are the 5-nitroimidazoles (overall cure rates ~95%), with metronidazole the most extensively used. If allergy reported consider metronidazole desensitization. Single dose has the advantage of ↑ adherence but has ↓ cure rate (by 6–12%), especially if partner(s) not treated simultaneously. Patients should be advised to avoid alcohol while taking treatment and for 48 hours thereafter because of a possible disulfiram-like (Antabuse®) reaction (similar reaction possible with tinidazole). ▶Vaginal metronidazole cream is not advised as cure rates only ~20% probably because of poor absorption and failure to penetrate infected Bartholin's and Skene's glands and urethra.

Although caution is advised in the use of metronidazole during pregnancy the manufacturers only warn against high-dose regimens (💷 Chapter 14, Management p. 210), which should also be avoided during breastfeeding.

Alternative 5-nitroimidazoles include tinidazole (2g orally as a single treatment). They have a longer half-life than metronidazole.

Spontaneous resolution is estimated at around 20–25%.

Treatment failure

- Non-adherence, reinfection.
- Absorption and local tissue levels: metronidazole is a small molecule which is well absorbed and does not bind to serum proteins. Conflicting data reported regarding vaginal levels following oral treatment ranging from only 50% of serum levels to ~100%.
▶Plasma levels achieved when administered rectally or vaginally are only 50% and 20%, respectively, of those of oral metronidazole (although this varies with the formulation). Body weight plays a role in drug excretion; therefore some fixed-dose regimens may be not be appropriate for all patients.
- Low plasma zinc (unusual): provide oral zinc supplement.
- 5-nitroimidazole deactivation by vaginal bacteria: no evidence to support this but theoretically aerobes and anaerobes, including β-haemolytic streptococci, could be implicated.
- Resistance (usually but not always to all 5-nitroimidazoles). 5% of all clinical strains estimated to have at least some metronidazole resistance. Generally aerobic but anaerobic resistance has also been reported. Resistance testing should be conducted in aerobic conditions but is not readily available. However, data suggest that repeated treatment failures are invariably related to resistant organisms.

Although metronidazole-resistant strains show ↓ susceptibility to oral tinidazole, the minimal lethal concentration is likely to be significantly ↓ and should be considered. There are no reliable alternatives to 5-nitroimidazoles.

Treatment options to consider in refractory cases

- Enhanced/extended oral metronidazole (effective in ~80% of these patients), e.g. 400mg 3 times daily for 7–14 days or 2g daily for 3–5 days.
- Other azoles (i.e. tinidazole): successful responses reported using 500mg 3 times daily orally for 7–10 days up to 2g twice daily for 2 weeks with or without intravaginal tinidazole. Cure rates of 92% reported in resistant TV infection.
- Although clear evidence is lacking, case studies have reported cure by providing antibiotics (either before re-treatment or concurrently) to cover bacteria which may deactivate 5-nitroimidazoles (e.g. oral amoxicillin 250mg 3 times daily, or oral erythromycin 250mg 4 times daily, both for 7–14 days).
- High-dose oral or IV metronidazole (up to 3–3.5g daily for up to 14 days.) ± amoxicillin/erythromycin for 14 days ± clotrimazole 500mg pessary daily for 14 days.
- High-dose oral metronidazole with intravaginal metronidazole 1g daily for ≥7 days, or metronidazole rectal suppository 1g daily for ≥7 days, or vaginal douches (zinc sulphate 1% or 3% acetic acid).
- Other treatments recorded in case studies but without consistent verification include:
  - 6% nonoxynol-9 pessaries (treatment for up to 7 months)
  - arsenical (acetarsol) pessaries (500mg daily for 10–14 days)
  - paromomycin sulphate pessaries (250mg once or twice daily for 14 days) or cream
  - vaginal clotrimazole (probably largely symptomatic relief)
  - povidone–iodine pessaries and douches
  - nifuratel (similar activity as metronidazole but role in resistant infection unclear)
  - hamycin (topical treatment used in India but has side effects).

Trichomoniasis and HIV infection

- HIV acquisition is associated with TV, probably related to genital inflammation
- Successful treatment of trichomonal urethritis in ♂ ↓ levels of HIV RNA

Genital candidiasis

Introduction

Also referred to as candidosis, moniliasis, or thrush. It is considered to be pathogenic activity by commensal yeasts in individuals with reduced local or systemic resistance. Association with vaginitis first described in 1849, although oral thrush was recognized in the 4th century BC.

Aetiology

Candida spp, especially *Candida albicans* responsible for 85–90% of infections and *Candida glabrata* responsible for 3–15%. Other yeasts rarely implicated include *C.tropicalis* (~4%), *C.parapsilosis* (~4%), *C.krusei* (~2%), *C.stellatoidea* and *C.gulliermondi*. Occasional cases of vaginitis reported include *Saccharomyces cerevisiae*, a yeast from the family Crypto-coccaceae (to which *Candida* also belongs) and *C.dubliniensis*.

All pathogenic *Candida* spp multiply by the production of buds from a blastospore (yeast cell), approximately 1–5.0µm in diameter.

C.albicans produces:
- hyphae—long tubes made up of multiple cell units divided by septa arising from blastospores or as branches of existing hyphae
- pseudohyphae—single elongated cells from blastospore buds with constrictions instead of septa. Each generation remains attached to its parent
- chlamydospores—large refractory bodies, with double-layered cell walls (probably a dormant phase).

The mycelium is the entire yeast aggregate (spores, hyphae, and branches).

C.glabrata does not produce hyphae or pseudohyphae.

Candida spp contain their own set of virulence factors which may contribute to their ability to cause infection. They include surface molecules that facilitate mucosal adherence, proteases when there is mucositis, and the ability to convert into a hyphal form. *C.albicans* has the greatest ability to adhere and invade the mucosa, enhanced by the production of germ tubes (also useful in species identification), where it may form a reservoir for recurrences.

Epidemiology and transmission

75% of ♀ have at least one episode of genital candidiasis with 40–50% having one or more recurrences. It is much less common for ♂ to present with symptomatic infection. However, in GUM clinics *Candida* spp colonization of the glans penis has been reported in 16% (unrelated to sexuality or the presence of a prepuce but associated with vaginal carriage in ♀ partners) with ~33% admitting to symptoms.

Candida spp can be found anywhere on the body but most commonly in the mouth (30–55% of young adults), vagina (8–32% of young ♀, 40% if pregnant), and anorectal canal (40–65%). *C.albicans* accounts for 80–90% of genital yeast isolates and 60–80% of oral carriage, although seldom recovered from normal skin (*C.parapsilosis* and *C.gulliermondi* are more prevalent).

Although penovaginal intercourse is a factor in the direct transmission of yeast infection, its role is unclear. However, it is generally accepted that, without predisposing factors, ♂ usually acquire infection sexually. In ♀ it seems that coitus is more likely to act as a trigger by introducing perineal organisms and causing microtrauma which breaches mucosal integrity. Hypothetically, vaginal intercourse following anal penetration is more likely to introduce infection, although there are no data to support this. However, there does seem to be an association with recent cunnilingus. This may be by direct transmission, with saliva promoting pathogenesis by moistening and irritating the vulval mucosa and altering the local immunity. Non-specific genital infection and other STIs have been shown to be associated with yeast infection in 39% of ♀ and 29% of ♂.

Frequently asked questions

What is thrush?
Thrush is an infection caused by a yeast, usually *Candida albicans*. *Candida* spp commonly live in small numbers in and around the genitals, especially the vagina. Asymptomatic until candida multiplies and penetrates the skin surface.

Is thrush sexually transmitted?
Usually not, especially in women. Partners do not need any treatment unless they have symptoms and signs of thrush themselves.

Predisposing factors

Reduction in local mucosal resistance
- Sexual contact causing microfissures.
- Inflammation (e.g. eczema related to contact irritants, other dermatoses, tight/non-absorbent clothing although evidence is inconclusive).

Diabetes mellitus
Produces a glucose-rich environment ideal for the growth of yeasts, especially in poorly controlled diabetes. Associated with a 20% ↑ in oral colonization by *Candida* spp

Hormonal factors
- Physiological: ↑ oestrogen raises the amount of glycogen in the vagina and ↓ cell-mediated immunity and progesterone (also immunosuppressive and stimulates germ tube formation). Therefore symptomatic candidiasis is uncommon before menarche and after the menopause. In the child-bearing years it is found most commonly:
  - in the luteal phase of the menstrual cycle
  - during pregnancy, especially the 3rd trimester (↑vaginal glycogen and immunological factors)—a large proportion of ♀ who subsequently present with recurrent vulvovaginal candidiasis (RVVC), first present with infection during pregnancy.
- Combined oral contraceptives: only associated with high-dose oestrogen (50mcg) preparations.
- Oestrogen replacement treatment: probable relative ↑.

Impaired immunity
Includes HIV, drugs (e.g. corticosteroids, chemotherapeutic agents).

Broad-spectrum antibiotics
↑ vaginal yeast carriage by 10–30%. Although there is an association with candidiasis, it is small, and the vast majority of ♀ on antibiotic treatment are unaffected.

Other contraceptives
Conflicting evidence of an association with the use of spermicides (cidal effect on lactobacilli), diaphragms, and caps (causing reinfection) and intra-uterine devices (IUDs). More likely to be carriage rather than disease.

Local factors
Lack of consistent evidence relating intimate hygiene practices or menstrual sanitation (use of external towels or pads) with genital candidiasis. Vaginal deodorants, disinfectants, and perfumed products may exacerbate candidiasis by causing dermatitis. No evidence to support reinfection by fomites such as underwear.

Clinical features

Women

Acute vulvovaginitis (90% of presentations)

Symptoms

Vulval pruritus, and burning, with external dysuria and dyspareunia being common. Usually starts or worsens from mid-menstrual cycle, often improving with menstruation.

Signs

Vulval erythema with fissuring is the most common finding. Usually localized to the vulval mucocutaneous margins but can spread to involve the labia majora, perineum, and perigenital skin where satellite lesions (small areas of erythema adjacent to but separate from the main body of inflammation), pathognomonic for candidiasis, may be seen. Vaginal erythema seen in 20% with a thick white curdy adherent discharge in 20%,↑ to 70% if pregnant, forming plaques on the vagina, cervix, and vulva. Discharge may be purulent or watery.

Recurrent vulvovaginal candidiasis

Definition

Four or more episodes of symptomatic candidiasis annually.

Frequency

Occurs in ~5% of ♀. Thought to be due to incomplete elimination of infection (usually identical strain), or inadequate treatment with a change in the protective vaginal mucosa cell-mediated host defence mechanisms leading to relapses.

Other factors

Hypersensitivity

Probably important as shown by associations with perennial allergic rhinitis and a family history of allergies. Compared with ♀ with isolated episodes, ♀ with RVVC cannot tolerate small numbers of yeast organisms.

Sex

Positive association between the monthly frequency of sexual intercourse and the incidence of RVVC. Asymptomatic penile colonization with *Candida* spp occurs 4× more commonly in partners of ♀ with candidiasis.

Clinical features

Recurrent candidiasis

Vulval pruritus with burning common, but signs (erythema, oedema, fissures, white curdy discharge) are found less commonly than in acute cases.

Chronic persistent candidiasis

Vulval lichenification and local oedema; more commonly found in older obese diabetics.

Men

In colonized ♂ most common symptom is post-coital itching or burning. Clinically presents as follows.

- Direct infection with inflammation of glans (balanitis) and/or prepuce (posthitis). More common in the uncircumcised, presenting as a glazed erythematous rash, sometimes with white papules/discharge and, if severe, fissuring, oedema, and 2° phimosis.
- Contact hypersensitivity reaction.
- Usually mild to moderate balanoposthitis within 24 hours of contact with vaginal candidiasis. Yeasts are often not detected from the penis.
- ~20% of ♂ contacts of ♀ with RVVC complain of soreness and irritation lasting for 24–48 hours starting shortly after intercourse.
- Rarely as non-gonococcal urethritis.

Chronic mucocutaneous candidiasis

Characteristically involves skinfolds, nails, skin in and around the mouth, and vulva/vagina. If present consider:

- anaemia
- auto-immune conditions, e.g.
  - Addison's disease
  - hypothyroidism
  - hypoparathyroidism
- thymomas.

▶ These conditions are not associated with simple genital candidiasis.

Diagnosis

Patient's self-assessment is not a reliable method of diagnosing candidiasis. Only pruritus and objectively gauged signs are reliable clinical indicators.

Sampling

- Women: specimens should be taken from any vaginal discharge and also the lateral vaginal walls, using a plastic loop or swab. In addition, material can be taken from inflammatory areas on the vulva or surrounding skin.
- Men: sampling for microscopy is more difficult and a variety of methods are used including dry or moistened swabs, plastic loops (which may also be moistened with normal saline), skin scrapings and a dry slide (or prepared with double-sided clear adhesive tape) pressed against the penis.

Laboratory culture

Gold standard Genital specimens are usually sent in transport medium (e.g. Amies, Feinberg–Whittington) and cultured on growth medium (e.g. Sabouraud). Culture allows speciation which may be important in the patient's management. Germ tube formation is used in the presumptive identification of *C.albicans* with an accuracy of 95–100%.

As yeasts are commensals, treatment is not required unless clinically indicated.

Direct microscopy

Pseudohyphae and/or spores (*C.glabrata* only produces spores) may be seen in vulvovaginal saline suspensions viewed as wet-mount preparations in 40–60% of women with symptomatic candidiasis. If 10–20% potassium hydroxide is used in the wet mount to lyse epithelial and blood cells, the sensitivity ↑ by ~10%. Alternatively, vulvovaginal material examined by Gram stain detects infection (Gram-positive spores/pseudohyphae) in ~65% of symptomatic cases (Plate 9).

Other investigations

- Latex agglutination test: limited value. Sensitivity ~75%, specificity ~97%.
- PCR: not routinely available. Doubts about sensitivity and specificity.
- Vaginal pH: remains normal at 4.0–4.5. pH >5 may suggest bacterial vaginosis (BV). *C.glabrata* grows at a higher pH than *C.albicans* and may be associated with BV.
- Urinalysis: for sugar to exclude diabetes (especially ♂ and ♀ with RVVC).

Recurrent vulvovaginal candidiasis

Requires clinical examination, culture with speciation as *C.glabrata* and also *C.krusei* are more resistant to azoles, and consideration of underlying disease. Penile colonization with candida occurs in ~20% of the uncircumcised partners of ♀ with RVVC, usually with identical strains.

Important to exclude pregnancy, diabetes, and other risk factors (e.g. immunodeficiency and repeated antibiotic or corticosteroid use).

Frequently asked questions

Why do I keep getting it?

Treatment of candidiasis may not eliminate it entirely from the vagina, and so remaining spores/hyphae may multiply again when the conditions are right and produce a recurrent attack of thrush. Certain situations make thrush more likely (e.g. pregnancy, diabetes, immunosuppression, corticosteroids, and antibiotics). Avoid precipitants and irritants such as bubble baths, perfumed soaps, vaginal douching, and tight-fitting synthetic underwear. About 5–10% of cases are due to *C.glabrata*, which may be resistant to azoles but should respond to nystatin pessaries.

Is there anything that I can take to prevent it from coming back?

Recurrent thrush is defined as four or more symptomatic episodes in a year. Some people seem to go through phases of recurrence, which is probably because of incomplete eradication. A longer course of topical or oral therapy may help. Women with frequent episodes can try prophylactic treatment such as a clotrimazole 500mg pessary weekly or oral fluconazole 100mg weekly for up to 6 months. Thrush is associated with recent cunnilingus. Therefore avoidance may prevent recurrence.

Does my Pill make my thrush worse?

The usual type of contraceptive pill prescribed contains low levels of oestrogen and is not related to ↑ rate of thrush.

Do I need to go on a yeast-free diet?

There is no evidence that yeast-free diets make any difference to vaginal thrush infections. Studies to eliminate *Candida* spp from the gut using long-term oral medication have shown that recurrent vaginal thrush is not prevented.

I am pregnant. Is thrush harmful to my baby?

Thrush is more common in pregnancy. Asymptomatic colonization rates are higher and symptomatic episodes are more common in pregnancy. Thrush can be treated with topical azoles in pregnancy but oral preparations are contraindicated. There is no evidence that colonization with candida in pregnancy affects pregnancy outcome.

Does yoghurt help?

Probably not, but we're not sure. Intravaginal use (by applicator or on a tampon) has been tried with varying degrees of success, although it may just sooth irritation. Daily oral ingestion of 8 ounces of active yoghurt has been shown to decrease both candidal colonization and infection, although this has not been confirmed in other studies.

Management

Acute vulvovaginitis: principles (see Box 16.1 for drugs)

Bathing in saline or sodium bicarbonate may provide symptomatic relief and if severe, analgesics (e.g. non-steroidal anti-inflammatory drugs) are beneficial.

Little difference in efficacy between the drugs available and their route of administration, although to aid compliance short-duration treatments are favoured. Therefore azole therapies are preferred with a 80–95% clinical and mycological cure rate in acute candidiasis (if non-pregnant). Cure rates for nystatin are slightly lower (70–90%). Oral treatments are contraindicated if pregnant or lactating. If severe, creams may be preferred as they are more soothing than pessaries. They may also produce more prompt relief of symptoms than oral treatment. Nystatin stains the underwear yellow. Although candidal vulvitis can be treated locally with cream, it is almost always associated with vaginal infection, which should also be treated.

Topical preparations may damage latex in condoms or diaphragms.

If the candidiasis is 2° to dermatitis or there appears to be a hypersensitivity reaction, an antimycotic–hydrocortisone combination should be considered.

Unless symptomatic, no action is required for ♂ partners.

Balanoposthitis: principles (see Box 16.1 for drugs)

Mild cases will respond to simple saline lavage. Moderate or severe inflammation usually requires antimycotic treatment, commonly prescribed as a cream although similar results are achieved with oral azoles. Consider hydrocortisone-containing topical combinations if underlying dermatitis or hypersensitivity.

♀ sexual partners should be offered screening ± epidemiological treatment.

Drug resistance

~50% of all *C.glabrata* strains have ↓ sensitivity to azoles and there are ↑ levels of resistance with *S.cerevisiae* and *C.krusei* (intrinsic resistance to fluconazole). Polyene resistance is rare.

Box 16.1 Standard antimycotics for acute genital candidiasis

Available in the UK
Azoles
Intravaginal
- Clotrimazole:
  - pessary—500mg single dose, 200mg for 3 nights, 100mg for 6 nights
  - cream—10% as a single 5g intravaginal dose
- Econazole: pessary—150mg single dose or 150mg for 3 nights
- Miconazole:
  - pessary—100mg for 14 nights (or 200mg for 7 nights)
  - ovule—1.2g single dose
  - cream—2% 5g dose (in applicator) daily for 10–14 days or twice daily for 7 days.
- Fenticonazole: pessary 200mg for 3 nights (or 600mg single dose).

External
- Clotrimazole cream: 1% and 2%—2–3 times daily
- Econazole nitrate cream: 1%—twice daily
- Ketoconazole cream: 2% once or twice daily
- Miconazole nitrate cream: 2% twice daily

Oral ▶ (avoid in pregnancy or breastfeeding)
- Fluconazole 150mg as a single dose
- Itraconazole 200mg twice daily for 1 day
- ⚠ Avoid terfenadine as there is risk of arrhythmias

Polyenes

Intravaginal nystatin has been discontinued

External
Nystatin cream: 100,000U/g 2–4 times daily.

Topical combinations with hydrocortisone
- Canesten HC®: clotrimazole 1% + hydrocortisone 1% cream
- Daktacort®: miconazole nitrate 2% + hydrocortisone 1% cream
- Econacort®: econazole nitrate 1% + hydrocortisone 1% cream
- Nystaform-HC®: nystatin 100,000U + hydrocortisone 0.5% cream

Azoles not available in the UK
- Butaconazole: 2% cream—5g daily for 3 days, intravaginal
- Terconazole:
  - 0.4% cream—5g for 7 days, intravaginal
  - 0.8% cream—5g for 3 days intravaginal
  - pessary—80mg pessary for 3 nights
- Tioconazole:
  - 6.5% ointment—5g single dose, intravaginal

Management of recurrent vulvovaginal candidiasis

Induction Topical treatment for 7–14 days or oral fluconazole 50mg daily (or 150mg every 3rd day for 3 doses). If azole resistance suspected use nystatin.

Maintenance

If a regular pattern is followed, consider maintenance treatment, usually for 6 months initially, e.g.

- fluconazole: 100mg oral weekly
- itraconazole: 400mg oral monthly
- clotrimazole: 500mg pessary weekly
- ketoconazole: 100mg daily (risk of hepatotoxicity)
- nystatin pessaries: 100,000U can also be considered in resistant cases although there are no data on regimens.

During maintenance 90% remain free from symptomatic recurrences. However, they may occur in 30–40% of ♀ after cessation.

No evidence of ↓ recurrences by:

- routinely treating asymptomatic ♂ partners; however, limited data suggest treatment benefit if ♂ are colonized (systemic route advocated because of the possibility of oral reservoir of infection)
- reducing intestinal colonization (e.g. with oral nystatin)
- zinc supplements (no evidence of association with zinc deficiency)
- special cleaning of underwear.

Other medications

To consider if persistence encountered (unlicensed preparations).

- Boric acid—600mg vaginally as a gelatin capsule once or twice daily for 10–14 days has shown promising results with mycological cure rates of around 75% for *C.glabrata*. A 300mg dose is suggested if mucositis develops. Contraindicated in pregnancy. Although maintenance has been used (twice a week or for the 5 days during menstruation), data are limited and because of potential toxicity nystatin pessaries are advocated.
- Flucytosine and/or amphotericin in cream or KY Jelly® for vaginal insertion.
- Gentian violet 1% solution—used widely in the past as a vulval and intravaginal paint but messy, may cause irritation, and associated with hepatocellular carcinoma in mice.

Other approaches

- Self-help measures: avoid products that may cause vulval irritation (e.g. vaginal deodorants, perfumed preparations) and wear loose cotton underwear. Avoid douching.
- Desensitization: studies have shown a significant reduction in the frequency of RVVC following immunotherapy with *C.albicans* extract. There are also limited data suggesting that zafirlukast, a leukotriene receptor antagonist, may be beneficial.
- Change from combined to progesterone-only contraception: limited data.

- Complementary treatment
  - Vaginal or oral lactobacilli are of no value in preventing post-antibiotic candidal vulvovaginitis.
  - Yoghurt and milk containing *Lactobacillus acidophilus*—intravaginal use (by applicator or on a tampon) has been tried with varying purported degrees of success. Daily oral ingestion of 8 ounces of yoghurt containing *L.acidophilus* has been shown to ↓ both candidal colonization and infection (not confirmed in other studies).
  - Reduce pH: acetic acid, gel, lactic acid, and vinegar washes (no clear evidence of benefit).
  - Tea tree oil on a tampon or towel (frequently causes severe allergic reactions).
  - Others, e.g. topical calendula (cream, gel, or pessary), garlic clove wrapped in gauze and inserted into the vagina overnight: lack of scientific data for benefit.

Candidiasis and HIV infection

- Carriage rates ↑: *C.albicans*—vagina (75–85%), oropharynx (90–95%)
- Although vaginitis due to *Candida* spp is more common and persistent in ♀ with HIV infection, it is clinically similar to that found in HIV-negative ♀ and can be treated with conventional therapy
- Recurrent infection is not in itself an indicator of HIV infection
- In AIDS, ↑ colonization with fluconazole resistant *Candida* spp

Tropical genital and sexually acquired infections

Chancroid

Aetiology: *Haemophilus ducreyi*

Small Gram-negative coccobacillus occurring in chains. Culture requires blood-enriched medium incubated in an atmosphere of 5–10% carbon dioxide. Most clinical isolates are β-lactamase producers.

Epidemiology and transmission

Highest incidence found in tropical and subtropical countries (especially Africa, Southwest Asia, South America, Caribbean) with occasional outbreaks in temperate climates. In endemic areas genital ulcer disease (GUD) attributable to *H.ducreyi* decreasing and being replaced by herpes simplex virus 2 (HSV-2). Co-infections of *H.ducreyi* with *Treponema pallidum* and HSV infection found in over 10% in African studies.

Sexually transmitted (including oral sex) but also auto-inoculated, especially locally by fingers. Infection rate following single exposure from ♂ to ♀, ~60%. Carriage of *H.ducreyi* without symptoms or signs has been reported in prostitutes, who may be an important infection reservoir. No evidence of congenital or perinatal transmission.

Associated with: the prepuce (uncircumcised twice as susceptible), prostitution, crack cocaine use (in USA), HIV infection (GUD enhances the transmission of HIV).

Clinical features

- Incubation period 3–7 days (range 1–14 days).
- Initial tender red papule which progresses to a pustule forming 1–3 tender ulcers after 2–3 days. Multiple ulcers are common, facilitated by auto-inoculation—'kissing' lesions (Plate 10). Usually 1–2cm in diameter, irregular margins, bleeding on touch, non-indurated (soft chancre or sore). May coalesce into giant ulcers. Main features:
  - ♂—prepuce (may cause phimosis), coronal sulcus, frenum, anus (♂ who have sex with ♂ (MSM))
  - ♀: vulva, vagina, perianal area, rarely cervix
  - extragenital: very unusual (fingers, breasts, conjunctivae)
  - inguinal lymphadenopathy: usually unilateral occurring in ~50% as a tender swelling which may develop into a unilocular abscess (bubo) in 25%.
- Disseminated infection not reported.

Complications

Bacterial superinfection with tissue destruction (phagedenic chancroid); chronic suppurative inguinal sinuses.

Diagnosis

Microscopy
Sensitivity 50–62%, specificity 99% (compared with culture). Smear from cleaned ulcer or bubo by rolling the swab through 180° on the slide and stain with Gram stain. Typically small Gram-positive rods running in parallel and forming chains; 'shoals of fish' seen (unreliable due to bacterial contamination).

Culture
Standard diagnostic tool from ulcer swabs with 60–80% positivity rates in those clinically considered to have chancroid. Pus aspirated from intact bubo has much lower yield.

Polymerase chain reaction (PCR)
Most sensitive technique—95% sensitive compared with culture (due to presence of polymerase inhibitors) but culture only 75% sensitive compared with PCR. Multiplex PCR test has been developed to detect *H.ducreyi*, *T.pallidum*, and HSV simultaneously.

Serology
Available, but only useful for epidemiological studies, not direct patient management.

Management
- Oral ciprofloxacin 500mg as a single dose or 500mg twice daily for 3 days (no effect against treponemes; therefore will not mask developing syphilis).
- Oral azithromycin 1g single dose.
- IM ceftriaxone 250mg single dose.
- Oral erythromycin 500mg 4 times a day for 7 days.

Fluctuant buboes should be aspirated (by needle) under antibiotic cover.

Partner notification
Sexual contacts within 10 days of disease onset should be examined and given epidemiological treatment as for a clinical case.

Lymphogranuloma venereum (LGV)

Aetiology: L1, L2, L3 serovars of *Chlamydia trachomatis*
Primitive obligatory intracellular bacterium (📖 Chapter 8, Aetiology p. 148).

Epidemiology and transmission

Classical areas: Africa, India, Caribbean, Central America, Southeast Asia. However, since 2003 outbreaks and epidemics in the UK, Western Europe and America in MSM. New cases peaked in the UK in 2005 but are maintained at an endemic level (UK has highest rates in Europe).

Traditionally sexually acquired in tropical and subtropical areas. Highest rates in 20–30 year age group and associated with prostitution, multiple sexual partners, other STIs, and social deprivation. Congenital infection does not occur but perinatal infection may be acquired from birth canal.

Western European/American cases almost entirely MSM with high levels of co-infection with HIV (up to 80%) and other STIs, although heterosexual and female cases have been reported. Cases caused by the L2 serovar. Most infections have been acquired following local sexual contact, and factors implicated include ♂ meeting ♂ partners at sex-on-premises venues or sex parties, Internet dating, unprotected anal sex, fisting, and use of enemas and sex toys. Mode of transmission unclear in view of the overwhelming predominance of rectal infection. Recent data indicate that new index cases report significantly fewer sexual partners, suggesting that LGV may be moving into MSM eith lower risk status. In the UK, this is currently being monitored by the Health Protection Agency as an enhanced surveillance programme.

Clinical features

1° *LGV*

Incubation period: 3–30 days. Small papule at site of infection progressing to pustule and asymptomatic ulcer that heals without scarring. 1° lesion reported by only 20–50% of ♂ with 2° LGV. Sites involved include coronal sulcus, prepuce, glans, scrotum, vulva, vagina, cervix (cervicitis). Rarely causes urethritis in ♂. Oral lesions after oral sex have been reported.

2° *LGV (inguinal syndrome)*

Usually 1–6 weeks (up to 6 months) after 1° infection. In ♂ usual presentation is unilateral lymphadenopathy (~70%). Only 20–30% of ♀ with LGV develop inguinal lymphadenopathy as lesions from the posterior vulva, anus, and vagina drain to the perirectal or pelvic nodes. Femoral nodes may also be involved (20%) and the 'groove sign' (enlargement of nodes above and below the inguinal ligament) is found in 15–33%. Lymphadenopathy progressing to multilocular abscesses (buboes), which may rupture producing sinuses, occurs in ~33%. Otherwise, they involute forming firm inguinal masses. Associated constitutional features include fever, arthritis, aseptic meningitis, hepatitis, perihepatitis, pneumonia, erythema multiforme, and erythema nodosum.

3° *LGV (anorectal syndrome)*

Usually seen in ♀ and MSM because of direct infection following anal intercourse or possibly lymphatic spread from the initial infection site (e.g.

posterior urethra). Proctocolitis and lymphorrhoids (hyperplasia of peri-rectal lymphatic tissue) produce anal discharge with bleeding, rectal pain, tenesmus, fever, and malaise. Chronic infection leads to perirectal fistulae, abscesses, strictures, and scarring. Destructive sclerosing lymphangitis, and oedema of external genitalia (esthiomène—Greek: 'eaten away') may occur with penile and scrotal oedema causing distortion which may produce the 'saxophone penis'.

W.Europe/American MSM LGV

Asymptomatic infection uncommon. Most cases present with symptomatic proctocolitis (especially discharge, pain and bleeding), with about 25% having systemic symptoms. Rectal discharge almost twice as likely compared to ♂ with non-LGV chlamydial rectal infection and correlates well with many pus cells. Lymphadenopathy is rare. ~2% are inguinal-genital cases and the rare condition, bubonulus (lymphangitis of the dorsal penis with a large, tender lymphangial nodule) has been reported as a 1° manifestation following the use of a 'cock ring'. Oral ulcers have also been reported.

Complications

Genital lymphoedema (elephantiasis), suppurative fistulae and sinuses, rectal strictures leading to intestinal obstruction, rectal carcinoma.

Diagnosis

Obtain samples containing cellular material from ulcer base exudate, rectal swabs, aspirated pus from lymph nodes or buboes in saline and urethral swab/first catch urine if LGV-associated inguinal adenopathy suspected. Test using:

- Quadriplex reverse-transcriptase real-time PCR assay—best available as detects individual LGV or non-LGV infection and mixed infections. Highly sensitive and specific.
- Other PCR tests LGV-specific DNA (currently provided by the Health Protection Agency in the UK, with serotyping/enhanced surveillance).
- Cell culture: sensitivity ~80% from ulcer, ~30% bubo pus. Not appropriate for urine testing.

Serology: less value and limited availability. Three techniques are used: complement fixation test (LGVCFT), single L-type immunofluorescence test, and micro-immunofluorescence, the most accurate. A 4-fold antibody ↑ during the suspected illness is diagnostic, and single titres of ≥1:64 with clinical features considered diagnostic as only invasive infection would achieve these levels. In addition, ↑ IgA antibodies to *C.trachomatis*, especially in older MSM, correlates with early LGV proctitis

Management

- Oral doxycycline 100mg twice daily for 3 weeks
- Erythromycin 500mg 4 times a day for 3 weeks
- Repeat needle aspiration of buboes may be required

As buboes are multilocular, surgical incision of fluctuant glands is contra-indicated. Surgery may be required for late manifestations.

Partner notification Sexual contacts within 30 days of disease onset should be assessed and fully treated if infected or offered epidemiological treatment with azithromycin 1g orally as a single dose or doxycycline 100mg twice daily for 7 days.

Granuloma inguinale (Donovanosis)

Aetiology: *Klebsiella (Calymmatobacterium) granulomatosis*
Human parasite (no animal model). Gram-negative pleomorphic bacterium
with a well-defined capsule 1–1.5µm long and 0.6µm wide.

Epidemiology and transmission

Main areas: Western New Guinea, South Africa, Caribbean, Southern
India, Brazil, Southeast Asia, aboriginal Australia.

Infection routes are unclear. Sexual transmission, especially anal
intercourse, most likely but accidental inoculation from skin contact and
faecal contamination possible. Mother to child transmission at birth.

In support of STI origin
- Most commonly affects sexually active adults aged <30 years
- Genital infection usual (including cervix as sole site, anus with
  receptive intercourse)
- Associated with concurrent STIs, including HIV

Against STI origin
- Occurs in young children (allegedly from sitting on lap of infected
  adult) and the sexually inactive
- Relatively uncommon in sex workers
- Rare in partners of those with open lesions
- An outbreak linked to a healthcare professional

Clinical features

- Incubation period: uncertain (1–360 days), probably ~50 days.
- Predilection for moist mucocutaneous and mucous surfaces with
  external genital involvement in 90%, cervix in 10%, inguinal area
  (including mons pubis) in 10%, extragenital (usually anal and oral)
  in 6%.
- Starts as a firm pruritic papule or nodule (diameter 5–20mm)
  which ulcerates. Typically granulomatous, beefy red, painless, and
  haemorrhagic (Plate 11). May become necrotic and locally destructive.
  Less commonly hypertrophic verrucous lesions, resembling warts and
  dry ulcers, followed by scarring.
- Lesions gradually spread locally with destruction of genital tissue and a
  relapsing course. Mean duration ~18 months.
- No regional lymphadenopathy (unless there is 2° bacterial infection).
  Haematogenous spread to bone, liver, and spleen rare.

Complications

Include lymphatic genital oedema (elephantiasis) in 15–20%, stenosis (anus, urethra, vagina), and local skin malignancy.

Diagnosis

- Surface debris smear (air-dried and fixed in 95% ethanol) or biopsy from lesion stained with Giemsa stain. Donovan bodies (bipolar, resembling 'closed safety-pins') within mononuclear leucocytes.
- Other methods reported include cell culture (following antibiotic pre-treatment to remove contaminants) and PCR (not readily available in the UK but has been developed and used in Australia).

Management

- Oral azithromycin 1g weekly for 4–6 weeks or 500mg daily for 7 days.
- Oral co-trimoxazole 960mg twice daily, doxycycline 100mg twice daily, ciprofloxacin 750mg twice daily (all minimum of 3 weeks or until lesions healed).

Pregnancy Oral erythromycin 500mg 4 times daily (minimum 3 weeks or until lesions healed) and Caesarean section if active cervical lesions (which may complicate delivery).

Partner notification Sexual contacts within 40 days of disease onset should be assessed and offered treatment as for a clinical case.

Other genital infections

Other non-sexually transmitted infections (mostly tropical) which may affect the genitalia

- Schistosomiasis (*Schistosoma haematobium*): from swimming in fresh-water lakes in Africa (e.g. Lake Malawi). Usual urinary symptoms include dysuria and haematuria. Other features:
  - urethritis, lumpy semen, haematospermia
  - friable polyps and ulcers of cervix, vagina, and vulva;groin/scrotal cutanea tarda.
- Bancroftian filariasis (E. Africa): spermatic cord inflammation (funiculitis), hydrocele, scrotal and vulval elephantiasis.
- Onchocerciasis (tropical Africa, Central and South America): itchy papules and nodules around genitalia similar to scabies.
- Guinea worm infestation (dracunculiasis)—remote parts of Africa, especially Sudan: presents as a blister from which the worm's head protrudes. Usually affects lower limbs but may involve the scrotum.
- Amoebiasis (*Entamoeba histolytica*), especially Africa, Asia, Central and South America: peri-anal, cervical, and penile ulceration especially in MSM.
- Leishmaniasis (Middle East, Indian subcontinent): genital ulceration and annular perigenital skin lesions.
- Cutaneous larva migrans (*Ancyclostoma caninum*, dog hookworm), tropical and subtropical countries: usually acquired from bare skin contact (e.g. nude sunbathing) with infected tropical beaches. Pruritic erythematous papules or tracts moving several millimetres a day may be seen affecting the glutei and genitalia.
- Myiasis (Central and South America). Infestation by the larvae of certain fly species, e.g. *Dermatobia hominis* (botfly): may rarely affect healthy external genital tissue, especially the scrotum. Presents as a nodular inflammatory lesion.

Endemic treponematoses

Introduction

Important differential diagnosis of reactive syphilis serology in those coming from countries where such infections are found. Currently available tests cannot distinguish them from venereal syphilis. Identification of scars from old healed lesions may aid diagnosis. However, if there is doubt about the possibility of underlying syphilis or active non-venereal treponematosis, the patient should be fully treated for syphilis.

There are close similarities to syphilis: initial lesions, 2° development, latency, and asymptomatic infection. However, transmission is by close non-sexual body contact. Found more commonly in remote areas with limited healthcare and associated with poor hygiene. Worldwide prevalence ↓ by 95% between 1950 and 1970 with global control programmes, but dismantling of these resulted in re-emergence. Renewed efforts in several countries in the 1980s, failed but some regional programmes in South and Southeast Asia since 1995 have ↓ local prevalence.

Yaws (framboesia, pian, buba)

- Causative organism: *Treponema pertenue*.
- Areas found: warm humid tropical areas of Africa, South America, the Caribbean, Southeast Asia, and some Pacific islands.
- Transmission: direct contact with infectious lesions, especially in children. Spread by flies (*Hippelates pallipes*) has been suggested. Not vertically transmitted.
- Clinical features:
  - 1°—proliferative papilloma, often ulcerating, at site of infection after an incubation period of 10–45 days or longer. Usually heals after 3–6 months with a scar. Found most commonly on legs.
  - 2°—rashes and mucosal lesions similar to 2° syphilis. First crop may appear before 1° lesion has healed but take 1–2 years to develop. Plantar lesions (hyperkeratotic, macular) may be combined with a papilloma. These are very tender, leading to a crab-like gait. Relapses common in first 5 years, but skin lesions heal without scarring. Painful (especially at night) osteoperiostitis with development of sabre tibia.
  - Late—gummatous skin lesions, hyperkeratosis, juxta-articular nodules, and nasal and palatal collapse from underlying tissue destruction (gangosa). No cardiovascular and neurological sequelae.

Pinta

- Causative organism: *Treponema carateum*.
- Areas found: warm semi-arid areas of central and northern South America.
- Transmission: direct skin contact, especially in children. No vertical transmission.
- Clinical features (only involves the skin):
  - 1°—initial papule that may form a plaque, especially affecting limbs, with local lymphadenopathy.
  - 2°—widespread coloured skin rashes and papules with generalized lymphadenopathy, sometimes persisting for years.
  - Late: patchy altered skin pigmentation (hyperpigmentation and leukoderma) with pruritus and skin atrophy. No neurological or cardiovascular involvement.

Endemic syphilis (bejel, dichuchwa)

- Causative organism: *Treponema endemicum*.
- Areas found: hot dry countries (e.g. Arabian peninsula and Saharan/sub-Saharan Africa).
- Transmission: skin contact, the use of shared eating and drinking utensils, especially in children. No vertical transmission.
- Clinical features:
  - 1°: rarely seen (mucous patches in mouth most common site).
  - 2°: mucocutaneous papules around mouth and genitalia, condylomata lata (may persist for years), painful osteoperiostitis.
  - Late: nasal and palate collapse because of underlying bone and cartilage destruction (gangosa), skin gummata, periostitis. No neurological or cardiovascular involvement.

Management of endemic treponematoses

IM benzathine benzylpenicillin 1.2g (or 600mg if <10 years old) as a single dose is curative although scars may remain. Alternatives include tetracyclines and erythromycin. Contacts should be treated similarly.

Proctocolitis and enteric sexually acquired infections

Introduction

Related to penetrative anorectal intercourse and analingus. Unusual, although when found in ♀ most arise in ♂ who have sex with ♂ (MSM). Information based on 2007 European Guideline (International Union against Sexually Transmissible Pathogens/World Health Organization).

Sexually transmitted causes and clinical features

Symptoms

Proctitis (rectal inflammation—Neisseria gonorrhoeae, Chlamydia trachomatis (D-K and LGV genotypes), Treponema pallidum, herpes simplex virus)

- Acute:
    - mucopurulent anal discharge
    - anorectal bleeding
    - constipation
    - feeling of rectal fullness or incomplete defecation
    - tenesmus
- Mild/chronic:
    - mucus streaking of stool
    - constipation
    - feeling of incomplete defecation (sometimes)

Acute proctocolitis (rectal and colonic inflammation)—Shigella spp, Campylobacter spp, Salmonella spp, Entamoeba histolytica, Cryptosporidium spp, cytomegalovirus

- Small-volume diarrhoea
- Lower abdominal pain
- Abdominal tenderness
- Anorectal bleeding
- Feeling of incomplete defecation

Enteritis (inflammation of the small intestine—Giardia duodenalis, Cryptosporidium spp

- Large-volume watery diarrhoea
- Mid-abdominal cramps
- Nausea ± vomiting
- Malaise
- Weight loss

Pruritus ani (anal irritation): Enterobius vermicularis

- Anal itching, especially at night

Signs
- Distal proctitis (i.e. distal 12–15cm of the rectum):
  - mucopus in rectal lumen
  - loss of normal vascular pattern (although may not be evident in distal 10cm of normal rectum)
  - mucosal oedema
  - contact bleeding
  - ulceration (sometimes)
  - inflammatory mass (sometimes, e.g. with syphilis and LGV)
- Proctocolitis:
  - as for distal proctitis but changes beyond rectosigmoid junction
- Enteritis:
  - normal rectal mucosa unless concurrent infection with organisms causing proctitis

No infection demonstrable

- Acute anorectal symptoms related to peno-anal intercourse or the insertion of a fist, forearm, or foreign body. May lead to:
  - prolapsed haemorrhoids
  - fissures, ulcers, tears, and rectal perforation
  - retained foreign bodies.
- Chronic symptoms (non-specific proctitis): possibly related to recurrent trauma associated with rectal coitus and associated with an 8-fold ↑ in HIV infection.

Infections usually sexually transmitted

- *Neisseria gonorrhoeae* (📖 Chapter 7, Clinical features p. 136)
- *Chlamydia trachomatis* (📖 Chapter 8, Clinical features p. 150)
- *Treponema pallidum* (📖 Chapter 6, Clinical features: early syphilis p. 116)
- Herpes simplex virus (📖 Chapter 21, Clinical features p. 264)
- Tropical STIs: chancroid, LGV (current epidemics and endemic outbreaks in MSM in Western Europe and America), and granuloma inguinale (📖 Chapter 17)
- HIV infection (📖 Chapter 40, Enteric diseases and Anal diseases p. 464).

▶Consider empirical treatment for *N.gonorrhoeae* and *C.trachomatis* if suspected clinically.

Infections not usually sexually transmitted

Bacteria

Bacillary dysentery: Shigella spp (usually S.sonnei and S.flexneri)

- Usual spread: hand to mouth, fomites, water, and food. Outbreaks reported in MSM.
- Incubation period 2–7 days. Apyrexial; frequent loose stools usually resolving in a week. Occasionally chronic proctocolitis develops. Reactive arthritis may complicate. Prepubertal ♀ may develop vaginitis, especially with S.flexneri.
- Diagnosed by stool culture.
- Treated conservatively with bed rest, fluid replacement, and anti-motility drugs if necessary. Unless severe or patient has AIDS, antibiotics should be avoided to ↓ risk of resistance. If required, drug choice informed by local antimicrobial resistance pattern.

Typhoid. Salmonella enterica serotype Typhi

- Usual spread: food or water contaminated with faecal material but clusters reported amongst MSM, considered to have been spread sexually. Non-Typhi serotypes have not been recognized as sexually transmitted despite their importance as a cause of bloodstream infection in those with HIV infection.
- Diagnosed by stool culture.
- Conservative treatment unless severe; then antibiotics depending on antimicrobial sensitivity.

Campylobacter infection: Campylobacter spp (usually C.jejuni)

- Usual spread: contaminated water, food, and milk. In MSM sporadic case reports and higher rates in those with proctocolitis (compared with asymptomatic controls).
- Incubation period up to 10 days. Sudden diarrhoea with abdominal pain, malaise, pyrexia, muscle and joint pains. Usually resolves in 10 days. Reactive arthritis rarely complicates.
- Diagnosed by stool culture and serology.
- No treatment unless severe; then oral erythromycin 500mg 4 times daily or ciprofloxacin 250mg twice daily, both for 7 days.

Helicobacter pylori infection

☛ It has been suggested that *H.pylori* may be transmitted by the ingestion of infected vomit and regurgitated food during sexual contact, although there is no firm evidence.

Virus

Cytomegalovirus

Only in severely immunocompromised patients in the context of HIV infection with CD4 counts <100/mm^3.

Protozoa

Cryptosporidiosis: Cryptosporidium spp (usually C.parvum)

- Usual spread: oral–faecal (in poor social conditions), by water or animal contact. Symptomatic disease more commonly associated with HIV infection, where outbreaks occur. Sporadic cases in immunocompetent MSM, associated with multiple contacts (especially at sex-on-premises venues) and anal sex.
- Offensive watery diarrhoea with abdominal pain, low-grade pyrexia, anorexia, and vomiting, which spontaneously resolve in 1–3 weeks.
- Diagnosed by:
  - detecting oocysts in faecal samples
  - jejunal, colonic, rectal biopsies showing various stages of the organism within enterocytes
  - cryptosporidial antigen detection using enzyme immuno-assay or direct immunofluorescence tests.
- No specific treatment, but anti-motility drugs as required.

Giardiasis: Giardia duodenalis

- Usual spread: water or food contaminated with faecal material. Sexual transmission recognized, especially in MSM but no ↑ risk with HIV infection.
- Incubation period 12–19 days. Sudden onset of foul-smelling diarrhoea, abdominal pain, and distension. Stools float due to steatorrhoea with malabsorption contributing to weight loss. Symptoms resolve in 3 months.
- Diagnosed by:
  - Microscopy of fluid stool samples for trophozoites and cysts or solid samples for cysts—repeated examinations (at least 3) are often required
  - Jejunal biopsy if clinical suspicion and negative stools.
  - Antigen detection tests (available and more sensitive than single-specimen microscopy but at least 2 samples should be submitted).
- Treatment: oral metronidazole 2g daily for 3 days, or 400mg 3 times daily for 5 days or tinidazole 2g orally as a single dose. Review: three negative stool samples taken not less than 24 hours apart.

Amoebiasis: Entamoeba histolytica

- Usual spread: from faecally contaminated water and food (infecting about 10% of the world's population). The non-pathogenic strain, reclassified as *Entamoeba dispar*, is commonly found in faeces of MSM.
- ~90% are asymptomatic. Symptoms include bloody diarrhoea, abdominal discomfort, weight loss, and fever with colitis in ~20%. Invasive disease includes hepatic abscess and granulating ulceration around the anus and genitalia but is rare in MSM.

- Diagnosed by:
  - detecting trophozoites on diarrhoeal stool samples, rectal exudate, or scrapings from rectal ulcers by microscopy as *E.histolytica* if trophozoites contain red blood cells and *E.histolytica* or *E.dispar* if no red blood cells
  - detecting cysts in diarrhoeal or formed stools by microscopy, differentiating between *E.histolytica* and the non-pathogenic *E.dispar* by PCR
  - serology (for invasive disease).
- Treatment:
  - oral metronidazole 800mg 3 times a day or tinidazole 2g daily, both for 5-8 days (for trophozoites)
  - simultaneous oral diloxanide furoate 500mg 3 times a day for 10 days (to eliminate all bowel infection).
  - hepatic abscesses may require aspiration if large.
- Review: negative stool samples post-treatment and at monthly intervals for 3 months.

Nematodes

Threadworms: Enterobius vermicularis

- Usual spread: by food or fomites contaminated by ova (especially in children). Associated with analingus in MSM.
- Rarely causes vaginal infection in prepubertal girls. Cause pruritus ani (or vulvovaginitis in young girls).
- Diagnosed by seeing the adult worm in the anal canal or detecting ova from the perianal skin by microscopy using material collected on transparent adhesive tape.
- Treatment: oral mebendazole single 100mg dose, or oral piperazine single 4g dose repeated in 14 days. Neither treatment is advised in pregnancy.

Strongyloides stercoralis infection

Reports of detection in faeces of MSM STI clinic attenders (probably sexually transmitted).

Urinary tract infection

Aetiology

Considerable geographical variation in cause but predominant organism is *Escherichia coli* in ~67% (range 32–86%) of confirmed infections.
Other community-acquired organisms include:
- *Staphylococcus saprophyticus*—10% overall and 15–30% of sexually active young ♀
- *Klebsiella* and *Enterobacter* spp
- *Proteus mirabilis*
- enterococci.

Bacterial factors

Some strains develop uropathogenic properties including adhesins (e.g. type 1 pili adhesive organelles), serum resistance, and cytotoxins (e.g. haemolysins). These are important in overcoming host resistance in uncomplicated urinary tract infections (UTIs), and uropathogenic bacteria have been shown to remain in the bladder epithelium for weeks.

Resistance patterns vary geographically but up to 50% of all isolates are resistant to amoxicillin and 10–25% are resistant to cefalexin and trimethoprim, although the latter is favoured as 1st line treatment in view of its high level in vaginal and peri-urethral fluids. Lower levels of resistance are found with nitrofurantoin (10–15%) and low levels (<5%) with fluoroquinolones and co-amoxiclav. Before prescribing, check local sensitivity patterns.

Women

Common, with up to 15% of women affected each year and 25% of those who have been infected experiencing a recurrence.

Host factors for those with recurrent UTIs

- Maternal history of UTI.
- Use of spermicides alone (by a factor of 2–3) irrespective of concomitant use with diaphragms or condoms.
- Shorter distance between urethra and anus (but on average only 0.2cm shorter than controls).
- New sexual partner during the past year.
- UTI before the age of 15 years.
- Sexual activity (coitus >4 times a month). Relative odds of acute cystitis increase by a factor of 60 during the 48 hours following intercourse.
- Non-secretors of blood group antigens and oestrogen deficiency (peri- and post-menopausal ♀).
- Diabetes mellitus.
- Pregnancy (pyelonephritis most common at end of 2nd trimester).

There is no consistent evidence that the following factors are implicated:
- voiding habits (e.g. pre- and post-coital micturition)
- lifetime number of sexual partners
- sexually transmitted infections
- personal hygiene (e.g. wiping back to front, tampon use, douching, use of panty liners as intended, type of underwear)
- bacterial vaginosis.

Clinical features

Cystitis
Dysuria, ↑ frequency and urgency of micturition, strangury (slow painful micturition) and suprapubic/low back pain, haematuria, change in urine smell.

Acute pyelonephritis
Fever, rigors, malaise, loin pain, and vomiting—onset typically rapid, with urinary symptoms.

Dysuria alone
May indicate urethritis (e.g. caused by *Chlamydia trachomatis*, *Neisseria gonorrhoeae*, herpes simplex virus) or vulvovaginitis (e.g. caused by *Candida* spp, *Trichomonas vaginalis*, vulval dermatitis, or atrophy).

Other conditions
- Urethral syndrome: cystitis symptoms but no underlying infection on urine culture (occurs in ~25%). May be caused by *C.trachomatis*, low count bacterial urinary pathogens, vulvovaginal inflammation/atrophy, previous urogenital trauma (e.g. following obstetric procedures).
- Interstitial cystitis: ↑ frequency, urgency, suprapubic pain without a diagnosable cause. Bladder histology shows chronic inflammation, commonly with mast cell infiltration which may progress to bladder contracture.

Men

UTIs uncommon in ♂ <50 years old but ↑ thereafter as a result of incomplete bladder emptying 2° to prostatism or catheterization.

In younger ♂, possible underlying urological abnormality but uncomplicated infection (usually cystitis) probably related to uropathogenic strains of *Escherichia coli*. May present as an acute urethritis (purulent urethral discharge and dysuria).

- Risk factors include:
  - calculi and other foreign bodies
  - non-circumcision (enhanced colonization of the glans and subpreputial sac by *E.coli*)
  - bacterial prostatitis, prostatic calcification
  - reflux nephropathy.
- Others that have been suggested include:
  - anal sex and urethral exposure to coliforms
  - sexual partner with vagina colonized by uropathogens.

Diagnosis

- Clinical features and urine appearance: urine is often cloudy but this may be produced by amorphous phosphate crystals which clear on acidification (addition of 5% acetic acid to an aliquot of the specimen). Persisting turbidity has 66.4% specificity and 90.4% sensitivity for predicting symptomatic bacteriuria. Small numbers of bacteria and white cells will not alter turbidity. A fishy-smelling urine is highly suggestive of infection but is unusual.
- Urine dipstick testing (essentially to exclude infection—combined negative tests for leucocytes and nitrites have a 92% negative predictive value):
  - leucocyte esterase (enzyme from neutrophil granules)—72–97% sensitivity and may be more accurate than microscopy as enzyme activity is retained after white cells have disintegrated.
  - nitrate reductase (enzyme reducing nitrate to nitrite)—present in coliforms but not other bacteria (e.g. *Staph.saprophyticus* and enterococci). Sensitivity 35–85% (high specificity). When combined with leucocyte esterase, sensitivity ↑ to 70–100% with only small ↓ in specificity.
  - protein—poor indicator of infection with high rate of false positives and negatives
  - haemoglobin—poor specificity and ascorbic acid may produce false negatives.

- Lab culture (midstream sample of urine): reliability of single +ve urine culture is only 80%. Traditionally >10^5CFU/mL (or less with ≥10–20WBC/mm^3) required. UTI can be diagnosed with a count between 10^2 and 10^5CFU/mL provided that a single organism is isolated and there is pyuria (20% of those diagnosed with UTI). Counts as low as 10^2CFU/mL are relevant in symptomatic ♀ when *Enterobacteriaceae* are isolated and 10^3 CFU/mL is considered as the lower limit of significance in symptomatic ♂ (see Box 20.1).
- Check β human chorionic gonadotrophin if pregnancy risk.

Box 20.1 Pyuria with no or low bacterial counts

Consider the following:
- Prior antibiotics
- Incorrect sampling (disinfectant contamination)
- Urine acidification or alkalinization
- Bacterial infection not growing on standard medium (e.g. *C.trachomatis, N.gonorrhoeae, Mycobacterium tuberculosis*)
- Genital tract infection/inflammation (including prostatitis)
- Renal tract neoplasia
- Foreign body (also important to consider in recurrent UTI):
  - indigenous—calculi, penetration from GI tract into bladder (chicken/fish bones, swallowed needles and pins)
  - iatrogenic
    - –catheterization
    - –objects inserted into the lower urinary tract for sexual stimula tion (more commonly ♂), e.g. needles, screws, wire, pencils, pens, ink cartridges, snails, ants, dog penis, decapitated snake, grasses, wood, and rarely into the bladder via the vagina, e.g. cucumber, hairpin, wooden shoe tree.
  - Invasive—the parasitic catfish *Vandellia cirrhosa* (found in the River Amazon) penetrates the urethra of bathers, especially if they urinate in the water (urinophilic organism), and clings to the urethral wall by spines from the gills and jaw.

Management

- Push fluids.
- Antibiotics (see Box 20.2): trimethoprim 200mg twice daily, cefalexin 500mg twice daily, amoxicillin 250–500mg 3 times daily (or two 3g doses 12 hours apart), co-amoxiclav 250mg 3 times daily, nitrofurantoin 50mg 4 times daily, ofloxacin 200–400mg daily (avoid ofloxacin in pregnancy and trimethoprim for the 1st trimester).
  - ♀: a 3 day course of antibiotics is similar to 5–10 days for the symptomatic relief of uncomplicated UTI, although it is less effective in achieving bacteriological clearance. Despite the higher rate of adverse effects, 5–10 days treatment should be considered for bacteriological eradication and in complicated infection (e.g. acute pyelonephritis). Although trimethoprim is commonly advocated as 1st line treatment this should be reviewed depending on the sensitivities of the organisms most commonly isolated.
  - ♂: 7–14 days antibiotics recommended, preferably lipid-soluble low-protein bound antibiotics covering prostatic involvement, e.g. fluoroquinolones and trimethoprim.
- Urological investigations in ♀ and young ♂ following isolated episode responding to antibiotics are usually unrewarding.

Recurrent UTIs

Prevention

If ≥3 episodes a year:
- self-administered standard treatment (at symptom onset)
- prophylactic low-dose antibiotic for 6–12 months (e.g. cefalexin 125mg, trimethoprim 100mg, nitrofurantoin 50mg) daily or thrice weekly; however, no evidence of benefit after completion
- post-coital (e.g. single-dose trimethoprim 200mg, nitrofurantoin, or a quinolone) if related to intercourse.

Cranberry juice

Cranberry proanthocyanidins have been shown to reduce the adherence of *E.coli* to cultured bladder epithelial cells and vaginal epithelial cells. Drinking 200–750mL cranberry juice a day reduces the risk of recurrent symptomatic UTIs in ♀ by 10–20% but there is no clear benefit for ♂, older ♀, and children, and no evidence of a therapeutic effect for those with established infection. High-strength cranberry capsules or tablets may be more convenient than juice.

Urology referral

Ultrasound, radiology, cystoscopy especially in ♂ or complications (e.g. acute pyelonephritis, persistent haematuria).

Box 20.2 Antibiotic caution if renal impairment

Urinary tract infection

- *Trimethoprim*: half normal dose after 3 days if creatinine clearance 15–30mL/min; half normal dose if creatinine clearance <15mL/min
- *Amoxicillin*: care with high doses (risk of crystalluria) and reduce dosage if severe renal failure
- *Co-amoxiclav*: care with high doses (risk of crystalluria) and reduce dose if creatinine clearance <30mL/min
- *Nitrofurantoin*: avoid as urine concentration inadequate
- *Cefalexin*: 3g (maximum) daily if creatinine clearance 40–50mL/min; 1.5g (maximum) daily if creatinine clearance 10–40mL/min; 750mg (maximum) daily if creatinine clearance <10mL/min
- *Ofloxacin*: mild, usual initial dose and then half normal dose; moderate, usual initial dose and then 100mg every 24 hours

Antibiotics for other conditions commonly used in GUM

- *Azithromycin*: caution with severe renal impairment
- *Erythromycin*: if severe, limit dosage to 1.5g daily (ototoxicity)
- *Tetracyclines*: avoid except for doxycycline or minocycline which may be used cautiously (avoiding excessive doses)
- *Cefixime*: if moderate, ↓ dose

Anogenital herpes

Introduction

'Herpes' is named from ancient Greek 'to creep or crawl' with the typical spreading skin lesions described by Hippocrates.

Aetiology

Herpes simplex virus (HSV) types 1 and 2 is a neurotropic virus, about 200nm in diameter, with a central DNA core covered by an icosahedral capsid and enveloped in a lipid membrane derived from the host cell. There are two viral types: HSV-1 (usually transmitted by contact with infected orolabial mucosa) and HSV-2 (usually transmitted by contact with infected genital mucosa sexually or at delivery). HSV is readily inactivated at room temperature and by drying; therefore fomite and aerosol spread are unusual. Previous oral HSV-1 infection protects against genital HSV-1 but not HSV-2 disease, although it reduces severity of first-episode genital herpes and makes asymptomatic seroconversion more likely.

Terminology

- 1° infection: first exposure to any type of HSV.
- Initial infection: first infection by one HSV type. Either 1° (~50%) or non-1° if there has been exposure to other viral type (which may be detected serologically). Generally less severe symptoms if non-1°.
- Latency: dormant HSV in sensory (dorsal root) ganglia of nerves serving affected sites—sacral ganglia (S2–S5) for anogenital herpes (AGH).
- Reactivation: process unclear but precipitating factors include local nerve stimulation (e.g. by trauma, ultraviolet light) and immunosuppression by other infections such as HIV, drugs and malignancy. Persistent stress implicated but association with menstruation unclear.
- Recurrence: occurs when latent virus is reactivated, causing a peripheral lesion to appear.
- Asymptomatic viral shedding: reactivated HSV at nerve periphery without visible lesions. Viral shedding more common with HSV-2 (18–55%) than with HSV-1 (10–29%). Occurs most commonly in first 6 months after infection (during a mean 6% of days) diminishing thereafter and falling by at least 66% after 10 years. Oral HSV-2 shedding is infrequent and usually asymptomatic.

Epidemiology and transmission

HSV-1 antibodies (usually indicating oral infection) ↑ with age up to ~80%, (more common in low socio-economic groups). ↑ prevalence rate at adolescence suggests transmission by sexual contact. HSV-2 antibodies (usually indicating anogenital infection) appear at puberty and correlate with sexual activity, with a lifetime seroprevalence rate of 10–80%, greater in ♀.

Only 5–20% of those with HSV-2 antibodies recollect previous symptoms. Over the past 20 years there has been a disproportionate ↑ in HSV-1 as a cause of initial AGH especially in young ♀, now with up to 80% affected, but lower rates are found (35–45%) in ♂. HSV-2 sexual transmission rate between discordant couples is about 15–20% per year (↑ from ♀ to ♂). Transmission follows direct skin contact rather than from genital fluids. In ♀ hormonal contraceptive use, bacterial vaginosis and high-density vaginal group B streptococcal infection have been reported as risk factors for genital HSV-2 shedding. Male circumcision may provide a weak protective effect against HSV-2 infection.

Frequently asked questions

How have I caught it if my partner does not have symptoms?

It is possible to be infected with HSV without knowing. Two out of three people who contract the virus catch it from someone who is asymptomatic. People who experience recurrent symptoms may also occasionally shed the virus asymptomatically, as may those who have never had symptoms. It is also commonly acquired from the lips through oral sex.

Can I catch herpes from a toilet seat?

HSV can only survive for a short time away from the body. The virus may live for a short time on a wet towel and theoretically can be passed on this way. It is not thought possible to catch herpes from a toilet seat.

How often will I get an attack?

Some people have no further episodes after their primary attack, a few get frequent recurrences (i.e. >6 episodes per year). If the infection is due to HSV-2, 90% have a recurrence within the first year with the frequency of attacks related to the severity of the initial infection. Frequency of attacks tends to decrease in the second and subsequent years. If the infection is due to HSV-1, 60% will have a recurrence within the first year, with recurrences unusual beyond the first year.

What brings on an attack?

A recurrence occurs when latent virus is reactivated, causing a peripheral lesion to appear. It is not clear why, but precipitating factors have been recognized. Local nerve stimulation (e.g. local trauma or UV light); immunosuppression (e.g. HIV, drugs, or malignancies); and persistent stress have been implicated. The association with menstruation is unclear.

Will all the attacks be this painful?

The first symptomatic attack of herpes is usually the worst. Subsequent attacks tend to be shorter and less painful. Patients are advised to use painkillers, e.g. codeine phosphate and/or salt baths. Urinating into a bath may be more comfortable, particularly for ♀ with painful sores around the urethral orifice.

Clinical features

Initial infection

~70% of new infections acquired from asymptomatic viral shedders. 25% of those presenting with a first clinical HSV-2 episode have HSV-2 antibodies, indicating previous asymptomatic acquisition (pre-existing genital herpes). Over 60% of newly acquired HSV-2 infections are asymptomatic (↑ in ♂). In those with symptoms, 13% have atypical clinical features.

Incubation period is variable but typically 3–14 days. Clinical features and course of HSV-1, HSV-2, and AGH are similar, although severity of symptoms (systemic and local) and complications ↑ in ♀.

Constitutional symptoms occur within firstst week in over 50% (fever, headache, malaise, and myalgia). Non-1° infections are less likely to have constitutional or severe symptoms.

Local symptoms include pain, irritation, regional tender lymphadenopathy, and discharge—vaginal and urethral (~33% of ♂ with 1° HSV-2). Typically, vesicles appear over a local area of erythema and may become pustular before breaking down to form multiple tender ulcers with local oedema being common (Plate 12). Persist for 4–15 days before being followed by crusting (if keratinized skin) and re-epithelialization. New lesions (crops) during episode occur in 75%, usually within first 10 days. Mean resolution time without treatment 17–20 days (but may take up to 6 weeks) and viral shedding time about 12 days.

Problems with micturition, including urine retention, more common in ♀ than in ♂. Cervicitis occurs in 70–90% (with HSV-2). ♂ may develop 2° phimosis.

Anal infection, usually related to anal sexual contact, if symptomatic presents with pain, irritation, discharge, tenesmus, and sacral autonomic dysfunction. External peri-anal lesions only seen in ~50%.

Extra-anogenital lesions occur around groin, buttocks, lips, fingers (whitlow), and eyes (keratoconjunctivitis), and by infecting eczematous skin (eczema herpeticum).

Complications

- Associated HSV pharyngitis (both HSV-1 and HSV-2). Occurs in ~10% with HSV-2 AGH.
- 2° bacterial and yeast infection.
- Adhesions (especially labial in ♀).
- Aseptic meningitis (symptoms/signs of meningeal involvement found in 36% ♀ and 13% ♂ with 1° HSV-2 AGH).
- Sacral radiculopathy: urine retention, constipation, sacral anaesthesia (in ~1% with HSV-2 AGH).
- Disseminated infection: very rare but more common in the immunosuppressed and pregnant.
- Psychological, including denial, anger, anxiety, loneliness, fear, poor self-image.
- HSV-2 infection associated with occurrence of bacterial vaginosis

Recurrent infection

Following initial AGH:

- HSV-2—90% of patients (↑ in ♂) have recurrences in first year (median recurrence rate 0.33/month). Frequency of recurrences related to severity of initial infection. Significant reduction in second year and thereafter (though marked individual variability).
- HSV-1—60% recur clinically in first year (median recurrence rate 0.11/month). Recurrences are unusual beyond the first year.
- factors increasing risk of symptomatic recurrences include severe initial episode, infection with HSV-2 within 3 months of initial episode, and immunodeficiency (e.g. HIV infection).

Signs and symptoms are confined to affected anogenital site. Prodrome (local skin tingling, sciatic nerve pain) occurs up to 48 hours before appearance of lesions in ~50%. Although symptomatic recurrences are more common in ♂, severity ↑ in ♀. Lesions similar to initial infection but area of skin involvement one-tenth and re-epithelialization occurs in 6–10 days with viral shedding about 4 days. Cervical infection only found in 15–30% of ♀.

Main complication is psychological, especially if recurrences are frequent, and include: shame, frustration, depression, and withdrawal from social and sexual interaction.

Rarely erythema multiforme.

Recurrent rectal/peri-rectal herpes in men more likely to be HSV-1.

Atypical AGH

Very common, especially when recurrent. May present as non-specific erythema, erosions, fissures, and even frenal tear.

Causes of anogenital ulceration

- Trauma
- Sexually transmitted infections:
  - anogenital herpes
  - 1° or 2° syphilis
  - chancroid
  - lymphogranuloma venereum
  - granuloma inguinale
- Herpes zoster
- Aphthosis
- Behçet's disease
- Drugs—fixed drug eruptions; nicorandil—anal ulceration
- Erythema multiforme
- Pyoderma gangrenosum
- Inflammatory bowel disease
- Cicatricial pemphigoid
- Lichen planus
- Lichen sclerosis
- Basal cell carcinoma
- Squamous cell carcinoma
- Melanoma

Diagnosis

- Clinical presentation: important for early initiation of treatment. However, sensitivity 40%, specificity 99%, and false-positive rate 20%.
- Viral cell culture: swabs from lesions including vesicle fluid (best source—sensitivity up to 90%, falling to 70% for ulcers and 25% for crusted lesions). 1° lesions twice as likely to yield positive cultures than recurrences. Standard transport medium should be retained at 4°C but systems not requiring refrigeration are commercially available.
- Real time polymerase chain reaction (PCR): preferred diagnostic method. Performed in a closed system (limiting risk of contamination), does not require post-amplification manipulation. Swabs from lesions including vesicle fluid. Most sensitive method (detects 3–5 times more cases than culture), rapid, and highly specific. ↑ cost of consumables compared with culture; offset by ↓ labour costs per sample.
- Immunofluorescent antigen detection: smears from lesions. Quick result but ↓ sensitivity.
- Antibodies: usually appear within 2–3 weeks of infection.
  - Non-specific serology—complement fixation test (CFT), IgM—not type-specific. Paired samples needed for CFT (antibody response may take 6 weeks). Limited value but may be of use in late presentations when material from lesions is not available. In initial AGH positive predictive value of IgM is 100% but sensitivity is only ~48% because of narrow window of positivity (9–21 days after infection).
  - Type-specific serology (Western blot)—response may take 8–12 weeks to develop. Not widely available. Care with interpretation as HSV-1 and 2 are not site specific and there is extensive cross reactivity between the two antibodies. HSV-2 serology has sensitivity and specificity of 91-99% and 92-98%, respectively, which limits value in low prevalence populations.
- Cervical cytology (multinucleate giant cells) - sensitivity ~60% compared to culture.

Management: discussion and support

For many patients diagnosis of AGH infection and implications of recurrence can provoke severe emotions often fuelled by misinformation. Although chronic psychological morbidity may have an adverse effect, acute anxiety situations and everyday stresses do not ↑ recurrences. Time spent discussing AGH and its implications is important in its management. Points to consider include accurate information on natural course of infection, recurrences (prodromes and their recognition); management and implications of current episode and possible future recurrences, the avoidance of sexual contact until a week after the lesions disappear, and in future recurrences from the onset of the prodrome (to cover the period of highest risk of viral shedding), relevance of infection to current and potential future relationships, balanced consideration of potential to transmit infection both with and without symptoms (understood by the patient and clearly documented), safe sex issues and condom information, and issues relating to pregnancy.

Information received initially may not be retained, so an information leaflet containing key points should be supplied. Useful website: Herpes Viruses Association (🖱 www.herpes.org.uk).

Frequently asked questions

Do I need to treat each attack?

Usually only the initial episode of genital herpes is treated with an antiviral preparation, as treatment of subsequent attacks has little influence on the symptoms and their duration. Therefore generally only symptomatic treatment is advised for recurrent attacks, e.g. saline baths and simple painkillers. If someone is experiencing symptomatic attacks >6 times a year they can consider suppressive treatment (e.g. aciclovir 200mg 4 times daily for 6–12 months).

How do I tell a new partner that I have herpes?

There is a small risk of passing on the infection between symptomatic episodes by asymptomatic shedding, so informing a new partner about having herpes is a difficulty to face up to. Some people find it easier to wait until a relationship has developed and strengthened before disclosing this sensitive information while at the same time being careful to practice safer sex.

Will I give it to a new partner?

The sexual transmission rate between discordant couples is about 10–15% a year. The risk of transmission is reduced by avoiding sex when active lesions are present, but asymptomatic shedding may occur with the subsequent risk of transmission.

Should my partner be seen?

Unless your partner has any symptoms there is little point. However, if your partner wants to discuss the implications of the infection in your relationship, an appointment may be useful. It is also important if there are concerns about other STIs.

Is herpes dangerous in pregnancy?

A 1° attack of herpes in pregnancy may be serious. In the last 6 weeks of pregnancy it is associated with ↑ risk of neonatal herpes infection. The woman should be treated with aciclovir and delivered by Caesarean section. If a ♀ has never had herpes but her partner has, they should use condoms during intercourse throughout the pregnancy. The ♂ partner can be offered suppressive treatment during the duration of the pregnancy to ↓ the risk of a 1° attack of herpes in the ♀ during her pregnancy. Recurrent attacks of herpes in pregnancy should be treated as though the ♀ were not pregnant. There is now evidence that Caesarean section is not necessary for a non-1° attack of herpes in pregnancy, even if the attack is in the last 6 weeks of pregnancy.

Management: treatment

Initial AGH

- Saline lavage (if severe dysuria, suggest urinating within bath water).
- Analgesia:
  - oral, e.g. codeine phosphate 30–60mg 4–6 hourly as required
  - topical, e.g. 5% lidocaine (lignocaine) ointment, with caution in view of local hypersensitivity risk.
- Rarely, hospital admission may be required for urinary retention (for suprapubic catheterization), meningitis, or other severe constitutional symptoms.
- Antiviral management:
  - start within 5 days of onset or while new lesions are appearing
  - always use systemic treatment (usually oral)
  - 5 days treatment adequate unless new lesions are still appearing
  - duration of symptoms reduced by 50% and viral shedding by ~60%
  - antiviral treatment does not seem to influence recurrence rate.
- Antiviral drugs (all 5-day courses):
  - aciclovir 200mg 5 times a day or 400mg 3 times daily
  - famciclovir 250mg 3 times daily
  - valaciclovir 500mg twice daily.

Recurrent AGH

Typically mild and self-limiting. Unless unusually severe, antiviral treatment is of limited benefit in reducing duration and viral shedding. General advice and support are often adequate.

Regular recurrences

Episodic treatment

May be considered for infrequent but regular recurrences. Should be commenced as early as possible, ideally at prodrome to reduce duration by a median of 1–2 days. Therefore patient-initiated treatment should be arranged by providing medication in anticipation of next episode to commence before signs appear. This approach may have a placebo effect as it gives reassurance that medication is available. Treatment regimens are same as for initial herpes except that famciclovir is reduced to 125mg twice daily. Short treatments have also shown to be effective, i.e. aciclovir 800mg 3 times daily for 2 days, famciclovir 1g twice daily for 1 day, valaciclovir 500mg twice daily for 3 days.

Suppressive treatment

Usually considered for >6 recurrences a year. Provide continuous treatment for 6–12 months and then discontinue for reassessment. If recurrences resume at a high level, further suppressive treatment may be required. >90% have a significant reduction in recurrences (mean recurrence rates of 12.8/year pretreatment falling to 1.8 during treatment). ~20% experience a reduction in frequency of recurrences after completion. Daily suppressive treatment with valaciclovir has been shown to reduce HSV-2 transmission among HSV-2 discordant couples by 75% for clinical disease and reduced acquisition (measured by serology) by 48%.

- Aciclovir 200mg 4 times daily or 400mg twice daily.
- Famciclovir 250mg twice daily.
- Valaciclovir 500mg daily.

Aciclovir resistance

Rarely found in immunocompetent patients but reported in ~6% of those with immunosuppression, including HIV infection. Resistant strains can be treated with foscarnet and cidofovir.

Herbal treatment

Extract from the plant *Echinacea purpura* has been advocated in treatment of genital herpes, but a double-blind trial in recurrent AGH showed no significant benefit when compared with placebo.

Transmission prevention

- Condoms: laboratory experiments indicate that latex is impervious to HSV-2. Data on effectiveness is conflicting, with only some evidence of partial prevention from infected ♂ to their ♀ sex partners. Studies of HSV-2 serodiscordant couples or those with ≥4 sex partners support condom use, but other studies of sex workers, their clients, and male heterosexual attenders at GUM clinics recorded no evidence of protection. One studied reported that female condoms are as effective as male condoms in preventing genital ulcer disease.
- Antiviral drugs: all ↓ asymptomatic shedding by 80–90% with small studies showing ↑ suppression with aciclovir (400mg twice daily) and valaciclovir (1g daily) compared with famciclovir. In serodiscordant couples suppressive valaciclovir has been shown to ↓ risk of acquiring symptomatic infection by 75%, although ~60 people require treatment to prevent one transmission.
- Circumcision: circumcised ♂ found to have a 25% ↓ risk of HSV-2 infection and wives of circumcised ♂ have ↓ risk of genital ulcer disease (generally herpes).

Pregnancy and neonatal infection

Clinical aspects

- *Epidemiology* Incidence of new HSV-1 or HSV-2 infection during pregnancy ~2%, relatively evenly distributed by trimester. About 10% ♀ HSV-2 seronegative have seropositive partners.
- *Woman* Clinical course of AGH in pregnancy similar to non-pregnant, with most new infections asymptomatic, except disseminated infection (visceral) more common with recurrences more frequent and severe. If ♀ have recurrent AGH, ~75% can expect one recurrence during pregnancy with ~14% having prodromal symptoms or clinical recurrence at delivery.
- *Pregnancy* Symptomatic 1° HSV-2 genital infection associated with ↑ in spontaneous abortion (1st trimester), preterm labour, and low birth weight (3rd trimester). Complications do not usually arise from recurrent herpes. Although the propensity for HSV-1 reactivation is substantially less, when it does occur during delivery it is much more likely to be transmitted to the neonate (relative risk ~60)
- *Neonate* Incidence of neonatal infection: in UK 1.65/100,000 live births annually from 1986–91; USA estimated average incidence is 1/15,000 with ~30–50% due to HSV-1. 80% of infected infants born to mothers with no history of AGH. Maternal neutralizing antibodies protect neonate so the highest risk of transmitting HSV is when acquisition occurs at or near labour. Risk of neonatal herpes with 1° AGH at term delivered vaginally from five studies is 41% falling to ~20% for initial HSV-2 infection with previous HSV-1 infection. Rate of neonatal transmission with maternal recurrent herpes is estimated at <1%. Transmission rate for ♀ with recurrent AGH and no visible lesions at delivery estimated to be 2/10,000. In 85% of cases neonatal infection occurs at delivery, 10% postpartum (from family or carers, e.g. *metzitzah*, the sucking of the circumcision wound to promote healing following religious circumcision) and only 5% antepartum.
- *Clinical features and natural course (without treatment)* Signs usually start towards end of the 1st week of life (up to 3 weeks) and infections classified as:
  - superficial (45%)—skin (vesicular) lesions (often protracted), conjunctivitis, and gingivo-stomatitis—low mortality
  - CNS disease (30%)—4% mortality
  - disseminated (25%)—multi-organ especially CNS, liver, lung, and superficial sites—mortality 30%.

Overall mortality has substantially ↓ in past 20 years but still ~20% of survivors have long-term neurological sequelae.

Diagnosis

- Pregnancy: as above. No value in taking serial swabs in late pregnancy from ♀ with recurrent herpes to detect viral shedding.
- Infant: if infection is suspected, or for babies born to ♀ with initial genital herpes test for HSV—urine, stool, oropharyngeal, and conjunctival swabs, skin vesicle fluid.

Management

Consult local guidelines (which may vary) ♠.

Prevention

Avoid intercourse during partner's recurrences. Advise about risk of acquiring HSV-1 through cunnilingus. Routine HSV screening of pregnant ♀ and routine antepartum HSV swabs in those with a history of AGH are not recommended. Consider type-specific serology if:

- ♂ partner has herpes and ♀ has no history (suppressive antiviral treatment is an option if pregnant partner is discordant)
- first episode in pregnancy, especially in final trimester
- suggestive clinical features and negative PCR or culture
- HIV seropositivity.
  Invasive procedures in labour should be avoided or minimized for ♀ with recurrent AGH.

Treatment

Aciclovir is well tolerated and has been shown to be safe in pregnancy (from Pregnancy Registry data up to 1999), but its use is not currently licensed. Therefore, although it is widely prescribed, this must be discussed with the patient and documented. Oral aciclovir should be pre-scribed as indicated for initial episodes and IV aciclovir for severe genital or disseminated infection with case reports demonstrating significantly improved survival. It is rarely indicated for the treatment of recurrences during pregnancy.

A systematic review of suppressive aciclovir prescribed in pregnancy (after 36 weeks of gestation) demonstrated a 75% ↓ in recurrences at delivery and a 40% ↓ in Caesarean section rate for recurrent AGH. Viral detection at delivery was reduced by 90% (although shedding was not completely eliminated), and there were no cases of neonatal infection. For ♀ with recurrent AGH, USA guidelines recommend offering suppressive treatment at or beyond 36 weeks and UK guidelines recommend discussing this with ♀ who opt for a Caesarean section if active lesions at delivery (although careful consideration is required with concomitant HIV infection). In addition, suppressive treatment may be considered for those with first-episode genital herpes in 1st and 2nd trimester (to ↓ risk of clinical recurrence at term), for those with HIV infection, and to male partners if pregnant ♀ is serodiscordant.

There are no documented adverse fetal effects because of medication exposure. There are insufficient data for the use of valaciclovir and famciclovir in pregnancy.

Caesarean section

Routinely advised for all ♀ with initial genital herpes at term and for those acquiring initial infection after 34 weeks gestation but not indicated for 1st and 2nd trimester acquisition. If vaginal delivery is unavoidable, the mother and baby should be treated with aciclovir. The use of Caesarean section for a recurrence at term is contentious, with UK guidelines recommending that the mode of delivery should be discussed with the ♀ and individual-ized based on the clinical circumstances and her preferences. However, in a large study of ♀ with recurrence at delivery neonatal herpes occurred in 1.2% infants delivered by Caesarean section compared with 7.7% delivered vaginally. Therefore US guidance recommends Caesarean section for those with prodromal symptoms or active lesions at delivery.

Caesarean section not advised for ♀ with history of AGH but no active genital lesions at delivery.

Infant with HSV infection
IV aciclovir 10mg/kg body weight 8 hourly for 10 days.

Herpes and HIV

- Strong association between HSV-2 and HIV infection, increasing transmission of both, with prevalent HSV-2 infection associated with a 3-fold risk of HIV acquisition among both ♂ and ♀ in the general population.
- Atypical lesions if immunosuppressed, e.g. extensive persistent ulceration, herpes vegetans (proliferative, verrucous), hyperkeratotic lesions.
- Viral shedding ↑ with low CD4 counts.
- Enhanced antiviral treatment is recommended, especially if immunodeficient.
  - *Initial:*
    —aciclovir 400mg 5 times daily for 7–10 days
    —valaciclovir 1g twice daily for 10 days
    —famciclovir 250–750mg twice daily for 10 days.
  - *Episodic:*
    —aciclovir 400mg 3 times daily for 5–10 days
    —famciclovir 500mg twice daily for 5–10 days
    —valaciclovir 1g twice daily for 5–10 days
  - *Suppressive*
    —aciclovir 400–800mg 2 or 3 times daily
    —famciclovir 500mg twice daily
    —valaciclovir 500mg twice daily
- In pregnancy ♀ are at increased risk of more frequent and severe AGH recurrences with increased replication of both viruses. Therefore genital reactivation of HSV may increase the risk of perinatal transmission of both HIV and HSV so serious consideration should be given to suppressive aciclovir.
- Aciclovir resistance (>1–3mg/L for inhibition). Found in 5-7% isolates from AGH lesions of those with HIV infection, usually due to thymidine kinase deficiency. Partially resistant strains may respond to high-dose IV antiviral treatment but fully aciclovir-resistant strains are also resistant to valaciclovir and ganciclovir, and most are resistant to famciclovir. Alternative treatments demonstrating benefit:
  - foscarnet—1% cream; 40mg/kg body weight IV every 8 hours until resolution
  - cidofovir—1% gel; 5mg/kg body weight IV weekly infusion with oral probenecid until resolution.

Anogenital warts

Introduction

References to anogenital warts date back to Roman and Hellenic periods, with Celsus observing, in the 1st century AD, that anal warts resulted from sexual intercourse.

Aetiology

Human papilloma virus (HPV) is a genus in the family of papilloma viruses with a double-stranded DNA structure. The virion is 55nm in diameter. The capsid (envelope) comprising 72 capsomeres has an icosahedral symmetry. Hybrid capture II and polymerase chain reaction (PCR) are highly sensitive in detecting HPV.

HPV is classified by the nucleotide sequence of the major capsid gene L1 into >100 types which are identified by a number and are usually site specific (Table 22.1). Types frequently detected in anogenital squamous cell carcinoma are described as oncogenic ('high risk') and the remainder as non-oncogenic ('low risk'). The 'low-risk' types HPV6 and HPV11 account for ~90% of anogenital warts; 'high-risk' HPV is found in >95% of cervical squamous cell carcinoma (HPV16 in 50%, HPV18 in 20%).

Infection begins in the basal stem cells of the epithelium. Active viral replication occurs in the well-differentiated layers near the surface with sudden amplification of virus to 100,000 genomes per cell. Virions are then released from desquamating cells.

Epidemiology and natural history

Genital tract HPV DNA is found in 10–20% of those aged 15–49 years. However, <10% have clinically apparent lesions, i.e. ~1% overall. The peak age of prevalence is 20–24 years in ♀ and 25–34 years in ♂. The infection rate is ↑ in smokers (>5-fold).

The median incubation period of exophytic warts is 3 months (range 2 weeks–9 months, but can be much longer). In the immunocompetent, warts eventually regress with immune response which usually begins after a period of 3–6 months of active growth. Response to E6 antigen leads to clearance but E7 results in persistent or relapsing infection. In ~95% HPV can no longer be detected 2 years after infection.

Transmission

Transmission is through contact with apparent or subclinical epithelial lesions and/or genital fluids containing infective virus, usually during sexual intercourse (including non-penetrative contact). Resultant micro-abrasions enable viral inoculation into the basal layers of the epithelium. Occasional reports of anogenital types at other sites (e.g. fingers) and non-anogenital types on anogenital skin suggest digital–genital trans-mission (including auto-inoculation). This may explain the absence of a history of genital–genital/anal or orogenital–anal sexual contact reported in ~1% of ♀ with anogenital warts (no data available for ♂). The finding of oral, laryngeal, conjunctival, and nasal lesions in those with anogenital warts (~5%), with the same HPV type, suggests orogenital transmission.

Mother-to-child transmission may occur during vaginal delivery, with a 10–70% rate of neonatal infection, and has also been reported following Caesarean section. In pre-pubertal children digital warts may be transmitted to anogenital regions, up to 20% of which may be due to skin types.

Table 22.1 HPV types in lesions

Lesion	HPV types (more common types in bold)
Skin warts	**1, 2, 3, 10, 7,** 4, 7, 26, 28, 29, 41, 49, 57, 60, 63, 65
Anogenital warts	**6, 11,** 16, 30, 40, 41, 42, 43, 44, 54, 55
Squamous intra-epithelial lesions*	**6, 11, 16, 18, 31,** 30, 33, 34, 35, 56, 57, 58, 59, 61, 62, 64, 67, 68, 69, 70
Anogenital squamous cell carcinoma	**16, 18, 31, 45,** 33, 35, 39, 51, 52, 54, 56, 66, 68
Oral warts	**2, 6, 11, 16** (7, 13, 18, 32 in HIV +ve)
Laryngeal papilloma	**6, 11**
Head and neck carcinoma	**16,** 18, 33, 57

*Cervical, vaginal, vulval, anal, or penile intra-epithelial neoplasia.

Clinical features

Symptoms

Usually little physical discomfort but disfiguring lesions may lead to psychological distress. Peri-anal or large growths may cause irritation and soreness. Urethral, anal, and cervical warts may cause bleeding and urethral warts may distort the urinary stream.

Signs (Plate 13)

Warts (usually multiple) appear most commonly at sites likely to be traumatized during sexual intercourse with HPV detectable in apparently normal surrounding skin. Peri-anal and anal warts (almost always below the pectinate line) may occur in both ♂ and ♀, more commonly but not only with receptive anal sex. May be found on the cervix and in the vagina, anal canal, urethral meatus, with rare involvement of urethra and bladder (Table 22.2)

Lesions are either pedunculated or sessile and sometimes pigmented. They may be:

- condylomata acuminata—soft/non-keratinized, 'cauliflower-like' in appearance, found on mucosae/warm moist non-hairy skin
- keratinized—resembling skin warts, usually on dry anogenital skin
- smooth papules on dry skin (e.g. penile shaft).

Subclinical infection may be detected as aceto-white patches with 5% acetic acid, better visualized through a colposcope (⚠ low specificity). Atypical balanoposthitis/vulvitis may be associated with HPV 🔊.

Giant condyloma of Buschke and Lowenstein

Usually associated with HPV6 and HPV11. Resembles a very large wart but invades the dermis and underlying tissue (e.g. corpus cavernosum). Starts as a keratotic papule and grows into a large cauliflower-like lesion. Most commonly located on the glans penis, but may occur anywhere on the penis, scrotum, vulva, vagina, rectum, and bladder. Does not metastasize but malignant transformation (verrucous carcinoma) develops in up to 50%. Diagnosed histologically. Liable to recur if not completely excised.

Diagnosis

- Usually on clinical appearance.
- Internal examination:
  - speculum for vaginal/cervical warts
  - proctoscopy for anal warts if peri-anal lesions present
  - urethral meatoscopy (with an otoscope) if meatal warts.
- Biopsy under local anaesthetic if in doubt, or lesion atypical or pigmented. This may be aided by the use of a colposcope.
- Routine DNA detection is unnecessary and is not cost effective.

Differential diagnosis

See Table 22.3

Table 22.2 Relative frequency (reported range) of location of genital warts

	% of cases (range)		% of cases (range)
Prepuce	65 (49–80)	Posterior aspect of introitus	73 (77–94)
Frenum, corona and glans	46 (22–70)	Labia minora/ majora, clitoris	32
Urethral meatus	34 (24–45)	Cervix	34 (6–64)
Penile shaft	27 (16–55)	Vagina	42 (32–52)
Scrotum	23 (2–25)	Urethra	8
Peri-anal area	8 (3–15)	Perianal area	18 (13–85)
		Perineum	23

Table 22.3 Differential diagnosis of external anogenital warts

Achrocordon (skin tag)	Molluscum contagiosum
Epidermal/melanocytic naevi	Condylomata lata (secondary syphilis)
Sebaceous glands	Seborrhoeic keratosis
Penile pearly papules	Dermatofibroma
Vulval papillae	Angiokeratoma
Ectopic sebaceous glands (Fordyce spots)	Epidermal cyst
Prominent hair follicles	Lichen planus
Nabothian follicles (cervix)	Psoriasis
	Penile/anal intra-epithelial neoplasia
	Giant condyloma of Buschke and Lowenstein
	Squamous cell carcinoma
	Basal cell carcinoma

Pregnancy and infection in the neonate and children

Warts may rapidly enlarge with pronounced vascularity during pregnancy (probably as a result of altered immunocompetence or ↑ oestrogen/ progesterone) and regress in the puerperium, often with complete resolution. Warts do not usually obstruct vaginal delivery.

Neonatal infection commonly clears within 6 weeks. Persistence is usually subclinical but may lead to recurrent respiratory papillomatosis or ano-genital or extra-genital warts. Recurrent respiratory papillomatosis incidence is 0.25% in children (3 months–5 years of age) born to mothers with warts. Mostly caused by HPV6 and HPV11. Usually located on the vocal cords and epiglottis (laryngeal papillomas), rarely on the entire larynx, tracheobronchial tree, or even the lungs.

Perinatal infection is the usual cause of anogenital warts in children up to 3 years of age. However, sexual abuse and non-sexual transmission should be considered in older children.

Management

General principles

The aim of treatment is essentially cosmetic or for symptomatic relief. Treatments have no direct effect against HPV and only limited impact on viral clearance and infectivity. Diagnosis of subclinical infection is of no practical benefit.

Optimal management is enabled by a treatment protocol with clear guidelines on the choice of treatment and arrangements for review (Algorithms 22.1 and 22.2). Treatment choice depends on the morphology, number, and distribution of warts and should be made after considering the available options and discussing side-effects, e.g. scarring, with the patient. Serial documentation of the number, size, appearance, and distribution of warts in genital maps gives a visual record of treatment response. If the wart area is >4cm^2 treatment under direct supervision of clinical staff is recommended. No treatment is an option particularly for vaginal/anal warts.

Condom use does not impact on anogenital HPV prevalence but may reduce the incidence of genital warts in ♂ and cervical neoplasia in ♀. Psychological distress may require referral for counselling. The possibility of a long incubation period should be discussed, especially if there are concerns about infidelity.

All treatments have significant failure rates. Soft non-keratinized warts respond well to podophyllotoxin (and podophyllin). Keratinized lesions are better treated with ablative methods e.g. cryotherapy, trichloroacetic acid (TCA), excision, or electrocautery. Imiquimod may be suitable for both types. Preferred initial treatment for small number/low volume warts of either type is ablation.

▶Risk of scarring and pigment changes should be discussed before treatment.

Frequently asked questions

How have I caught them?

Genital warts are usually sexually transmitted by direct skin-to-skin contact. It is thought that ~90% of people who are infected with HPV have no visible warts. After infection it takes a mean of 3 months for warts to develop, but may extend to months or years.

Will they go on their own?

Warts left untreated may disappear on their own (usually within 18 months) but they can also grow and spread, becoming unsightly and more difficult to treat.

Will I ever get rid of them?

When warts are treated they should clear, but HPV may persist, depending on the host's immunological response. Therefore the patient should be warned that they may recur. Recurrences are more likely within 3 months of treatment. HPV usually clears within 24 months although this may be longer, especially if the patient is immunocompromised.

Am I infectious?

Someone infected with HPV is infectious until it clears. The level of infection is probably greater when warts are present as viral shedding is likely to be greater.

Can I have sex?

It is often recommended that if visible warts are present condoms should be used during sex, although there is no clear evidence of benefit. Friction associated with coitus may spread warts. However, it is likely that the regular partner of someone who has warts will also be infected with the wart virus whether they have visible warts or not.

Do warts cause cervical cancer?

There are many strains of HPV, but those causing genital warts are different from the types associated with cervical cancer. It is recommended that a ♀ attends for routine smear tests which will detect abnormalities associated with the HPV strains that may be related to cervical cancer. ♀ with warts do not need extra smears.

My partner does not have warts. Does he/she need to be seen?

Only if there are concerns about possible warts or other STIs.

Specific treatments

- *Podophyllotoxin* (self-applied) The active lignan ingredient of podophyllin resin and an antimitotic agent causing local tissue necrosis. Available as 0.5% solution or 0.15% cream. Should be applied twice daily for 3 consecutive days, repeated at weekly intervals for a total of up to 4–5 three-day treatments. Clearance rate 42–88%. Recurrence rate 10–91%. In ♀ 0.15% cream is more effective than 0.5% solution (81% vs 50%).

- *Cryotherapy*. Liquid nitrogen spray (–180°C), swab (–20°C) or probe (–196°C), nitrous oxide probe (–75°C), or carbon dioxide snow (–79°C) may be used to freeze (for ~20 seconds) the wart(s) and a margin ('halo') of 1–3mm of surrounding epithelium. The depth of freezing achieved is variable and operator dependent. Local anaesthetic is usually not needed, but may be required depending on pain tolerance and extent of warts. Adequate cryotherapy causes immediate erythema followed in a few hours by blistering due to cytolysis of the epithelial cells. Healing takes 7–10 days with minimal scarring. If the treated area is large, severe ulceration may occur causing wound-care problems and scarring. Cryotherapy may be repeated at 1–2 week intervals. Clearance rate 63–88% after 1–10 (average 3) weekly treatments. Recurrence rate up to 39%.

- *Trichloroacetic acid (TCA)* Caustic agent causes chemical coagulation leading to necrosis. Applied once a week as a 80–90% solution (unlicensed), ensuring protection of surrounding epithelium with petroleum jelly Treatment-induced pain, ulceration, irritation, and scarring limit its use. Clearance rate 50–81%. Recurrence rate 36%.

- *Imiquimod 5% cream* (self-applied) Stimulates innate and acquired immune responses. Applied once a day, 3 times a week, for up to 16 weeks. Clearance rate 50–62% with partial clearance (≥50% reduction) in 59–81% of the remainder. Recurrence rate 13–19%. More effective in ♀ than ♂ (64–72% versus 33–42%) and in uncircumcised than circumcised ♀ (62% versus 33%). Also used as an adjunct to ablative treatment. Erythema, burning, irritation, and tenderness are common side-effects, reflecting effective immune response, and do not warrant cessation of treatment unless severe.

- *Podophyllin 15–25%*. A resin extracted from *Podophyllum peltatum* dissolved in alcohol or benzoin. In addition to the active ingredient podophyllotoxin, it contains quercetin and kaempherol which are mutagenic. (Teratogenic and oncogenic effects in animal experiments but no evidence in humans.) As there are safety concerns regarding the preparation of the solution and podophyllotoxin preparations are more effective with less toxicity, this preparation is no longer in general use.

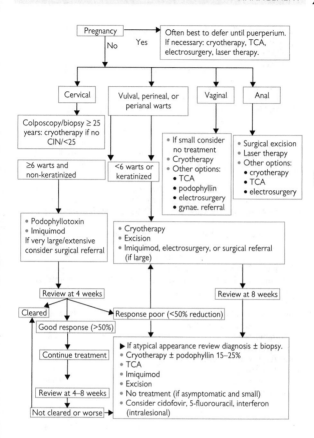

Algorithm 22.1 Treatment algorithm for genital warts in ♀

- *Electrosurgery* Tissue destruction by electrically produced heat. Common methods:
  - Electrocautery—application of heat to warts and surrounding tissue under local anaesthesia.
  - Hyfrecation—high-frequency (0.5–3MHz) low-power (1–30W) electricity heats the tissue causing necrosis. Patient return electrode ('diathermy pad') is not needed since low power is used. Two techniques are used: electrofulguration (current sparks across an air gap) and electrodessication (electrode in contact with and penetrating warts). Requires local anaesthesia.
  - Surgical diathermy—high-frequency (0.5–3MHz) high-power (up to 400W) electricity (requiring 'diathermy pad') to produce coagulation or cutting. More suitable for large warts. Requires general anaesthesia.
  Clearance rate ~94%. Recurrence ~24%.
- *Excision* Excision using scalpel, curette, or scissors under local or general anaesthesia. Clearance rate 89–93%. Recurrence rate up to 29%.
- *Laser therapy* Vaporization of warts under local or general anaesthesia. Clearance rate 27–89%. Recurrence rate 7–45%. Adverse effects include pain, itch, bleeding, and scar formation.
- *Cidofovir 1% cream* (self-applied) Unlicensed for routine use. Applied daily for 5 days, repeated fortnightly (i.e. after 9 treatment-free days) for a total of up to 6 five-day treatments. Clearance rate 27–89%. Recurrence rate 7–45%.
- *5-Fluorouracil 5% cream* Pyrimidine analogue inhibiting RNA/DNA synthesis. Applied twice a week for up to 10 weeks. Not recommended for internal warts (especially urethral). Clearance rate 13–43%. Recurrence rate ~50%.
- *Interferon* Various regimens have been described using interferon α, β, or γ as intralesional or systemic injection (also as self-applied cream). However, its use is limited by a variable response rate, systemic side-effects, and expense. Clearance rates: intralesional 19–62%, systemic 7–51%, and topical 6–90%. Recurrence rates: intralesional up to 33%, systemic up to 23%, and topical ~6%. Cyclical low-dose injection used as an adjunct to laser therapy has been reported to reduce relapse rate.
- *Isotretinoin* Conflicting results when used to treat genital warts. A recent study using oral isotretinoin 0.5mg/kg/day showed efficacy in the treatment of recalcitrant cervical warts. However, because of its teratogenicity, its use as first-line therapy for genital warts in ♀ is unacceptable.

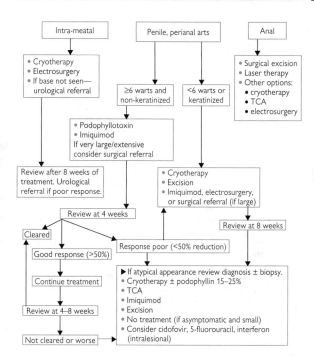

Algorithm 22.2 Treatment algorithm for genital warts in ♂

Management: sexual partners

Current sexual partner(s) may benefit from assessment for undetected genital warts and other STIs, and there may be a need for explanation and advice about disease process.

Special situations

- **Pregnancy** Treatment does not reduce perinatal transmission and is better deferred until the puerperium. Very rarely Caesarean section may be indicated because of obstruction. Cryotherapy, TCA, electrocautery, and laser vaporization are suitable if necessary. Excision may cause severe haemorrhage and diathermy of large lesions may cause intense postoperative pain. Imiquimod is not approved but has been used in exceptional circumstances (after discussion of risks and benefits with the patient and registration with 3M, the manufacturers).
- ⚠ Podophyllin, podophyllotoxin, 5-fluorouracil, cidofovir, interferon, and isotretinoin are contraindicated because of possible teratogenic effects or lack of safety data.
- **Vagina** Treatment may not be necessary especially if warts are small. Cryotherapy is the usual first-line therapy. Electrosurgery, TCA, podophyllin (total area treated <2cm^2), or gynaecological referral are other options.
- **Cervix**
  - Cervical warts—cryotherapy, electrosurgery, or TCA. If ≥25 years of age colposcopy ± biopsy best practice to exclude cervical intra-epithelial neoplasia (CIN) before treatment
  - Cytology—no changes to routine screening intervals necessary.
- **Urethral meatus** If base of lesions seen, preferred treatment iscryotherapy or electrosurgery. Other options are podophyllotoxin or imiquimod, but use with caution. Deeper lesions require surgical ablation under direct vision.
- **Anal canal** Surgical excision or laser preferred. If small and accessible—cryotherapy, TCA, electrosurgery.
- **Immunosuppressed patients** Poor treatment response, ↑ relapse, and dysplasia more likely with ↓ cell-mediated immunity, e.g. following renal transplant or HIV infection. Careful follow-up required.

Vaccine

Virus-like particle (VLP), the capsid without DNA, is immunogenic but non-infectious. Two vaccines using VLP to induce immunity have been shown by trials to be effective. Gardasil® is a tetravalent (quadruple) vaccine containing recombinant VLP from HPV types 6, 11, 16, and 18, and a transformed *Saccharomyces cerevisiae* (yeast) cell line complexed with a conventional aluminum adjuvant. Cervarix® is a bivalent vaccine containing HPV types 16 and 18 VLPs derived from a recombinant baculovirus vector expression system using *Trichoplusia ni* (cabbage looper moth) cell line. Cervarix®, and to a lesser degree Gardasil®, provide some cross-protection against HPV types 31, 33, 45, and 58 (92%, 52%, 100%, and 65% with Cervarix®). Based on available evidence these vaccines are likely to prevent 70% of invasive cervical cancers and 60% of high-grade CIN if given to all girls before the onset of sexual activity. The quadrivalent vaccine is likely to be effective in preventing 90% of ano-genital warts if given to both sexes before the onset of sexual activity. While the HPV vaccination programme in the UK has chosen the bivalent vaccine for girls aged 12–13 (with an initial 2-year 'catch-up' of 13–18-year-old girls) programmes in some other countries have chosen the quadrivalent vaccine. An observational study in Australia has shown a reduction in the number of cases of anogenital warts in women and heterosexual men since the introduction of the quadrivalent HPV vaccine programme for girls. There is no evidence to support the use of HPV vaccines in those who have already acquired HPV vaccine, and studies to assess the effect of the vaccines in those already sexually active or HPV infected are being conducted. There is an anecdotal report of cessation of recurrence of recurrent respiratory papillomata in infants given the quadrivalent vaccine after initial surgical removal of the papillomata.

Frequently asked questions

Can I treat warts myself?

It is advisable not to treat warts at home with over-the-counter preparations. These preparations are designed for use on hands or feet and may damage genital skin.

There are special prescription-only preparations (podophyllotoxin and imiquimod) for home use, although the treatments recommended depend on the position, number, and appearance of the warts.

Can I pass them to my children?

The HPV types that usually cause genital infection almost exclusively favour this site and so are sexually transmitted. However, occasionally other types, such as those causing warts on the hands, can be spread to the genitals and have been found in children.

I am pregnant. Are the warts harmful to my baby?

Warts are common in pregnancy, often grow more quickly, and are more difficult to manage as certain treatments cannot be used. They often resolve spontaneously after the pregnancy is over. Although HPV can be transmitted to babies at delivery it is unusual. Treating the warts will not remove the underlying infection.

HPV and HIV

- HPV infection has not been associated with ↑ risk of HIV acquisition.
- Those with HIV infection appear to be at greater risk of acquiring or reactivating HPV.
- Oral warts (due to HPV types 7, 13, 18, and 32) are more common in those with HIV infection.
- Duration and natural history of concurrent HPV infection may be altered, leading to ↑ incidence of cervical and anal neoplasia.

Molluscum contagiosum

Introduction

First described in 1817. Viral origin discovered by Juliusburg in 1905.

Aetiology

Molluscum contagiosum virus (MCV), genus *Molluscipoxvirus*, a poxvirus. A benign self-limiting skin infection caused by a large DNA virus replicating in cytoplasm of epithelial cells. There are four major subtypes: MCV1 (↑ in children) and MCV2 (↑ in adults and those with HIV infection) are the most common, and two further subtypes (MCV3 and MCV4) are described although these remain rare. Humans are the only natural host.

Epidemiology and transmission

Worldwide, more common in warm climates. Linked to poor hygiene and overcrowding. Equal sex distribution. Transmitted by direct skin-to-skin contact. Microscopic abrasions (trauma) and a warm moist environment facilitate transmission. The period of infectivity and viral shedding is thought to be equal to the duration of lesions.

Both sexual and non-sexual spread occurs. The latter is more common especially in:

• pre-adolescent children (17% in those aged <15 years)
• individuals with impaired cellular immunity
• sports involving skin-to-skin contact
• those using gyms, swimming pools, and saunas (including fomites, e.g. shared towels)

If sexually acquired, lesions are usually found around the anogenital area and in:

• sexually active adults aged 20–29 years
• those with a history or presence of other STIs
• those whose partner has molluscum contagiosum

There are no documented cases of maternal–fetal transmission. HIV testing is recommended in those presenting with facial lesions.

Clinical features

Incubation period usually 2–12 weeks, up to 6 months. Smooth pearly coloured umbilicated lesions growing over several weeks to a diameter of 2–6mm, occasionally larger (Plate 14). In adults, when sexually acquired, found in pubic region, thighs, buttocks, lower abdomen, and less commonly external genitalia sparing mucous membranes. Usually up to 10–20 lesions unless immunosuppressed. May appear during pregnancy and generally resolve after delivery. Typically asymptomatic but may cause pruritus (10% develop dermatitis around lesions), leading to auto-inoculation through excoriation. In children lesions are characteristically found on face, upper limbs, and trunk but 10–50% have genital lesions.

Spontaneous resolution within 2–3 months is common, but recurrences occur in 15–35% over 8–24 months.

Diagnosis

- Characteristic appearance
- Histology: enlarged epithelial cells with intra-cytoplasmic molluscum bodies.

Frequently asked questions

Where have I caught it?
Molluscum contagiosum is a viral infection spread by skin-to-skin contact. If lesions appear around the genitals they have probably been sexually transmitted.

How long has the infection has been there and how long will the lesions stay?
Lesions usually appear after an incubation period of 3–12 weeks (although this can be longer) and usually disappear spontaneously within 2–3 months. Clearance depends on the body mounting a suitable immunological response against the causative poxvirus.

Does it need treating?
As molluscum resolves spontaneously, treatment is offered for cosmetic purposes only. Generally people with genital lesions want them cleared up as soon as possible.

Can it be treated?
The usual treatment is by cryotherapy, but curettage, diathermy, and piercing with an orange stick followed by applyication of iodine or phenol have also been used. There are limited data on podophyllotoxin cream and imiquimod cream (currently unlicensed).

Will it recur?
33% of people will experience recurrences over the next 1–2 years.

Management

As molluscum contagiosum frequently resolves without treatment, the benefits of treating lesions must be balanced against the possible risk of post-treatment scarring.

Treatment options include:
- curettage, cryotherapy, electrocautery, puncture with sharpened orange stick dipped in 80% phenol
- imiquimod cream 5%
- podophyllotoxin 0.5% (reported but very limited data on efficacy)
- oral cimetidine (conflicting results on efficacy)
- adapalene.

Partner notification

Unnecessary. No evidence that treating partner prevents reinfection.

HIV infection

Molluscum contagiosum is found in up to 20% of those with HIV. Lesions may become widespread in those with low CD4 counts and high viral loads (commonly affecting the face) and hypertrophic. Use of HAART may lead to resolution of lesions, but conversely may present following an immune reconstitution inflammatory syndrome (IRIS) (📖 Chapter 53, Immune reconstitution p. 592)

Sexually acquired viral hepatitis

Hepatitis A virus (HAV) infection

Aetiology

A highly infectious RNA picornavirus. Identified in 1972 but condition had been known for a long time as epidemic jaundice, yellow jaundice, or infectious hepatitis.

Epidemiology and transmission

Common in developing countries (poor sanitation) and with close personal contact. Prevalence in USA and Western Europe 10–33%. Transmission usually faeco-oral (contaminated food/water). Associated with urine contamination and contact with infected urine (e.g. urophilia). Most commonly affects children, but outbreaks reported in ♂ who have sex with ♂ (MSM) (possibly through faecal contact), injecting drug users (IDUs), and institutions. Batches of contaminated blood products have been found. Patients are infectious for 2 weeks before and 1 week after the onset of jaundice. After infection immunity is lifelong.

Clinical features

Incubation period

Usually 2–6 weeks.

Symptoms

Most children and up to 50% of all adults are either asymptomatic or have mild non-specific symptoms with no obvious jaundice. It is an icteric illness with jaundice, anorexia, nausea, and fatigue usually lasting 1–3 weeks (up to 12 weeks) which is preceded by prodromal flu-like symptoms (malaise, myalgia, fatigue, nausea), often with right upper abdominal pain lasting 3–10 days. Pyrexia usually disappears at the beginning of the icteric phase with symptomatic improvement at onset of jaundice.

Signs

Jaundice (hepatitic and/or homeostatic) often with pale stools and dark urine. Liver tenderness and dehydration may occur.

Complications

Fulminant hepatitis in ~0.4% (more common in those with hepatitis C). Up to 15% of symptomatic patients may require hospitalization with 25% having severe hepatitis. HAV-associated mortality is very low (<0.2%). Chronic infection does not usually occur.

HAV in pregnancy

Associated with ↑ rate of premature labour and miscarriage proportional to severity of illness. Vertical transmission rarely reported.

Diagnosis and investigations

- HAV-IgM: positive within 5 days of illness (up to 6 months)
- HAV-IgG: indicates past exposure or response to vaccination
- Alanine aminotransferase (ALT)/aspartate aminotransferase (AST) and bilirubin can ↑ to 10,000 IU/L and 500μmol/L, respectively.
- Alkaline phosphatase (ALP) ↑ modestly but higher with cholestasis.
- Prothrombin time prolongation of >5 seconds suggests decompensation.
- Screen for other hepatotropic infections and STIs if appropriate.

Management

Provision of information and advice (avoid alcohol; stop food handling and unprotected sexual intercourse until non-infectious). Most cases managed on an outpatient basis. Follow-up only necessary for patients whose ALT or bilirubin does not settle within 4–8 weeks.

HAV infection is a notifiable disease with contacts requiring follow-up by public health authorities including partner notification for sexual partners. Human normal immunoglobulin (HNIG) or early HAV vaccine may be considered for non-immune close contacts including neonates. Breastfeeding can be continued.

Vaccination (Box 24.1)

Active vaccination recommended for travellers to endemic countries and in outbreak situations (e.g MSM) and those with chronic liver disease, IDUs, and HIV infection.

Schedule

Two doses at 0 and 6–12 months gives 95% protection for 5–10 years. Vaccination provides protection for up to 25 years. Combination vaccine with hepatitis B follows same schedule as hepatitis B vaccination. HAV vaccine response may be lower in HIV/immunocompromised patients.

Hepatitis B virus (HBV) infection

Aetiology

Hepadna DNA virus first reported in 1965 (Australia antigen). Six genotypes (A–F).

Epidemiology and transmission

Occurs endemically with high chronic carriage rates (up to 8%) in Southeast Asia, China, Africa, Southern and Eastern Europe, and Central and South America. Low carriage rates in North America, Western Europe, and Australia. UK rate <0.04% but ↑ in IV drug users (IDUs), MSM, commercial sex workers, and heterosexual HBV contacts.

In MSM sexual transmission is associated with multiple partners, unprotected anal sex, and oro-anal sex. Mother-to-child transmission is common; its frequency depends on maternal antigen status (90% if HBeAg +ve, 10% if eAg –ve). Other transmission routes include parenteral (IDU, tattoos, blood products, acupuncture). Sporadic infections may occur in healthcare professionals (HCPs) and institutions.

Clinical features

Incubation period

Usually 6 weeks to 6 months.

Symptoms

infants and children usually have asymptomatic acute infection. 10–50% of adults are asymptomatic. Symptoms more likely if HIV infected. Prodromal and icteric phases are similar to HAV but may be more severe and prolonged.

Signs

- Acute: similar to HAV.
- Chronic: usually no physical signs. After many years signs of chronic liver disease, signs including spider naevi, finger clubbing, gynaecomastia, and palmar erythema may emerge. In endstage disease jaundice, ascites, liver flap, and encephalopathy may appear.

Complications

- Acute infection: mortality due to fulminant hepatitis is <1%.
- Chronic infection (defined as >6 months of HBsAg positivity) develops in 5–10%. More common in HIV infection, chronic renal failure, the immunosuppressed, and >90% of vertically infected children. Immunosuppression can also lead to HBV reactivation. ↑ mortality rate in cirrhosis due to decompensating liver disease and progression to liver cancer. Concurrent infection with hepatitis C virus can lead to more progressive chronic liver disease. Co-infection with hepatitis D (delta agent), usually IDU associated, may lead to rapid deterioration and its response to treatment is poor.
- HBV ↑ rate of miscarriage and premature labour.

Diagnosis (Table 24.1)

- HBsAg (surface antigen) is positive in acute and chronic infection and disappears in resolved/immune infection. Usually appears within 3 months of infection (rarely up to 6 months).
- HBcAb (core antibody) is a marker of acquired infection and remains positive in resolved infection but is negative in vaccinated patients.
- HBeAg (envelope antigen) is a marker of high viral activity/high infectivity.
- HBV DNA identifies the amount of virus present and correlates with infectivity and hepatic activity.
- HBsAb (surface antibody) is a marker of successful vaccination and its titre determines the level of protection. It may be positive in those with resolved/immune hepatitis B.
- Liver function tests may be normal, but are often of variable level and are usually ↑ during hepatic 'flares'.

Table 24.1 Serological, virological, and liver enzyme tests at different stages of viral hepatitis A, B, and C

	HAV	HBV	HCV
Acute infection	• HAV IgM +ve • ALT ↑ usually	• Usually HBsAg +ve • Anti HBc IgM +ve • ALT ↑ usually • HBV DNA present	• HCV IgG +/−ve • ALT ↑ often • HCV-RNA +ve (usually)
Chronic infection	Does not usually occur	• HBsAg +ve • HBeAg +/−ve • HBc IgG +ve • ALT ↑ ↓ • HBV-DNA +/−ve	• HCV IgG +ve • ALT ↑ ↓ • HCV-RNA +ve
Recovered infection	• HAV IgG +ve • Normal ALT	• HBs IgG +ve • HBc IgG +ve • ALT normal	• HCV IgG +ve • HCV-RNA −ve • ALT normal
Successful vaccination	HAV IgG +ve	• HBs IgG +ve • HBc IgG −ve	• Not available

Management

Information and advice, including avoiding unprotected sexual intercourse until non-infectious or partner successfully vaccinated. Stop (or ↓) alcohol consumption. Refer to specialist unit if acute deteriorating liver disease.

Notifiable disease

Partner notification and screening of close family contacts are important with public health involvement for non-sexual contacts. Consider specific HBV immunoglobulin 500 units IM and rapid vaccination of contacts.

Newborn

Vaccination (rapid schedule) and HBV-specific immunoglobulin 200 units IM ↓ vertical transmission by 90%. Breastfeeding can continue.

Chronic infection

Specialist referral recommended. High level HBV viraemia predicts progressive liver disease. Some HBeAg –ve patients may also progress. Lamivudine, adefovir, pegylated interferon, tenofovir, telbivudine, and entecavir are licensed for the treatment of HBV infection.

Decision to treat depends on patient's age, severity of liver disease, and co-pathologies. Patients with active liver disease and high viral load (HBV-DNA >10^{5}copies/mL) should be considered for:
- either long-term viral suppression with lamivudine 100mg daily (duration not defined but a minimum of 1 year usual)
- or an attempt at inducing HBV seroconversion (only in eAg +ve with high ALT) by using sequential lamivudine/interferon or pegylated interferon monotherapy (unlicensed).

In the UK adefovir is currently limited to lamuvidine-resistant virus. Treatment primarily ↓ risk of liver cirrhosis and liver cancer.
In decompensated liver disease interferon is absolutely contraindicated.

Vaccination (Box 24.1)

Apart from contacts, vaccination should be considered for those at ↑ risk, e.g. MSM, sex workers, association with endemic areas, prisoners, IDUs, those sexually assaulted, occupational/needlestick risk. Protection of vaccinated patients is assessed by HBsAb level: >100U/L is ideal but even with levels >10U/L subsequent HBV infection is very rare. It has been suggested that memory cells provide protection as immunity appears to be maintained even if HBsAb ↓ provided there has been a good initial response.

Schedules

- Ultra-rapid course: of recombinant vaccine schedule: 3 doses and booster at 0, 7, 21/28 days plus 12 month booster.
- Rapid course schedule: 3 doses and booster at 0, 1, 2 months plus 12 month booster.
Note these schedules are not licensed for neonates.
- Standard schedule: three doses at 0, 1, and 6 months; booster dose if protective antibody level <100mIU/mL.

Protective antibody level in 80–95% after a full course of vaccination but lower response rates if aged >40 years or immunocompromised, e.g. HIV infection, particularly if CD4 < 200cells/µL (but even <500cells/µL).

Combined hepatitis A and B vaccine has an overall lower response rate but may sometimes be useful. Newer types of vaccines (pre-S formulations, not widely available) or ↑ dosage of HBV vaccine may effect seroconversion.

Box 24.1 Active hepatitis A and B vaccines

Hepatitis A vaccine

- Havrix monodose®: suspension of formaldehyde-inactivated hepatitis A virus.
- Adult dose: 1mL with the deltoid region the preferred site (subcutaneous can be used in those with bleeding disorders).

Hepatitis B vaccine

- Engerix B®, HBvaxPRO®: both suspensions of HBV surface antigen prepared from yeast cells by recombinant DNA technology.
- Adult dose: 1mL with the deltoid region the preferred site (subcutaneous may be used in those with bleeding disorders). Should not be injected into the buttocks (efficacy reduced).

Combined hepatitis A and hepatitis B vaccine

- Twinrix®: inactivated HAV and recombinant HBV surface antigen.
- Adult dose: 1mL with the deltoid region the preferred site (subcutaneous may be used in those with bleeding disorders, although immune response may be reduced). Should not be injected into the buttocks (efficacy reduced).

Hepatitis C virus (HCV) infection

Aetiology

RNA virus of the family Flaviviridae discovered in 1989. Six predominant genotypes. In the UK genotype 1 (G1) is the most common (~50% of cases) followed by G2/G3 (together 40–50%). G1 is relatively more common in those infected through blood products and G2/G3 in injecting drug users (IDUs).

Epidemiology and transmission

High prevalence rates found in Egypt (up to 29%), Southeast Asia and Eastern Europe. UK has a rate of ~0.5% with a higher prevalence in IDUs (20–50% IDUs) and people who received a blood transfusion before September 1991 and blood products prior to 1986.

Transmission mainly parenteral through shared needles/syringes/equipment. ~67% are ♂ (more IDUs and haemophiliacs are ♂). Found in up to 1% of GUM patients, although <2% of infections are sexually acquired. Outbreaks described in HIV-positive MSM and there is ↑ prevalence in ♀ sex workers. Vertical transmission occurs in up to 6%.

Clinical features

Incubation period

4–20 weeks.

Symptoms

Acute hepatitis occurs in 20% and is less likely to be followed by chronic infection.

Signs

Similar to HAV and HBV.

Complications

Aacute fulminant hepatitis is rare but can occur in HCV patients with acute HAV infection.

Natural history

>80% become chronically infected with HCV; most are unaware. High alcohol intake, coexisting HBV, HIV, and other chronic liver diseases can lead to a more rapid progression to cirrhosis and liver cancer. Progress to cirrhosis in ~20% after 20 years. Thereafter annual rate of developing cancer ~5%. ►ALT may be normal despite severe liver disease.

Diagnosis

- Antibody testing with confirmation by polymerase chain reaction (PCR) test for viral RNA. Antibodies usually appear within 3 (rarely 6) months of infection.
- Genotype testing. Influences duration of treatment and estimates response rate.
- Liver function, clotting tests, and exclusion of other viral hepatotropic infections and liver-related diseases are helpful.
- Screening for other blood-borne infections including HIV advised.
- Abdominal ultrasound and α-fetoprotein monitoring recommended.

Screening should be offered to:
- all IDUs (past and present)
- in the UK recipients of
  - blood prior to September 1991
  - blood products pre-1986
  - tissues/organs before 1992
- regular sexual partners of those with HCV infection
- HCP exposure to blood/needlesticks
- those with HIV infection
- people with tattoos/skin piercing where there is poor infection control
- children of mothers with HCV infection.

It may be advised for prisoners/ex-prisoners, those sexually assaulted, and MSM if outbreak identified.

Management

A notifiable infection with partner notification and public health implications. Provide information and advice (IDU risk of sharing, risks of sexual transmission). Stop (or ↓) alcohol consumption. Consider discussion of insurance issues. If patient amenable to further management refer to specialist.

Acute infection

Consider high-dose α-interferon (pegylated/non-pegylated) and/or ribavirin.

Chronic infection (persistent HCV-PCR positive)

Based on genotype and degree of liver disease (biopsy, if indicated). Current guidelines recommend combination treatment:
- ribavirin 800mg–1.2g divided into two doses daily by mouth
  (dependent on genotype, weight, and type of pegylated interferon)
- pegylated interferon once a week by subcutaneous injection:
  - α-2a: 180mcg
  - α-2b: 1.5mcg/kg body weight.

Duration depends on genotype. People infected with G2, G3 should be treated for 24 weeks. Those with G1, G4, G5, or G6 should be treated for 48 weeks (unless VL <10^6 pre-treatment and undetectable at week 4 when 6 months is possible) but tested for response at 12 weeks. If there is an undetectable viral load (VL) or ↓ in VL drop (of at least 2-log) then treatment should be continued for full 48 weeks; otherwise it should be stopped.

Combination treatment has multiple side-effects and requires close monitoring of haematology, liver function, and thyroid function, with psychiatric support if needed. Ribavirin may cause haemolytic anaemia which may require dose reduction or its cessation. Sustained viral response rates vary between 40% and 70% for G1 and G2/3, respectively. Interferon may benefit liver fibrosis independently of viral clearance.

Prevention and prophylaxis

No vaccine available. Currently no treatment for needlestick injuries recommended. Newly employed HCPs with high risk exposure must declare their HCV status or undergo pre-employment testing.

Other viral infections

Epstein–Barr virus (EBV)

Aetiology

A DNA herpesvirus consisting of types EBV1 and EBV2. Infects >90% of humans, persisting for life. Probably evolved from a non-human primate virus.

Epidemiology and transmission

Virtually all children infected in developing countries (especially with socio-economic deprivation).

In developed countries most infections are acquired by those aged 15–25 years. Characteristically spread by ingestion of infected saliva from a seropositive carrier during kissing. Although unproven, reports of EBV isolated from a vulval ulcer, semen, and cervical secretions suggest the potential for sexual transmission.

Clinical features

Incubation period: 20–50 days. Infection in children usually asymptomatic. In adolescents and young adults >50% present with infectious mono-nucleosis (glandular fever):

- fever
- lymphadenopathy
- pharyngitis
- >10% develop hepatosplenomegaly and palatal petechiae (Forscheimer spots).

Other less common features include anaemia (haemolytic and aplastic), thrombocytopenia, myocarditis, hepatitis, genital ulcers, Guillain–Barré syndrome, encephalitis,and meningitis.

Non-specific diffuse central rashes may be found in up to 50% with an immune complex macular rash and in >70% of those taking ampicillin or amoxicillin.

Investigations

- Haematology: leucocytosis of $(12–25) \times 10^9$/L, lymphocytosis of $(4.5–5) \times 10^9$/L with 20% of cells atypical. May also be thrombo-cytopenia.
- Biochemistry: elevated liver enzymes in up to 100% from week 2–5.
- Antibody testing
  - Monospot test: heterophil antibodies (sensitivity ~80% in adults)
  - EBV antibody tests: IgM to viral capsid antigen IgM (transient). Most reliable test is paired IgG showing >4-fold titre rise. IgG to EB nuclear antigen appears in convalescence.

Management

Bed rest, analgesics, antipyretics. Antibiotics (not ampicillin/amoxicillin) if 2° bacterial infection. Steroids if airways obstruction.

Prognosis

Self-limiting although associated with persisting tiredness and possible relapses during the first 6–12 months. Not associated with chronic fatigue syndrome.

Other conditions associated with EBV

These include:
- Burkitt's and Hodgkin's lymphomas
- Nasopharyngeal carcinoma
- Lymphoproliferative disease
- In HIV infection
  - Oral hairy leukoplakia
  - Some non-Hodgkin's lymphomas

Cytomegalovirus (CMV)

The largest known DNA herpesvirus; host-specific, with four human/ higher primate subtypes.

Epidemiology and horizontal transmission

Worldwide distribution favouring developing countries and low socio-economic classes. Spread through contact with infected saliva (kissing↑ infection rates in adolescence), urine, genital fluids (cervical, vaginal seminal), breast milk (via lactation), and blood. Infection with multiple strains reported in sexually active. ↑ rates found in those with history of STIs, bacterial vaginosis, and seroprevalence proportional to number of lifetime partners. In STI clinics prevalence of CMV antibodies in ♂ who have sex with ♂ (MSM) is about 1.5 times that of heterosexual ♂.

Epidemiology and vertical/neonatal transmission

Most common vertically transmitted viral infection. Worldwide incidence of fetal CMV acquisition during pregnancy 0.8–4%. In UK ~50% ♀ becoming pregnant are CMV seronegative, with ~3% becoming infected during their pregnancy (largely from young children). 30–40% with 1° infection and about 1% with recurrent CMV will infect their fetus (overall congenital infection rate 0.5–1%).

Acquired by fetal ingestion of infected intra-amniotic material, haematological transplacental spread, and lactation.

Clinical features

Horizontal transmission

- Generally causes asymptomatic infection unless immunosuppressed.
- Only 10% of 1° infections cause an infectious mononucleosis type illness consisting of fever, myalgia, cervical lymphadenopathy, and less commonly pneumonitis and hepatitis.
- Illness self-limiting, although lifelong viral persistence often with extended periods of asymptomatic viral shedding (e.g. during pregnancy).

Vertical transmission

Severity of neonatal symptoms/signs less if mother seropositive (neutralizing antibodies). Range from none (in about 80%) to the classical congenital syndrome—hepatosplenomegaly (with jaundice) and thrombocytopenia (with purpura), which are self-limiting. Less common but permanent CNS features include microcephaly, chorioretinitis, aprogressive sensorineuronal deafness.

Diagnosis

- Immunocompetent adults—serology; 4-fold ↑ in IgG CMV antibodies from paired blood samples taken 10–14 days apart or IgM from single specimen (persists up to 20 weeks).
- Fetal infection: CMV detection from amniotic fluid by PCR after 21 weeks gestation.
- Congenital/neonatal infection: CMV culture or PCR from urine and pharynx.

Management

Symptomatic treatment (as for EBV infection).
For CMV associated with HIV infection see 📖 Chapter 44, Opportunistic infections, p. 514.

Human T-cell lymphotropic virus 1 (HTLV-1)

Single-stranded RNA retrovirus.

Epidemiology and transmission

Endemic in Japan and parts of the Caribbean, South America, and sub-Saharan Africa. Main transmission routes are breastfeeding and sexual intercourse (mostly heterosexual), but also from blood products and sharing injecting drug equipment.

Diagnosis

Serology: enzyme immunoassay or gelatin particle agglutination.

Clinical features

Most infected individuals remain healthy carriers but up to 5% develop adult T-cell leukaemia/lymphoma and ~2–3% develop myelopathy.

Adult T-cell leukaemia/lymphoma

Leukaemic involvement in 80% with wide-ranging skin lesions in ~40%. Other manifestations include hepatosplenomegaly, lymphadenopathy, hypercalcaemia, and sometimes immunosuppression.

Myelopathy (tropical spastic paraparesis)

Demyelination of long motor neurons of spinal cord producing lower-extremity weakness, spasticity, urinary incontinence, and erectile dysfunction.

Management

Adult T-cell leukaemia/lymphoma has poor prognosis (median survival without treatment <1 year). Besides conventional chemotherapy and allogeneic stem cell transplantation, other therapeutic approaches include interferon-α plus zidovudine, arsenic trioxide, and retinoid derivatives. The use of monoclonal antibodies and proteasome inhibitors is currently under development.

Human herpes virus-8 (HHV-8)

Herpes virus with five major variants (A–E). Variants B and C predominate in Europe and the USA.

Transmission

Sexual contact, particularly oro-anal sex, and also mouth-to-mouth contact as HHV-8 is found in saliva. Implicated in close family contact in endemic areas (Africa), especially when associated with poor hygiene. In developed countries ↑ rates among MSM. Transmission does not appear to be related to pregnancy or breastfeeding.

Clinical features

- Associated with >95% of cases of Kaposi's sarcoma with immunosuppression an important co-factor, although now uncommon with use of antiretroviral treatment (☐ Chapter 52, Kaposi's sarcoma p. 567)
- Associated with Castleman's disease—nearly all HIV cases (☐ Chapter 52, Introduction p. 566) and ~50% of non-HIV cases.

Scabies (*Sarcoptes scabiei var hominis*)

Introduction

Discovered in 1687 by Bonomo, arthropod class Arachnida, subclass Acari, family Sarcoptidae.

Aetiology

A parasitic mite with no natural enemies. The ♀ penetrates the stratum corneum constructing short burrows where it lays 1–3 eggs daily during its lifespan of 4–6 weeks. Eggs are oval and 0.1–0.15mm long. Six-legged larvae hatch in 3–4 days and then moult to form an eight-legged nymph. After a further moult the adult develops. The total time to maturity is 10 days with females becoming gravid within 14 days.

The adult is tortoise-like in shape with 8 legs (Fig. 26.1). The two sets of anterior legs end in stalked pulvilli (suckers) which allow the mite to grip the host's skin, aiding its movement. Spines and bristles cover the body. Mites are blind with no eyes. The adult female measures $0.4 \times 0.3mm^2$; the male is smaller and dies after mating. It has no spiracles, trachea, or body armour and obtains its oxygen through its surface. Mites can move rapidly on warm skin at ~2.5cm/min. Burrows are created at variable rates (0.5–5.0mm per day) and are lined with scar tissue to prevent them collapsing, thus allowing the mite to breathe and larvae to escape. Mites feed on the lymph and lysed tissue. Survival of the mite away from its host is contentious, but is unlikely to be >48–72 hours and is probably much less. However, there are occasional reports of infection after 96 hours ♠.

Classification

Classical scabies

Found in immunocompetent people with an average of 5–10 mites.

Norwegian scabies (crusted scabies)

Found in the immunocompromised and elderly, and may be related to failure of sensitization to mite antigen. Highly contagious, with honeycombed cavities in the skin containing many thousands of mites. Extensive crusted lesions with thick hyperkeratotic scales ('bread-crumb') develop over the elbows, palms, knees, and soles of the feet.

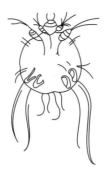

Fig. 26.1 *Sarcoptes scabiei*

Frequently asked questions

Is scabies always sexually transmitted?

No. The majority of cases are not sexually transmitted. It commonly occurs in people living closely together and is spread by prolonged skin contact, including holding hands.

Do I just need to treat my body from the neck down?

No. Although this may still be suggested, we advise that all skin surfaces are treated, taking care around mucous membranes. Even the scalp should be treated if you are bald. Relapses occur because of failure to treat all sites that may be infected.

Does anyone else require treatment?

Treatment is advised for current sexual partners and intimate household contacts.

I finished the treatment 2 weeks ago but still have some itching. Do I need to repeat it again?

No, not if you have used it properly and not been reinfected. Symptoms often take 4–5 weeks to resolve as they are due to a hypersensitivity reaction stimulated by mite products. It usually takes this time for them to be expelled from the skin and for the reaction to settle. If relief is required, topical crotamiton or antihistamines should help.

Epidemiology

Appears as sporadic outbreaks, especially in families, schools, dormitories, institutions, and nurseries. Epidemics occur in 15–30 year cycles. Mammals such as domestic cats, dogs, pigs, and horses may be infected with other sarcoptidae (mange) which may be transferred to humans, resulting in irritation without infestation.

Associated with previous or concurrent STIs.

Transmission

Holding hands is the most likely route of transmission. The more parasites on a person the greater is the risk of transmission. Prolonged skin-to-skin contact is necessary; however, the parasites may remain viable on inanimate objects for 2–5 days but this is less likely. Mites are transferred after about 10–20 minutes of close contact and can penetrate the epidermis within 30 minutes. Not vectors of other infections.

Clinical features

In 1° infection patients may be asymptomatic for the first 4–6 weeks. Intense irritation only occurs after immunological reactivity develops (less common in Norwegian scabies). In reinfestation signs and symptoms become evident in 24–48 hours because of previous sensitization.

- Symmetrical polymorphic lesions appear, most commonly on hands (especially finger webs), wrists, axillae, genitals, buttocks, and extensor aspect of elbows (Fig. 26.2). They are usually eczematous and associated with burrows (fine short serpiginous grey/black channels 5–10mm long, often with a small associated papule or vesicle).
- Indurated nodules (nodular scabies) are commonly found affecting the scrotum, penis, and groin. Mites cannot usually be recovered from these lesions.
- Urticarial papular rash, without mites, may be found in the axillae, upper abdomen, loins, and inner thighs.

Excoriation may lead to 2° bacterial infection.

Diagnosis

Clinical appearance

Burrows may be identified as follows.
- Staining the suspected site with a washable felt-tip marker. After removal by washing, the ink will be found to have delineated the burrow.
- Applying topical tetracycline to the skin and washing off the excess. Burrows retain tetracycline which will fluoresce under Wood's light.

Material for microscopy can be obtained by:
- extraction of mites (or eggs) from their burrows with a needle
- scraping the skin using a scalpel blade, following local application of liquid paraffin.

Mites can be recovered from the wrists (63%), extensor aspect of elbows (11%), feet and ankles (9%), genitals (9%), buttocks (4%), and axillae (2%).

Other possible methods of diagnosis include videodermatoscopy, epiluminescence microscopy, or skin biopsy.

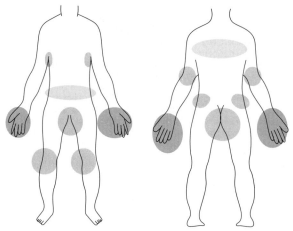

Fig. 26.2 Distribution of scabies

Management

Patients should be told that irritation may last for several weeks following treatment (antigenic material in the dermis and epidermis). Antihistamines, crotamiton 10% cream, or calamine 15% lotion may give symptomatic relief. Contaminated clothes or bed linen should be washed at >50°C.

Norwegian scabies is best treated in isolation to prevent nosocomial spread.

Treatment

Current opinion recommends that topical preparations be applied head to toe (except for the scalp unless bald) and left for a period of not less than 12 hours. Generally a single application is advised for common scabies (except for benzyl benzoate), although the British National Formulary now advises repeating the treatment after 1 week (based on expert opinion). Aqueous rather than alcohol preparations are recommended because of ↑ irritation of excoriated skin, especially around the genitalia. Patients should be advised not to apply an acaricide following a hot bath as this may remove it from its site of action by ↑ absorption into the bloodstream. If hands are washed within 8 hours of treatment, a repeat application is required. There are some reports that tea tree oil is effective as an acaricidal in the face of emerging resistance to conventional treatment.

Common scabies
• Permethrin 5% cream
• Malathion 0.5% aqueous lotion
• Benzyl benzoate: leave for 24 hours (2–3 applications on consecutive days).

Norwegian scabies
• Topical: repeat applications required for all products
• Ivermectin (named patient basis): 200mcg/kg body weight (single dose) in addition if no response to topical agents alone. Recommend second dose after 2 weeks (results in 95% cure). First choice in those with eczema or unable to tolerate topical preparations.

Pregnancy/breastfeeding

Permethrin is the treatment of choice.

Partner notification

Advise patients to avoid close body contact until sexual and household contacts have been treated.

Pediculosis

Pediculosis

Introduction

Pthiriasis (pediculosis) is an ancient disease. Nits (eggs of lice) have been discovered on the pubic hair of a 2000-year-old Chilean mummy, and also in fossilized form dating back 10,000 years. Despite a rise in other sexually transmitted infections in recent years, it is now seen with less frequency in sexual health clinics. It has been suggested that the trend for pubic shaving has resulted in the dramatic decline in the number of cases of pediculosis pubis recorded.

Aetiology

Belonging to the sub-order of Anoplura (sucking lice), the families of Pediculidae (body lice) and Pthiridae (pubic lice) are wingless insects unable to fly or jump. *Pthirus pubis* (the crab louse) (Fig. 27.1) is classified as a species of the genus Pthirus. *Pediculus humanus capitis* (head lice) and *Pediculus humanus humanus* and *corporis* (body lice) are morphologically similar and easily distinguished from pubic lice (smaller and squatter). The life-cycle of pubic lice is ~15–25 days occurring in three stages.

The nit

- White oval egg <0.8mm attached to the hair base by a chitinous envelope.
- It is encased by a proteinaceous sheath except for the operculum, allowing ventilation.
- It appears to move up the hair and away from the skin as hair grows.

The nymph

- Resembles a pubic louse but is smaller.
- Hatches in 7 days by releasing itself from the egg with air expelled from its anus.
- Migrates back to the hair base to suck blood and mature.

The adult

- ~1–2mm in length, dark grey to brown in colour. The ♂ is smaller and has a more pointed tail.
- Three distinct pairs of legs, each with claw-like appendages whose grasp is designed to match the diameter of pubic or axillary hair in contrast with the finer scalp hair. Can move ~10cm in a day.
- Sensory antennae detect human smell and tactile hairs on its body determine surface type. Eyes are faceted; it is almost blind but photophobic.
- Buries sharp mouthpiece stylets inside a pubic hair follicle to obtain a constant blood supply. Ingests several times its own weight in blood during each feed. May feed at the same place for days.
- Single pair of spiracles allow gaseous exchange and prevent dehydration.
- ♀ will lay 2–3 eggs during a 24-hour period and 15–50 eggs over a lifetime.

Diagnosis

Identify lice, eggs, or maculae caeruleae with the naked eye. Low-power microscopy of the louse may show movement, sucking pumps in the head, and a blood-filled oesophagus.

Management

Offer full screening for STIs and advise avoidance of close body contact until patient and partner(s) complete treatment. Clothes and bed linen should be washed at 50°C or dry-cleaned.

Because of the delicate nature of the genital skin aqueous rather than alcohol-based preparations are recommended. Lotions are more effective than shampoos. All body hair should be treated (not just groins and axillae) and left for 12 hours (or overnight). A second application after 7 days is advisable to kill lice emerging from any surviving nits. Dead nits may continue to adhere to hairs for several weeks following treatment and can be removed with a fine-tooth comb.

Suggested treatments

- Malathion 0.5%
- Carbaryl 1% (unlicensed for pubic lice)
- Permethrin 1% (recommended in pregnancy or during lactation)
- Phenothrin 0.2%

Eyelashes

- Permethrin 1% lotion, ensuring patient keeps eyes closed throughout the procedure and for the following 10 minutes
- Aqueous malathion (unlicensed for eyelashes)
- Pilocarpine hydrochloride 4% (Pilogel®)
- Physostigmine
- Application of yellow soft paraffin or Vaseline® which kills the lice by occluding their spiracles
- Removal of lice with forceps

Partner notification

Sexual partners within the previous 3 months should be advised to seek screening and treatment. Those sharing the same bedding may also require treatment.

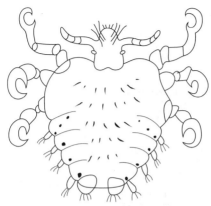

Fig. 27.1 Pthirus pubis

Frequently asked questions

How have I got them?
The crab louse is transmitted by close body contact and hence during sexual contact. More rarely infestation can be spread through contact with an infested person's bed linen, towel, or clothes.

Do I need to treat all my body hair?
Yes, a lotion should be applied to all of the body hair including a beard and moustache if necessary.

Will shaving get rid of the lice?
Lice are treated with carbaryl, malathion, or permethrin preparations. All the body hairs need to be treated, not just the pubic hair. Therefore shaving is not recommended as treatment.

Do I need to wash all my bedding?
Yes, it is recommended that all clothes and bed linen are machine washed on a hot water cycle.

Does my partner need treatment?
Yes, current sexual partners need treatment. Avoid close body contact until partner(s) have completed treatment. Contact tracing of all partners in the previous 3 months is recommended.

Pthirus or Phthirus?
Spelling varies, with both Pthirus and Phthirus widely used. Although the name is derived from the Greek *phtheir* (louse), the former spelling is used more widely.

Epidemiology

- Essentially a human parasite, although reported to infest higher apes.
- Does not occur in epidemics, although more common in the cooler months of the year (unlike body and head lice which occur more often in the warmer months).
- Considered to be usually sexually transmitted because:
  - found most commonly in sexually active adults (aged 16–25 years)
  - associated with other STIs, especially chlamydia.
- Related to crowded living conditions, poor personal hygiene, and low socio-economic status.
- Infestation of the scalp is rare (about 1% of louse infestation) but occurs more often in red-headed people, who have fewer hairs per unit area than others.
- Rarely reported in the scalp and eyelashes of children, in whom sexual abuse may need to be considered. However, acquisition from nipple hairs during breastfeeding has also been reported.
- Not known to be vectors of human disease (unlike body and head lice which may carry organisms responsible for epidemic or louse-borne typhus, trench fever, and louse-borne relapsing fever).

Transmission

- Usually by skin-to-skin contact with up to 95% of sexual contacts of an active carrier developing an infestation.
- Occasionally by clothing, bedding, or towels.
- It is unlikely that lice can survive for more than 24–48 hours if removed from the host.

Clinical features

~76% complain of intense irritation in the genital area because of hypersensitivity, with ~40% of patients experiencing erythema. In the hirsute, infestation may spread to the thighs, perineum, trunk, abdomen, or axillary hair. Eyebrows and eyelashes (pthiriasis palpebrarum) may also be infested with the possibility of 2° conjunctivitis.

Blue macules (maculae caeruleae) caused by an enzyme secreted from the salivary glands of the lice may be visible at feeding sites. They are 0.2–0.3cm in diameter, with an irregular outline, painless, do not disappear on pressure, and appear to be in the deeper tissues. They become apparent some hours after the louse has fed, and last for several days. 'Black spots' on underwear or in the genital area usually indicate insect faecal matter or blood spots.

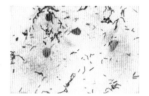

Plate 1 Gram-smear lactobacilli

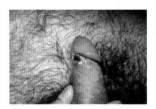

Plate 2 Classic primary chancre

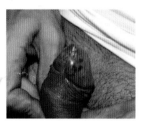

Plate 3 'Contemporary' chancre

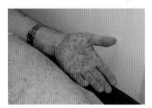

Plate 4 Secondary syphilis

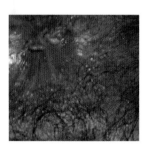

Plate 5 Condolymata lata

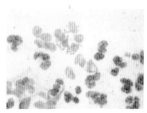

Plate 6 Gram-smear gonorrhoea

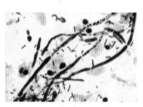

Plate 7 Gram-smear BV

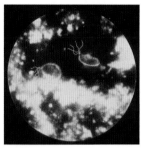

Plate 8 Dark-ground trichomonas vaginalis

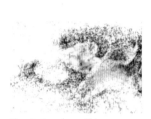

Plate 9 Gram-smear candidiasis

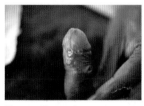

Plate 10 Chancroid

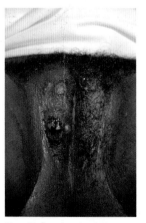

Plate 11 Granuloma inguinale

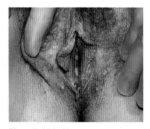

Plate 12 Vulval herpes

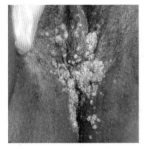

Plate 13 Anogenital warts

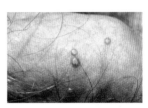

Plate 14 Molluscum contagiosum

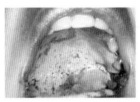

Plate 15 Oral candidiasis and HIV

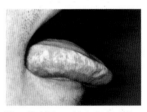

Plate 16 HIV—oral hairy leukoplakia

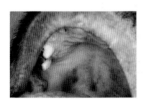

Plate 17 Oral Kaposi's sarcoma

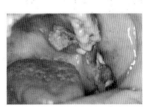

Plate 18 Oral lymphoma and HIV

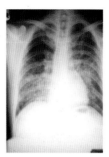

Plate 19 Chest x-ray—PCP

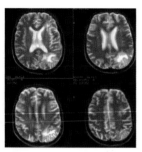

Plate 20 Brain scan—progressive multifocal leukoencephalopathy

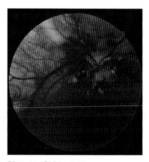

Plate 21 CMV retinitis

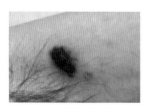

Plate 22 Cutaneous Kaposi's sarcoma

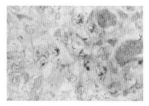

Plate 23 Mycobacteria in lymph node biopsy (Ziehl–Neelsen stain)

Anogenital dermatoses

Common benign lesions/anomalies

- *Angiokeratomas* Purple/dark red papules on labia majora, scrotum, and penile shaft. ↑ in those aged >50 years. Benign hyperkeratosis with dilated capillaries. Rarely associated with Anderson–Fabry disease.
- *Ectopic sebaceous glands (Fordyce spots)* Tiny yellow grouped papules. Occasionally form larger nodules. Usually found on the mucosal surface of the prepuce and inner labia minora.
- *Epidermoid cysts* White or creamy coloured nodules commonly found over scrotum and labia majora. Hair follicles blocked with keratin and filled with sebaceous matter. If required remove surgically.
- *Epidermal naevi* Epidermal outgrowths present at birth (50%) or developing during childhood.
- *Haemangioma* Red macule up to 3–5 mm in diameter on glans penis or vulval mucosa.
- *Idiopathic calcinosis of the scrotum with multiple nodules* Starts in the teens and may be mistaken for cysts. Surgery may be necessary for troublesome lesions but should be avoided if possible
- *Melanocytic naevi (moles)* Genital lesions (keratinized skin) are found in ~15% of the population
- *Nabothian follicles* Bluish or yellow coloured translucent lumps on cervix. Retention cysts from cervical 'glands'.
- *Pearly penile papules* White dome-shaped papules found at the corona and adjacent to the frenulum. Sometimes confused with warts. Reported in 20–50% ♂, usually <1mm in size, may extend to 3mm. Consist of connective tissue core with central thinned epidermis. Removal generally not recommended, but clearance possible with cryosurgery and carbon dioxide laser ablation.
- *Pigmentary changes*
  - Vitiligo: depigmentation (may also affect hair). Association with autoimmunity, especially thyroiditis.
  - Mucosal melanosis (genital lentiginosis): more commonly in ♀.
- *Prominent hair follicles* Found on penile shaft, scrotum, labia majora.
- *Seborrhoeic keratosis* Domed heavily pigmented papule usually ~ 1cm in diameter. Commonly found on mons pubis, penile shaft, labia majora usually in those aged >50 years. If removal required, cryosurgery or curettage.
- *Skin tags (achrocordon)* Common around the groin and thighs especially in those aged >50 years and more common if obese.
- *Vulval papillae* Fleshy filiform papules commonly found within the labia minora and often confused with warts. Typically soft, symmetrical, linear, and pink with separate bases.

Degenerative condition

Ovarian failure, usually 2° to the menopause, leads to urogenital atrophy, symptomatic in >50%. Symptoms include vulvovaginal dryness with discomfort, irritation, and dyspareunia. Often associated with other systemic symptoms which may influence management. Treat with oestrogen-based hormone replacement therapy which can be administered by various routes (oral, transdermal, subcutaneous, vaginal, and intranasal). Uro-genital symptoms may take some months to respond.

Infective conditions

Tinea cruris

Dermatophytic fungal infection commonly due to *Trichophyton rubrum* or *Epidermophyton floccosum*. Found in those sharing communal facilities (e.g. towels) and auto-inoculation from tinea pedis. More common in ♂. Pruritic plaques in the groin, spreading out to the thigh, with well-defined erythematous scaly edge and central clearing.

Diagnosis

Appearance, scraping from margins for microscopy (de-keratinize with potassium hydroxide), and culture.

Management

Topical imidazoles twice daily for 2 weeks or topical terbinafine for 1–2 weeks; oral terbinafine 250mg daily for 2–4 weeks or itraconazole 100mg daily for 15 days or 200mg daily for 7 days.

Erythrasma

Chronic infection of crural folds (especially axilla and groin) caused by *Corynebacterium minutissimum*. Associated with hyperhidrosis, diabetes mellitus, and living in crowded conditions. Dull red or brownish uniform scaly patch with little or no pruritus.

Diagnosis

Coral-pink fluorescence with Wood's light makes culture of scale unnecessary.

Management

Topical imidazoles for 2 weeks are usually effective. Sodium fusidate ointment 2%, topical erythromycin gel 2% twice daily for 2 weeks, or oral erythromycin are alternatives.

Inflammatory conditions

Irritant and contact dermatitis (see Box 28.1)

- Irritant: direct response to noxious agent, e.g. urine, chemicals, soaps, disinfectants.
- Allergic: idiosyncratic hypersensitivity reaction, e.g. spermicides, semen or its contents (e.g. antibiotics), local anaesthetics, latex, deodorants, fragrances, lubricants, and body lotions containing propylene glycol or glycerin, anti-mycotic creams, or other topical medications.

Erythema, excoriation, pruritus

Thin mucosal skin is more prone to react to contact agents. May become chronic (lichen simplex chronicus) with excoriation producing lichenification and erythema or hyperpigmentation).

Diagnosis

History, appearance, exclude infection. For contact dermatitis patch testing can be considered although positive results are often not relevant. Radio-allergosorbent and skin-prick tests can be performed for suspected Type I immediate hypersensitivity.

Management

Advice on avoiding irritants. If moderate to severe, low-potency topical steroids. If lichenified or failure to respond, moderate-potency topical steroids.

Box 28.1 Genital allergic contact hypersensitivity

- Seminal fluid or its contents (e.g. antibiotics)—often associated with systemic symptoms.
- Spermicides and lubricants (may cause irritant or contact dermatitis).
- Latex or products used in condom manufacturing (e.g. carbamates). Polyurethane is safe.
- Topical skin preparations or chemicals (e.g. steroid preparations, anaesthetics, imidazoles). May cause irritant or allergic contact dermatitis).
- Perfumes and cosmetic preparations:
  - female hygiene sprays or wipes
  - bubble baths, scented soaps, hair shampoos.
- Sanitary pads and towels (may be chemically treated).

Seborrhoeic dermatitis

Scaly inflammation of sebaceous skin. More common with HIV infection. Presents as dry erythema with yellow scale (labia minora, sub-preputial sac, and glans penis).

Diagnosis

Appearance of erythematous lesions covered with greasy yellowish scales at other typical sites (scalp, eyebrows, nasolabial folds, sternum, axillae, umbilicus, natal cleft).

Management

Combined imidazole plus hydrocortisone cream, ketoconazole shampoo (can use as shower gel), low-potency topical steroids and oral itraconazole if severe and extensive.

Fixed drug eruption

Reaction at the same site in an individual to repeated use of a systemic agent. Over 500 drugs implicated including tetracyclines, barbiturates, phenolphthalein (laxative chocolate), sulphonamides, paracetamol. Preferentially affects genitals (especially glans penis). Sudden onset of erythematous macule or bulla with irritation or pain.

Diagnosis

History and appearance.

Management

Stop drug. Spontaneously resolves but may leave hyperpigmentation.

Psoriasis

Affects ~2% of UK population, 30% familial incidence, ↑ severity with HIV infection. Anogenital/perigenital lesions common which may be:
- well-demarcated erythematous scaly papules or plaques. Usually found on skin around genitalia, labia majora, scrotum, penile shaft, and occasionally glans penis.
- flexural—macular erythematous non-scaly moist patches arising in perigenital flexures, peri-anal, labia minora, sub-preputial sac, and glans penis.

Diagnosis

Appearance, lesions in more classic sites (knees, elbows, scalp, nails with pitting), and histology.

Management

Moderate-potency topical corticosteroids, coal tar preparations. Systemic treatment (methotrexate, acitretin, ciclosporin) may be necessary if disease is severe or extensive.

Lichen planus

Polygonal violaceous papules (2–10mm) or annular lesions which may be covered by white streaks (Wickham's striae). Usually found around flexor aspect of wrists but genital involvement common and may cause erosions on mucous epithelium. May lead to scarring with narrowing of introitus. Reticulate network over the buccal mucosa is characteristic. Itchy on skin; may be painful on mucous membranes. Has been associated with the development of squamous cell carcinoma (SCC) of the vulva.

Diagnosis

Appearance, classic sites, and histology showing a band-like lymphohistio-cytic infiltrate in the upper dermis, cytoid bodies, and basal cell hydropic degeneration.

Management

Potent topical corticosteroids. Topical tacrolimus has been shown to be of benefit.

Plasma cell balanitis (of Zoon)

Condition of middle-aged/older uncircumcised men. Moist shiny area of speckled erythema on glans or mucosal aspect of prepuce and often on adjacent surfaces. Half of cases have multiple lesions. Relatively asymptomatic despite striking appearance.

Diagnosis

Histology with heavy plasma cell infiltration; lozenge-shaped keratinocytes.

Management

Topical corticosteroids often combined with antimicrobials, e.g. Trimovate®, Betnovate C®. Persistent cases respond well to circumcision.

Plasma cell vulvitis

Similar histopathological features but more symptomatic; occasionally found in ♀. Clinically resembles erosive lichen planus.

Lichen sclerosus (LS)

Associated with autoimmune conditions especially thyroid abnormalities in women and with trauma (Koebner phenomenon). Anogenital skin involvement common, but may also occur in extragenital sites. May be asymptomatic or cause pruritus, discomfort, and painful intercourse and defaecation.

Although there may be signs of acute inflammation, typical finding is ivory-white appearance associated with atrophy, purpura, erosions, or lichenification. ♂ may develop 2° phimosis and meatal strictures and ♀ labial adhesions with fusion and anal fissuring or stenosis and a loss of clitoral architecture. LS may simulate signs of sexual abuse in pre-pubertal girls, although it has been alleged that abuse may be related to its aetiology through trauma. May also cause phimosis in pre-pubertal boys.

▶ Penile carcinoma rarely reported with LS, but up to 5% ♀ with LS develop SCC of the vulva.

Diagnosis

Histology shows atrophic epidermis, hyalinization of the upper dermis, and a lymphohistiocytic infiltrate.

Management

If active, potent or very potent topical corticosteroids for 3 months then ↓ frequency of application, titrating against response. Topical tacrolimus has been helpful in some cases. Lubricants may help with intercourse. Potassium permanganate soaks are useful for moist inflamed lesions, especially in ♀. Acitretin has been shown to be of benefit, but is rarely necessary. Surgical intervention may be required for urethral stenosis and circumcision for phimosis. Circumcision may be curative in boys.

Hidradenitis suppurativa

Chronic inflammatory disorder of apocrine glands Associated with acne, obesity, familial predisposition. Painful nodules which may progress to abscesses, sinuses, fistulae, and scarring. Found in axillae, groin, buttocks, perianal skin.

Diagnosis

Clinical appearance. Exclude Crohn's disease.

Management

Weight reduction, chlorhexidine wash, topical clindamycin, long-term tetracyclines, and other antibiotics used for acne, local or systemic steroids, and surgery for severe disease. A non-controlled study of oral clindamycin combined with rifampicin showed benefit. Biological drugs including infliximab and etanercept have been used with benefit in severe cases.

Ulcerative conditions

Aphthous ulcers

Common condition of unknown aetiology. Recurrent oral ulcers, rarely genital (especially vulva and scrotum). May be familial. Shallow painful ulcers about 1–10mm in diameter with no systemic symptoms.

Diagnosis

Clinical features. Exclude HSV infection and Behçet's disease.

Management

Local anaesthetic gel, very potent topical steroids (if severe).

Behçet's disease

Multisystem disease of unknown aetiology but more commonly found in the Middle and Far East (Silk Route). Associated with certain HLA types, especially B51.

Diagnosis

Based on defined clinical features according to the International Study Group for Behçet's Disease.

- Recurrent oral ulceration (as aphthosis) at least three times a year and two of the following:
  - genital ulcers (including epididymitis)
  - eye lesions (iritis, uveitis, cells in vitreous on slit-lamp examination, retinal vasculitis)
  - skin lesions (erythema nodosum, folliculitis, or papulopustular lesions, acneiform nodules in post-adolescents not on corticosteroids).
  - positive pathergy test (papule/pustule over 2mm developing at site of hypodermic needle puncture; read at 24–48 hours).
- Neurological (meningoencephalitis, nerve palsies, brainstem, and spinal cord lesions), psychiatric changes, arthritis, thrombophlebitis and gastrointestinal (diarrhoea, abdominal pain) features may appear.

Management

Local topical steroids. Severe disease—systemic steroids, azathioprine, colchicine, dapsone, thalidomide. Anti-TNF therapy shows promise.

Erythema multiforme (EM) and Stevens–Johnson syndrome (SJS)

Acute skin reaction of unknown aetiology but precipitated by infection (e.g. herpes simplex virus, *Mycoplasma pneumoniae, Histoplasma capsulatum*), drugs (e.g. sulfonamides, phenytoin, penicillin), autoimmune diseases (e.g. polyarteritis nodosa), sarcoidosis, malignancy, ↑ frequency of SJS with HIV infection. Non-pruritic maculopapular circular lesions with a deep red centre (may form bullae) and erythema producing target or iris lesions, typically found around the hands and feet. The severe bullous form (SJS) includes orogenital bullae with ulceration, urethritis, conjunctivitis and keratitis, pyrexia, and multisystem disease. Secondary infection and death may occur.

Diagnosis

Clinical features and histopathological changes with necrotic epidermal cells.

Management

EM resolves without scarring in 2–3 weeks. Systemic steroids have been used for severe SJS, but recent studies have suggested that this may increase mortality. The role of IV immunoglobulin is still controversial.

Pyoderma gangrenosum

Associated with many conditions, particularly inflammatory bowel disease, seropositive and seronegative arthritis, and blood dyscrasias. Initial pustule progressing to a painful necrotic ulcer, occasionally affecting the vulva, penis, or scrotum.

Diagnosis

Appearance of ulcer with black undermined edge and associated pathology. Histology usually non-specific.

Management

Treat underlying condition. Topical or systemic corticosteroids, topical tacrolimus, ciclosporin. There are case reports of other immunomodulatory agents and biological drugs including infliximab and adalumimab being of value in treatment.

Pemphigus vulgaris

Most common type of pemphigus. Autoimmune condition. Age group 50–60 years usually affected. Cutaneous lesions appear as flaccid bullae which burst to form painful ulcers. The mucosae, especially the mouth, are commonly involved. Genital ulcers are slow to heal but only occasionally scar. Finger pressure on skin may cause epidermis to separate because of its poor attachment .

Diagnosis

Histology with direct or immunofluorescence to show intercellular deposits of IgG and complement and serology to show circulating anti-epidermal antibodies.

Management

Local or systemic corticosteroids, tetracyclines, immunosuppressants (dapsone, azathioprine, mycophenolate mofetil). Biological drugs, especially rituximab, look promising in refractory cases.

Premalignant conditions

Extra-mammary Paget's disease

Most commonly found around anus and genitals, especially labia majora, typically presenting as well-defined erythematous scaly plaques which may be itchy. May be associated with underlying adnexal carcinoma, possibly of sweat glands. A significant proportion have a primary carcinoma of other organs, particularly rectum, urethra, cervix, or breast.

Diagnosis
Histology shows typical large clear Paget cells in the epidermis

Management
Excision where possible, but recurrence is common as it is often multifocal. Topical imiquimod and photodynamic therapy have been reported to be helpful. Patients should be investigated for other carcinomas as above.

Vulval, penile, and anal intra-epithelial neoplasia (VIN, PIN, AIN)

These pathological descriptive names encompass and replace other terms used to describe dysplasia and squamous cell carcinoma in situ, including Bowen's disease, bowenoid papulosis, and erythroplasia of Queyrat. Intra-epithelial neoplasia (IN) is commonly associated with LS, high-risk HPV infection and ↑ risk of neoplasia elsewhere (e.g. cervical and vaginal IN), and is also found more frequently in those who are immunosuppressed (including with HIV infection). Patients should be screened for HIV infection. The International Society for the Study of Vulvovaginal Diseases regraded VIN and abandoned VIN1, since minimal dysplasia may be insignificant and combined 2 and 3 as usual or differentiated type. Therefore diagnosis is made on histology.

VIN
Usually ♀ aged 30–40 years, 70% current or past cigarette smokers, 50–90% association with HPV (especially type 16). Clinical appearance varies but often presents as white plaques or nodular lesions, which may be pigmented, with multifocal involvement

PIN
Associated with HPV (especially type 16), smoking and possibly agricultural chemicals. High-grade lesions found most commonly in the 6th decade. Usually presents as multiple lesions which may be:
• flat (grey/red, well demarcated with increased vascularity)
• small plaques of leukoplakia (hyperkeratinized)
• papular and pigmented.

In addition, usually in older uncircumcised ♂ there may be mucosal erythroplastic lesions (shiny friable moist red lesions on glans penis or mucosal surface of prepuce).

AIN
Found most commonly in men having sex with men, especially those with HIV infection, and in ♀ with a history of anal sex. Human papilloma virus 16 is associated with anal SCC.

Management of external anogenital IN

There is little evidence-based data on the management of this group of conditions. Current practice depends on the grading and extent of the pathology, influenced by clinical factors such as appearance and symptoms. Patients should be screened for HIV infection. If HIV +ve review should be maintained indefinitely. Grade 3 IN carries a 5–10% risk of subsequent SCC; therefore treatment is usually advised. This includes topical imiquimod, surgical excision, and destructive methods including laser and electrodessication. Review after treatment required as ~30% recur within 5 years.

Malignant conditions

Rarely seen in the GUM clinic but require urgent referral elsewhere.
- SCC: associated with IN and LS.
- Melanoma: rare on penis but genital lesions reported to account for 2–3% of melanomas in ♀.
- Basal cell carcinoma rare on surfaces not commonly exposed to the sun. However, genital lesions have been reported, especially scrotal.

HIV infection

Conditions exacerbated by or found more frequently with HIV infection
- Seborrhoeic dermatitis
- Psoriasis
- Stevens–Johnson syndrome
- Anogenital intra-epithelial neoplasia

Cervical neoplasia

Introduction

The vagina and ectocervix are lined with stratified squamous epithelium and the endocervix with columnar epithelium. The position of the squamo-columnar junction (SCJ) varies throughout life. Hormonal changes in puberty and pregnancy (or the use of hormonal contraception) lead to eversion of the endocervical columnar epithelium, moving the SCJ distally. This is counterbalanced by squamous metaplasia (the normal process of reversion to squamous epithelium). The area between the original and receding SCJ is known as transformation zone (TZ), which is susceptible to malignant change when exposed to oncogenic stimuli, especially high-risk human papilloma virus (HPV).

- *Atypia* Cells in the epithelium show nuclear or cytoplasmic abnormalities not considered to be malignant or premalignant. Koilocytotic atypia or koiloctytosis refers to the presence of cells with a perinuclear halo associated with HPV infection.
- *Cervical intra-epithelial neoplasia (CIN)* Squamous cell premalignant lesion also known as dysplasia. Identified by architectural and cytological changes in the epithelium with the underlying basement membrane intact (essential feature). Three grades of CIN based on the level of epithelial involvement:
  - CIN1—lowest third (mild dysplasia)
  - CIN2—lower two-thirds (moderate dysplasia)
  - CIN3—more than two-thirds (severe dysplasia or carcinoma *in situ*).
- *Cervical glandular intra-epithelial neoplasia (CGIN)* Columnar cell premalignant lesions. Less common than CIN. Identified by nuclear, nucleolar, and gland structure abnormalities. Low-grade (LCGIN) is also known as endocervical gland dysplasia (EGD) and high-grade (HCGIN) as adenocarcinoma *in situ* (AIS).
- *Invasive cervical carcinoma (ICC)* Penetration of the basement membrane by malignant epithelial cells. 85–90% are squamous cell carcinoma (SCC) and the remainder are adeno/adenosquamous.

Epidemiology

Cervical carcinoma is the second most common malignancy in ♀ worldwide. ~80% of cases arise in developing countries (rates 25–45/100,000). Variations between and within countries occur because of differing HPV infection rates, other aetiological factors, and uptake of screening (2%of all ♀ cancers in UK). Most frequently diagnosed in those aged 40–50 years. The reciprocal association between vaginal/anal and cervical SCC demonstrates the multifocal nature of high-risk HPV infection.

Natural history

Untreated, 25–60% of CIN3 will progress to ICC over 20 years, and ~20% of CIN1 and ~30% of CIN2 to higher-grade lesions. 25–50% of CIN1 may regress to normal, especially in younger ♀. Persistence of high-risk HPV infection is associated with progression to CIN2–3 (10–40% in 2 years).

Risk factors

- Infection
  - Human papilloma virus (HPV): high-risk HPV in >99% of SCC (usually 16 (50%) and 18 (20%), also 31, 35, 39, 45, 51, 52, 56, and 58). The relative risk of SCC is ↑ ≥15×. However, the probability of an individual with high-risk HPV developing SCC is <2% with other factors important for malignant transformation. In adeno/adenosquamous carcinoma HPV 18 (50%), 16 (30%).
  - Other genital infections: cervicitis is considered to be a reason for the association between *Chlamydia trachomatis* and CIN3/SCC (2-fold ↑). Conflicting evidence implicating herpes simplex virus 2, *Neisseria gonorrhoeae* and *Trichomonas vaginalis*.
- Sexual activity: age of coitarche is linked to ↑ risk of SCC, e.g. relative risk 2.5 if <18 years compared with >21 years. Risk ↑ by multiple sexual partners e.g. ↑ 14-fold if >5 lifetime partners.
- Parity: incidence of SCC ↑ with parity independent of other risks. Young age at first pregnancy also appears to be a risk marker.
- Male factor: ↑ incidence of CIN and ICC in partners of ♂ with high-risk HPV infection or a history of multiple sexual contacts.
- Smoking: appears to ↑ risk of CIN and SCC.
- Oral contraception: long-term use (>5 years) is associated with ↑ risk of ICC/CIN (3× if >5 and 4× if >10 years).
- Immunosuppression: ↑ risk with immunodeficiency, e.g. HIV infection, Hodgkin's disease, treatment causing immunosuppression.

Condoms offer some protection especially in delaying CIN progression.

Clinical features

- CIN is typically asymptomatic but is important to exclude in those with post-coital bleeding (PCB) or intermenstrual bleeding (IMB).
- ICC diagnosed in up to 4% of ♂ with PCB and 1.5% with post-menopausal bleeding. If symptomatic, it is usually more advanced so signs are generally evident (pronounced cervical contact bleeding, hard, irregular, and enlarged or ulcerated cervix, profuse offensive vaginal discharge) but subtle signs of early stages may be missed.
- In advanced ICC:
  - bimanual and rectal examination may demonstrate a fixed uterus and parametrial/posterior pelvic induration
  - general examination may show hepatosplenomegaly or inguinal/supraclavicular lymph node enlargement.

Screening

Cervical cytology: Papanicolaou smear (Boxes 29.1 and 29.2 and Table 29.1)

Introduced in the 1940s to screen for premalignant exfoliated cervical cells. Adequate sampling of TZ is achieved by visualizing the full circumference of the cervix. If incomplete, it can lead to false-negative results (2–25%). 'Unsatisfactory' results are due to insufficient epithelial cells or presence of blood or pus cells (~10% with slide preparations, <2% using liquid-based cytology).

Exfoliated cells display nuclear and cytoplasmic characteristics which correspond to the underlying pathology. Dyskaryosis is the nuclear abnormality of exfoliated cells, graded as mild, moderate, and severe. This indicates the minimum degree of cin likely to be present as 1, 2, and 3, respectively. Cells suggesting possible invasive carcinoma show coarse chromatin clumps and extensive keratinization with bizarre forms. False-negative results may be found in established icc because of cell necrosis. Closer correlation between cytological and histological findings occurs with higher degrees of abnormality.

▶Cytology laboratories will advise on the correct management and follow-up of abnormal cytology.

High-risk HPV DNA detection

Role in 1° screening unproven although more sensitive than cytology in predicting CIN2/3. Low specificity, especially in those <30 years, because of the high prevalence of transient HPV infection.

Box 29.1 Cervical cytology guidance

A computerized call–recall system is used to invite ♀ who are registered with a GP for screening every 3 years if aged 25–49 and every 5 years if aged 50–64. (♀ aged 65+, only if not screened since age 50 or have had a recent abnormality).

It is important not to commence routine screening below the age of 25 because much of the low-grade abnormality due to high hpv prevalence resolves spontaneously and the rate of cervical carcinoma is extremely low, with cytology screening not having any impact. Screening is best provided in primary care but if taken in gum, arrangements should be made for a copy of the result to go to the patient's GP.

Table 29.1 Cervical cytology—comparison of classifications by British Society for Cervical Cytology (BSCC) and Bethesda system (2001)

BSCC	Bethesda system (2001)
Borderline nuclear changes	Atypical squamous cells of uncertain significance (ASCUS)
Borderline nuclear changes with koilocytosis Mild dyskaryosis	Low-grade squamous intra-epithelial lesion
Moderate dyskaryosis Severe dyskaryosis	High-grade squamous intra-epithelial lesion
Suspected invasive carcinoma	Squamous cell carcinoma
Borderline nuclear changes, endocervical	Atypical glandular cells (endocervical/endometrial/glandular)
Suspected glandular neoplasia (in Scotland 'adenocarcinoma' if invasive adenocarcinoma suggested, otherwise 'glandular neoplasia')	Atypical glandular cells (endocervical/glandular) favour neoplastic
	Endocervical adenocarcinoma *in situ*
	Adenocarcinoma (endocervical, endometrial, extra-uterine, other)

Box 29.2 Cervical cytology technique

- Take cervical smear before cleaning the cervix and taking endocervical swabs for *N.gonorrhoeae* and *C.trachomatis*.
- Note the macroscopic appearance of the cervix. Defer cytology if in menses or there is marked cervicitis.
- Sweep 360° around the cervix, being sure to sample the transitional zone:
  - liquid-based cytology—the end of the sampling brush is rinsed or broken off into the preservative medium
  - alcohol-fixed smear—Aylesbury spatula (if the SCJ is within the endocervical canal, a spatula/endocervical brush combination is recommended).

Diagnosis

CIN

Colposcopy is an essential investigation of cervical premalignancy. Using up to 40× magnification and acetic acid ± iodine, it enables visual grading of CIN and highlights optimal sites for biopsy.

- Cytological indications for colposcopy:
  - ⚠ suspected invasive carcinoma or glandular neoplasia—urgent.
  - moderate/severe dyskaryosis or borderline endocervical changes
  - mild dyskaryosis/borderline nuclear changes—indicated if any repeat cytology at 6, 12, or 24 months is abnormal (if mild dyskaryosis, initial colposcopy rather than repeat cytology may be advised)
  - unsatisfactory/inadequate samples—indicated if three consecutive unsatisfactory smears (3 monthly intervals)
  - any dyskaryosis with a history of CIN.
- Clinical indications for colposcopy/gynaecological assessment:
  - symptoms raising suspicion of carcinoma after excluding infection (e.g. postcoital/intermenstrual bleeding in ♀ >40 years, post-menopausal bleeding).

ICC

- Biopsy, loop, or needle excision depending on appearance.
- For staging:
  - bimanual vaginal and rectal examination under anaesthesia (EUA) with proctoscopy and sigmoidoscopy if rectal spread suspected
  - chest and skeletal radiographs, IV urogram, and barium enema.
- Routine general haematological assessment and other investigations to exclude or gauge metastases, e.g. MRI with a transvaginal coil, lymph node dissection.

Management

CIN

CIN should be managed by accredited colposcopists following clear policies and protocols. Multidisciplinary links are essential. ♀ with CIN should receive clear information and have access to appropriate counselling. Treatment options are as follows.

- Ablation: by cryotherapy (only for small size CIN1) or laser vaporization (unless suspected invasion, glandular disease, SCJ not visualized, or previous treatment for CIN).
- Excision: has largely replaced ablation because of better results, greater applicability, more rapid treatment with less bleeding, and lower cost of equipment.
- Cone biopsy: preferred method for AIS.

Histology report should indicate if any excision is complete. If not, repeat is required. Cytological follow-up is recommended, with repeat colposcopy for abnormal results (at 6 and 12 months followed by annual repeat for 10 years after treatment of CIN2/3 and 2 years after CIN1).

Carcinoma

Histological diagnosis and clinical staging are the basis of treatment deci-sion ranging from cone biopsy to surgery, radiotherapy, and chemo-therapy in various combinations. Age, fertility requirements, and general fitness are individual factors influencing management. 5 year survival rates vary from ~100% (≤3mm micro-invasion) to 5–15% (extension beyond pelvis).

Pregnancy

Routine cervical cytology should be postponed until after delivery, but repeat following a previous abnormality may be taken in mid-trimester. Incidence of ICC is low and pregnancy does not have an adverse impact. Management of CIN (biopsy and treatment) can be deferred until the postpartum period, but colposcopic suggestion of ICC requires urgent biopsy. Treatment of ICC will entail termination or preterm delivery.

Prevention

- Screening prevents ~5000 cases a year in the UK by reducing the lifetime risk of SCC from 1.7% to 0.7%.
- Recently introduced bivalent and quadrivalent vacaccines against types 6, 11, 16, and 18, if given before the onset of sexual activity and exposure to HPV, are expected to prevent ~70% of invasive cervical cancers and ~60% of high-grade CIN. However, the introduction of the immunization programme does not remove the need for cervical screening since there are no data on the long-term efficacy of the vaccines and the epidemiological impact of immunization on the less common oncogenic HPV types and cervical cervical cancer incidence is not known.

HIV and cervical carcinoma

- ↑ high-risk HPV infection and persistence
- ↑ in incidence (>4-fold) of CIN2/3
- Annual cervical cytology recommended
- Colposcopy and biopsy recommended for borderline changes, mild dyskaryosis
- ↑ recurrence of CIN after treatment (which should be by excision)
- Cervical carcinoma is an AIDS-defining condition

Vulval pain syndromes

Introduction

Vulval pain has many causes—inflammatory, infectious, and neoplastic. This chapter describes vulvodynia.

Definition

Vulvodynia is described as 'vulval discomfort, most often described as burning pain, occurring in the absence of relevant visible findings or a specific, clinically identifiable, neurological disorder' (International Society for the Study of Vulval Diseases).

Vulvodynia is classified as follows:
- provoked: pain occurs on touch
- spontaneous: pain can occur at any time
- mixed: occurs on touch, but can also be spontaneous.

It is then divided into;
- local: an isolated area of pain (vestibulodynia)
- generalized: it is more widespread over the vulval area.

Vulvodynia is a clinical diagnosis without identifiable pathology. It is important not to diagnose someone with vulvodynia unless other causes of vulval pain are excluded, or pathology and treatment options may be missed. Descriptions such as vestibulitis and vulval dysthaesia should be avoided as they can lead to confusion.

It is not uncommon for women to have experienced many years of symptoms before a diagnosis is reached. They have often self-treated for candida infection and thought that their symptoms were attributable to other causes such as the menopause. Recognition and appreciation of a defined clinical entity is important and reassures the patient.

Vulvodynia can have a devastating effect—it can affect intimate relationships, and lead to social isolation and depression. Both the physical pain and the psychosocial consequences of the pain need management.

Aetiology

About 50% will have a trigger factor, e.g. childbirth, chronic candida infection, major stressful life event. The remaining cases develop gradually with no identifiable provoking factor.

Several aetiological factors have been proposed including pelvic muscle floor hypertonicity, genetic factors, bacterial inflammatory processes, and altered CNS function. It is likely to be multifactorial.

Clinical features

Neuralgic type vulval discomfort characterized usually by burning, stinging, irritation, rawness. Symptoms may be hyperaesthetic (exaggerated) or described as allodynia (when sensation different to that applied). Symptoms worsen while sitting and towards the end of the day for those with spontaneous pain. Associated with intolerance of tampon insertion because of local pain. Those with localized pain, symptoms confined to a specific area of the vaginal vestibule (usually 3–9 o'clock) with pain on touch or attempted vaginal entry (superficial dyspareunia).

Management

Management should be a team approach. Involve the GP, women's physiotherapist, psychosexual therapist (if relevant), and pain team in addition to the vulval specialist.

History-taking

- Explore the site and extent of pain, psychosexual and relationship issues, and possible features of depression
- Ask the patient what the pain prevents them from doing
- Ask the patient to scale the pain from 0 to 10 (10 is the worst pain imaginable)
- Check if pain is provoked by sitting and relieved by standing, which can be a sign of pudendal neuralgia (refer to pain team for assessment and pudendal nerve block)

Examination and investigations

No visible signs usually, but can be associated with varying degree of erythema. However, a light touch with a cotton bud can produce pain. This can be useful to map out the area of pain experienced and determine whether it is local or generalized.

- Exclude other causes: do a full STI screen for chlamydia, gonorrhoea, trichomonas, and candida, and microscopy. Some women will not be able to tolerate speculum examination, so self-taken swabs may be required.
- Look at the vulval skin for signs of genital dermatological conditions.
- In cases of diagnostic uncertainty, a biopsy or a second opinion may be helpful.
- Pelvic MRI for unprovoked pain is not routinely recommended.

Patient information

- Establish the diagnosis. If it is uncertain, refer to 'vulval pain of unknown cause' until diagnosis is clear.
- Provide verbal and written advice on vulvodynia.
- Give details of Vulval Pain Society for further information and telephone advice (℡ www.vulvalpainsociety.org.uk).
- Advise correspondence with her GP because of the many emotional and psychological consequences.
- Provide leaflet *Smears without Tears* available from Vulval Pain Society website.
- Avoid skin allergens and advise washing with a soap substitute such as aqueous cream.
- Advise those who experience pain on sitting to purchase a doughnut-shaped cushion.

Topical treatment

- Lidocaine ointment or gel can be used for those with provoked pain prior to sex (apply 15 minutes beforehand and advise condoms to prevent transfer to the partner—however, lidocaine will erode condoms so check family planning method). It can also be used by those with spontaneous pain for temporary relief or if they have a social engagement etc.
- A trial of topical steroids can be beneficial—although irritancy can be a problem in some.

Oral treatment

- Useful for managing unprovoked pain. Evidence for provoked pain less clear.
- Tricyclic antidepressants: amitriptyline 10mg/day gradually increasing to 75–100mg/day for 3–6 months (47% improved in one study).
- Anticonvulsants: gabapentin 300mg daily building up to four times daily for up to 3 months. Data limited but >80% response reported. Pregabalin can also be used. These can be used instead of or in addition to tricyclics.
- Carbamazepine has also been advocated.

Physiotherapy

- Good evidence for provoked pain, but not for unprovoked pain. Use biofeedback technique to help relax pelvic floor to lessen pain (sensor is placed in vagina and contraction results in light change or computer image).
- Massage and vaginal trainers can also be used.
- 70% of women have complete response or notice improvement.

Clinical psychology

- Can use cognitive behavioral therapy and teach pain coping mechanisms.

Psychosexual therapy

- Ideally with their partner. Can help with secondary complications (e.g. vaginismus, loss of libido, anorgasmia, poor lubrication) and improving non-coital sexual contact.

Surgery

- Can be used for local provoked pain if other methods have failed.
- Modified vestibulectomy works best, with 90% having complete or partial response.
- Vestibuloplasty and laser vaporization are not recommended.
- Surgery works best when combined with clinical psychology and psychosexual therapy pre- and postoperatively.

Other treatments
- Reduce urinary oxalate concentration—low oxalate diet and calcium citrate without vitamin D. Evidence lacking, but some patients find helpful.
- Apply white soft paraffin over vulva for swimming.
- Antihistamines—if patient has dermographism.
- Acupuncture—some women with unprovoked pain have had benefit.
- Botox® injection into affected areas—to date use is limited but looks promising.
- Massage affected skin with vibrator (acts like a local TENS machine).

Prognosis

Partial relief of symptoms occurs in 40–50% of cases (regardless of approach) and 50% improve spontaneously within a year of diagnosis. If triggered by an infection, prognosis is better.

Streptococcal and staphylococcal infections

Streptococcal infections

Group A: Streptococcus pyogenes
- Unusual cause of acute purulent vaginitis, generally related to obstetric or other trauma. May lead to necrotizing fasciitis.
- Recognized cause of acute vaginitis in pre-pubertal girls.
- May rarely cause balanitis (e.g. pyoderma following fellatio).

Management

Simple infections pending antibiotic sensitivities:
- phenoxymethylpenicillin (penicillin V) 500mg 4 times daily for 7–10 days.

Group B β-haemolytic streptococci (GBS): *Streptococcus agalactiae*

Found in 12–37% of ♀ attending GUM clinics. Usually not pathogenic (except in pregnancy) but associated with bacterial vaginosis.

Pregnancy

Carriage rate is 6–28%. Intra-amniotic infection and postpartum endometritis if heavily colonized. ~35% of babies of carriers become colonized, with ~1% developing invasive neonatal infection with an incidence of 1 in 2000 births. GBS is the most frequent cause of any severe infection in infants aged <7 days. Septicaemia, meningitis, pulmonary infection, and shock may follow in up to 50% of infected infants with a mortality of 6% if full term and 18% if preterm.

Risk factors for neonatal infection are:
- labour <37 weeks
- prolonged rupture of membranes (PROM) >18 hours
- intrapartum pyrexia
- GBS bacteriuria in current pregnancy
- previous infant with GBS.

In the UK, women identified with these risk factors are offered intrapartum antibiotics to prevent neonatal infection (Box 31.1). Recommended regimen is iv benzyl penicillin 3g (5mu) at onset of labour, then 1.5g (2.5mu) 4 hourly until delivery. Clindamycin 900mg should be given iv 8 hourly to those allergic to penicillin.

Practice varies worldwide, e.g. US guidelines recommend that all women are screened (vaginal/rectal swabs) at 35–37 weeks for GBS and prophylactic intrapartum antibiotics offered to those testing positive (or not tested). This results in 30-50% of women receiving IV prophylactic antibiotics during labour. Risk-factor-based approach is estimated to ↓ early onset of GBS disease of the neonate by 50–69%, while prophylaxis based on routine swabs may ↓ it by 86%.

Men

Urethral colonization in 38–46% of ♂ attending GUM clinics. GBS may cause balanitis, usually mild but rarely progressing to cellulitis. GBS also occasionally implicated in balanitis.

Box 31.1 Current recommendations by the Royal College of Obstetricians and Gynaecologists (UK) for prevention of neonatal GBS

- Intrapartum prophylaxis should be offered to those ♀ with risk factors.
- Intrapartum prophylaxis is not indicated if GBS carriage was detected in a previous pregnancy.
- Routine screening for antenatal GBS carriage is not recommended.
- Intrapartum antibiotic prophylaxis should be considered if GBS is incidentally detected in a vaginal/rectal swab. However, treatment before labour is not recommended (recolonization likely).

Staphylococcus aureus

Vaginal carriage rate is ~10%.

- Folliculitis.
- Local genital or peri-genital infection, including abscesses, especially in traumatized skin (e.g. excoriation with scabies). Cases of community-associated meticillin-resistant *Staph. aureus* (MRSA) infections transmitted heterosexually have been reported, presenting as abscesses or folliculitis involving the pubic, vaginal, or perineal region. These have been documented without any evidence of nasal colonization in 75% of people with active genital/peri-genital infection or colonization.
- Toxic shock syndrome. Caused by an exotoxin produced by phage group 1 *Staph. aureus* colonizing the vagina. It usually arises midway through menstruation and is associated with super-absorbent tampons (now discontinued), infrequent tampon change, or rarely the use of the contraceptive diaphragm. Typically sudden onset of sore throat, pyrexia, headache, myalgia, vomiting, diarrhoea, abdominal pain, and vaginal irritation, followed by a generalized rash, inflammation of oral and vaginal mucosae, vasoconstriction, hypotension, and shock. Skin desquamation and necrosis are common sequelae. Tampons should be changed regularly and diaphragms should not be left in situ for longer than the contraceptive needs dictate.

Management

- Simple infections pending antibiotic sensitivities: flucloxacillin 250–500mg 4 times daily for 5 days.
- Toxic shock syndrome: supportive treatment (for shock), removal of retained tampon or diaphragm, and treatment with high-dose anti-biotics.

Genital anomalies

Men

Epispadias Absence of upper wall of urethra. Frequency ~1 in 30,000. Urethra opens onto the dorsum of the glans penis or penile shaft as an epithelial-lined groove.

Hypospadias Termination of urethra ventral and posterior to its normal opening. Frequency 1 in 160–1800. Orifice found anywhere from the usual site (with backward extension) to the perineum. Often associated with other local anomalies (e.g. redundant prepuce, absent frenum, meatal stenosis).

Lymphocele Non-tender cord-like firm swelling in coronal sulcus. Probably related to sexual trauma (prolonged or frequent intercourse). May be associated with preputial oedema. Self-limiting (usually within days, up to 3 weeks); just requires reassurance.

Paraphimosis Strangulation of the glans penis by retracted prepuce. Usually results from partially phimotic prepuce which has been retracted and cannot be reduced. However, may follow trauma with swelling of the glans (e.g. from vigorous sexual activity) with a retracted normal calibre prepuce. Requires urgent intervention either by manual reduction (using anaesthetic cream and ice to reduce oedema) or by surgical intervention to prevent 2° infection and gangrene.

Peyronie's disease Fibrous infiltration of the penile intracavernous septum. Leads to plaque formation, causing curvature and angulation of the erect penis. Cause unknown but associated with trauma, diabetes mellitus, and Dupuytren's contracture. Medical treatments with proven control-matched benefit include intralesional collagenase, verapamil, interferon, and oral acetyl/propionyl-L-carnitine, colchicine. There are no data to support the use of vitamin E, para-aminobenzoate, intralesional corticosteroids, or laser therapy. If severe, the plaque can be removed surgically (but reduction in penile length).

Phimosis Tight constriction of the prepuce preventing retraction over the glans penis. Aetiology includes the following.
- Congenital (physiological in 1st year of life).
- Acute: 2° to underlying infection, e.g. syphilis (sub-preputial chancre), genital herpes, candidiasis.
- Chronic and progressive: 2° to repeated trauma (physical, chemical, repeated infections), skin disorders (e.g. lichen sclerosis), local malignancy.

Surgical referral for circumcision may be required.

Priapism Pathologically prolonged erection without libido. May be associated with blood disorders (e.g. sickle-cell disease, leukaemia), drugs used to manage erectile dysfunction, and rarely infection (e.g. gonorrhoea). ▶Failure to achieve detumescence using ice packs requires urgent urological referral.

Spermatoceles and epididymal cysts Commonly detected as incidental findings or raised by concerned patient, especially those aged >40 years. Usually <1cm in diameter and filled with spermatozoa (spermatoceles) or serum (epididymal cysts); therefore they transilluminate well. They arise from the epididymis (not testis) and generally reassurance can be given. If large or painful, they can be aspirated by needle, but surgical removal is not advised as there is a risk of sterility. Ultrasonography is recommended for intrascrotal lumps or swellings where malignancy is considered.

Urethral channels (accessory) Open dorsal or ventral to urethra and are usually rudimentary blind tracts, although they may terminate in bladder or posterior urethra. Accessory peri-urethral ducts are commonly found in ♂ opening into or around the meatus and are blind tracts extending from 2 to 10mm.

Varicocele Dilatation and tortuosity of the veins of the scrotal pampini-form plexus (along the spermatic cord). 10–17% of young ♂ affected, with spontaneous regression common. Swollen veins within the scrotum are bluish and feel like a 'bag of worms'. Most commonly diagnosed because of sterility in ♂ but ~67% of ♂ with varicoceles are fertile. Generally no treatment is required, although further assessment and surgical intervention should be considered if clinically apparent and concerns about infertility.

Women

Bartholin gland cyst and abscess Cysts arise following obstruction of the drainage duct, whereas abscesses are caused by local pathogens, most commonly *Neisseria gonorrhoeae* (up to 80% of abscesses) but also *Chlamydia trachomatis*, staphylococci, streptococci, and Gram-negative enteric bacteria. Found most commonly in ♀ aged 20–29 years with abscesses occurring about 3× as commonly as cysts. Most small abscesses respond well to appropriate antibiotics, although needle aspiration may be required. Chronic or recurrent cysts may require duct catheterization or marsupialization. In ♀ >40 years cyst edges should be examined histologically to exclude carcinoma. Recurrences may occur in up to 20%.

Cervical polyp Often an incidental finding during routine examination but may present with post-coital or intermenstrual bleeding. Red fleshy cervical projections, ~1–2cm long, containing both squamous and columnar cell epithelium. Found more commonly in multiparous ♀ >20 years, and may be associated with chronic local inflammation. 1.7% are malignant and 27% are associated with an endometrial polyp. Usually removed by gently twisting the base (which should be sent for histology to exclude malignancy). Excision with basal electrocautery or laser vaporization may be required for larger lesions.

Developmental anomalies Seen uncommonly in ♀ at GUM clinics. Epispadias is rare and usually severe; diagnosed in childhood. Abnormalities in vaginal development, unless minor, are likely to present at a younger age, including puberty if the menstrual flow is impeded (e.g. atresia or septal obstruction). It is estimated that vaginal malformations arise in 1/4000–10,000 ♀ births. Septa may be seen which are vertical (transverse) or lateral (longitudinal).

Vertical defects May be found anywhere along the length of the vagina. Usually present in the teens with cryptomenorrhoea, cyclical abdominal pain, and haematocolpos. Partial vertical septa may be seen as an incidental finding but can obscure the cervix and may cause dyspaerunia.

Lateral fusion disorders More common and often asymptomatic. The septum may create two vaginal passages (one usually larger) leading to a didelphic uterus with twin uterine cavities and cervices opening to each vagina. Important to sample both cervices when screening.

Female genital mutilation (fgm) or circumcision Illegal in the UK. It is estimated that 74,000 first-generation immigrant ♀ have undergone FGM, especially those from Africa, north of the equator excluding Arabic speaking countries other than Egypt. Although associated with some Muslim communities, it is not exclusively linked with Islam.

There are three forms of FGM.
- 'Clitoridectomy'—partial or complete removal of the clitoris.
- 'Excision'—removal of both the clitoris and labia minora.
- 'Infibulation' (pharaonic circumcision)—as above with stitching of raw labial surfaces to produce a small hole to allow urine and menses to escape. Found in ~15% of circumcised ♀.

Contraception including contraception in HIV infection and infection reduction

Introduction

Despite the availability of wide variety of contraceptive methods termination of pregnancy (TOP) rates remain high (UK data: 1 in 3 ♀ have TOP with a third having a repeat). Annually >200,000 TOPs are performed in England and Wales. At least 60% of these ♀ report having used a contraceptive method at the time of conception, usually oral contraceptives or condoms which require correct and consistent use. Table 33.1 compares failure rates for pills, condoms, and natural methods with typical and perfect use. At the first contraceptive consultation the healthcare professional (HCP) should:

- Consider the importance of efficacy and reversibility (is an unplanned pregnancy acceptable?).
- Find out if there is a particular interest in a contraceptive method?
- Take a comprehensive medical and sexual history. Dysmenorrhoea or heavy menstrual loss may indicate that a combined hormonal method, an injectable method, or a levonorgestrel intra-uterine system (IUS) would be ideal, offering therapeutic benefits.
- Dispel any contraceptive myths, e.g. the Pill makes you put on weight, injectables cause infertility, intra-uterine devices (IUDs) give you infections.
- Address the ♀'s worries and concerns and explore why any previous contraceptive methods have been discontinued
- Discuss all options, focusing on lasting and reliable contraceptive methods (LARCs).
- Explain how individual methods work, the advantages of each method, how to use the method, and any nuisance side-effects which may occur and how they may be resolved.
- Provide accurate and up-to-date advice, including information on help lines and follow-up appointments.

Table 33.1 Summary table of contraceptive efficacy

Method	% ♀ having unintended pregnancy within 1st year of use		% ♀ continuing use at 1 year[‡]
	Typical use*	Perfect use[†]	
No method	85	85	–
Spermicides	29	18	42
Withdrawal	27	4	43
Ovulation awareness	25	3	51
Sponge—parous ♀	32	20	46
Sponge—nulliparous ♀	16	9	57
Diaphragm	16	6	57
Condom—♀	21	5	49
Condom—♂	15	2	53
Combined and progestogen-only pill	8	0.3	68
Evra® patch (transdermal combined hormone)	8	0.3	68
NuvaRing® (vaginal combined hormone)	8	0.3	68
Depo-Provera®	3	0.3	56
Intra-uterine T380A (copper T)	0.8	0.6	78
Intra-uterine (LNG-IUS)Mirena® system	0.2	0.2	80
Implanon®	0.05	0.05	84
♀ sterilization	0.5	0.5	100
♂ sterilization	0.15	0.1	100

*Among *typical* couples who initiate use of a method (not necessarily for the first time), the percentage who experience an accidental pregnancy during the first year if they do not stop use for any other reason.

[†]Among couples who initiate use of a method (not necessarily for the first time) and who use it *perfectly* (both consistently and correctly), the percentage who experience an accidental pregnancy during the first year if they do not stop use for any other reason.

[‡]Among couples attempting to avoid pregnancy, the percentage who continue to use a method for 1 year.

Source: Trussell J (2007). Contraceptive efficacy. In Hatcher RA, Trussell J, Nelson AL, Cates W, Stewart FH, Kowal D. *Contraceptive Technology: Nineteenth Revised Edition*. Ardent Media, New York.

Combined hormonal contraceptives (CHCs) including the combined pill, vaginal ring, and patch

CHCs are highly effective and quickly reversible with failure rates of <1% per year when taken consistently and correctly (Table 33.1). ~3 million ♀ (18% of all in their reproductive years) in the UK take combined oral contraception (COC). >90% of sexually active ♀ have used the pill by the time they reach 30. COC is suitable from menarche to menopause if no contraindicating risk factors or coexisting illnesses are identified.

Mechanism of action

- Inhibit ovulation
- Alter cervical mucus, inhibiting spermatozoa penetration
- Produce characteristic changes in the endometrium preventing implantation of the blastocyst
- Modify sperm function and motility

Advantages of combined hormonal contraceptives

- Effective, reversible, convenient, non-intercourse related.
- Under the user's control.
- Regulates and ↓ menstrual loss, thereby improving iron-deficiency anaemia.
- ↓ dysmenorrhoea and relieves ovulation pain.
- May help premenstrual symptoms.
- May improve acne.
- Helps protect against ectopic pregnancies as it inhibits ovulation.
- ↓ incidence of benign breast disease.
- Long-term users are less likely to develop fibroids and functional ovarian cysts.
- Protects against pelvic inflammatory disease (PID) and ↓ the risk of hospitalization for the disease.
- ↓ incidence of endometriosis and a useful treatment and maintenance therapy for sufferers.
- Possible ↓ in the risk of developing rheumatoid arthritis.
- ↓ risk of ovarian cancer by about 50% even with low-dose COC. This protection ↑ with duration of use (5% ↓ with each additional year of use) lasting up to 30 years after the CHC is discontinued.
- Protects against endometrial cancer by about 50%, continuing for at least 15 years after the CHC is stopped.
- ↓ incidence of large bowel cancer by up to 40%.

Disadvantages of combined hormonal contraceptives

- Require correct and consistent use to be effective.
- Side-effects may occur in the first few months, e.g. headaches, breast tenderness, breakthrough bleeding (although these tend to resolve quickly).
- Patches may cause a local skin reaction in up to 20% of users with 2-3% discontinuing for this reason. 5–14% of ♀ using the vaginal ring complain of vaginitis.
- Potential drug interactions decrease the efficacy of these methods, e.g. use of liver-enzyme-inducing agents, broad-spectrum antibiotics.
- No protection against sexual transmitted infections (STIs).
- May be associated with ↑ risk of breast cancer. The re-analysis data published in 1996 reported that current COC use ↑ the risk of developing breast cancer by 24% but this fell back to background level 10 years or more after discontinuing the pill. However, four recently published studies have found no ↑ risk.
- After 5 years of use there may be ↑ incidence of cervical intra-epithelial neoplasia and cancer of the cervix. COC appears to be a cofactor leading to persistence or repeated replication of oncogenic human papilloma virus. Regular cervical screening as indicated by the NHS Cervical Screening Programme should be advised.
- Very small ↑ in the risk of myocardial infarction (MI) in non-smoking low-risk ♀. However the risk may ↑ up to 20-fold in heavy smokers.
- Possible small ↑ (up to 2-fold) in the risk of ischaemic stroke in users, with about 3 ischaemic strokes occurring in 100,000 ♀ under 35 each year. Risk factors include hypertension, smoking, diabetes, and family history of stroke. No ↑ in the risk of haemorrhagic stroke in low-risk non-smoking ♀ with normal blood pressure.
- ↑ risk of venous thromboembolism (VTE) with recent evidence suggesting a further additional risk for patch users. Background risk of VTE in young ♀ is now thought to be about 44 per 100,000 ♀ each year and 90 per 100,000 in low-dose pill takers. Only ~1% of these ♀ die as a result of this event. Increasing age, obesity, surgery, family history of VTE, and immobility ↑ risk of developing a VTE.

Choice of CHC

Although all CHCs have the same mode of contraceptive action and similar efficacy they may have different side-effects or benefits (e.g. less breakthrough bleeding or an improvement in acne). The first pill prescribed should be effective, suit the majority of ♀, have a proven safety record and be inexpensive. A monophasic 30mcg levonorgestrel pill (Microgynon30® or Ovranette®) fulfils these criteria. 40% of ♀ may complain of side-effects or perceived associated problems and request a change.

Combined hormonal contraceptive transdermal patch (Evra®) and vaginal ring (NuvaRing®)

These longer-acting combined methods avoid daily pill taking but have a similar efficacy as COC. Both give a regular monthly withdrawal bleed and are advantageous in ♀ who cannot remember to take a daily pill or who have gastrointestinal problems affecting pill absorption. The patch needs changing every 7 days with a patch-free week every 4th week. The vaginal ring is worn for 3 out of every 4 weeks. Minor and potentially serious, but rare, side-effects are similar to those with COC.

Pill choice
- *First choice*: 30mcg levonorgestrel, monophasic preparation (Microgynon30® or Ovranette®).
- To control poor cycle: 30mcg gestodene or 35mcg norgestimate pill or vaginal ring once pathology, drug interaction, or poor compliance are excluded (Femodene®, Cilest®, NuvaRing®).
- *Oestrogen side-effects* include headaches, nausea, breast tenderness or leg cramps:
  - ↓ the dose of oestrogen to a pill containing 20mcg ethinyl oestradiol (Femodette®, Loestrin20®, Mercilon®) or oestradiol (Qlaira®), or change to a progestogen-only pill.
- *Progestogen side-effects* include mood change, bloating, and greasy skin.
  - Change the progestogen in the pill. Cyproterone acetate and drospirenone in COCs are useful in ♀ with acne (Dianette®, Yasmin®).

Starting regimens for combined hormonal contraceptives

Circumstances	Start when?	Extra precautions for 7 days?
Quick start	At any time if it is reasonably certain not pregnant	Yes
Menstruating	Up to and including day 5	No
	After day 5	Yes
Amenorrhoeic	At any time if it is reasonably certain not pregnant	Yes
Post-abortion or miscarriage	Within 5 days	No
	After 5 days	Yes
Postpartum		
Not breast-feeding	Until day 21 postpartum	No
	From day 22 onwards	Yes
Breastfeeding	If > 6 months and amenorrhoeic, treat like other amenorrhoeic ♀	Yes
	If >6 months and menstruating, treat like other menstruating ♀	No

Circumstances	Start when?	Extra precautions for 7 days?
Switching from other hormonal methods (other than IUS)	Immediate start	No
	If previous method was DMPA, switch when next injection is due	No
Switching from a non-hormonal method (other than IUD)	Up to and including day 5 of cycle	No
	After day 5	Yes
Switching from an IUD or IUS	Start up to and including day 5 of cycle. IUD/IUS can be removed at the same time	No
	CHC can be started at any other time, if it is reasonably certain she is not pregnant	
	If she has been sexually active	Start CHC and then remove IUD/IUS at next period or after 7 days
	If she has not been sexually active	Start CHC and then remove IUD/IUS after 7 days or at next period
	If she is amenorrhoeic or has irregular bleeds	Start CHC. If unprotected sexual intercourse (UPSI) has occurred in preceding 7 days advise IUD/IUS removal 7 days after pill start.

Missed pill rules for COCs containing ethinyl oestradiol (as per COC packet insert)

- If missed a pill <12 hours:
  - take forgotten pill, take next pill when due.
- If missed a pill/pills >12 hours:
  - take forgotten last pill
  - take next pill when due
  - use a condom for 7 days
  - if pill-free interval in next 7 days do not stop pills, but start new packet straight away.

Progestogen-only pill (POP)

Taken by ~6% of ♀ in the UK. It is very effective when taken properly with quoted failure rates of 1%.

Mechanism of action

- Ovulation may be suppressed in 15–40% of cycles by POPs containing levonorgestrel, norethisterone, or etynodiol diacetate, but in 97–99% by those containing desogestrel.
- All POPs alter the cervical mucus to reduce sperm penetration.
- POPs induce changes in the endometrium to prevent sperm survival and implantation of the blastocyst.
- Sperm motility and function is affected, preventing fertilization.

Cervical mucus effect peaks within 2–3 hours of oral ingestion and then slowly wanes. Desogestrel-containing POPs differ from more traditional POPs in that no extra contraceptive cover is required until 12 hours after a missed pill compared with 3 hours for other POPs.

POPs have frequently been restricted to ♀ who are breastfeeding or who have contraindications to taking synthetic oestrogen. However, users from all age groups may be interested in taking a POP, particularly if the 'forgiveness window' is similar to that of a combined pill.

Advantages of progestogen-only pills

- Non-intercourse-related contraceptive.
- Simple and convenient to use.
- POPs are safe for ♀ who are breastfeeding.
- Ideal for ♀ who suffer from oestrogenic side-effects when using CHCs, e.g. breast tenderness, headaches, fluid retention, or nausea.
- Suitable for ♀ over 35 years who smoke.
- Can be used in grossly obese ♀ with no dose adjustment for those taking a desogestrel POP.
- Can be taken by ♀ with medical illnesses contraindicating the use of synthetic oestrogen, e.g. those with hypertension, migraine with focal aura, or a previous personal history of VTE.
- No evidence of ↑ risk of cardiovascular disease, thromboembolism, or stroke
- Minimal alteration in carbohydrate and lipid metabolism. Therefore they are ideal for diabetics even with neuropathic or nephropathic complications.

Disadvantages of progestogen-only pills

- POPs, excluding the desogestrel POP, are thought to be less effective than combined pills in practice as they are very reliant on regular pill taking.
- May cause nuisance side-effects such as breast tenderness, mood changes, headaches, and acne.
- Possible ↑ in ectopic pregnancy in the event of POP failure.
- Can alter ovulation, thereby disrupting the menstrual bleeding pattern, with users reporting ↑ in spotting, breakthrough bleeding, and amenorrhoea
- Functional ovarian cysts may develop in a small number of women. However, these tend to be transient and rarely require surgical intervention.

Starting regimens for progestogen-only pills

Circumstances	Start when?	Extra precautions for 48h
Quick start	Any time if it is reasonably certain that she is not pregnant	Yes
Menstruating	Up to and including day 5	No
	After day 5 of the cycle	Yes
Amenorrhoeic	Any time if it is reasonably certain that she is not pregnant	Yes
Post-abortion or miscarriage	Within 5 days	No
	After 5 days	Yes
Postpartum		
Breastfeeding or bottle-feeding	Day 21 postpartum	No
	From day 22 onwards	Yes
Switching from other hormonal methods (other than IUS)	Immediate start	No
	If previous method was DMPA, switch when next injection is due	No
Switching from a non-hormonal method (other than IUD)	Up to and including day 5	No
	After day 5	Yes
Switching from an IUD or IUS	Start up to and including day 5 of cycle. IUD/IUS can be removed at the same time	No
	POP can be started at any other time, if it is reasonably certain she is not pregnant:	
	If she has been sexually active	Start POP and then remove IUD/IUS at the next period or after 48h
	If she has not been sexually active	Start POP and then remove IUD/IUS after 48h or at the next period
	If she is amenorrhoeic or has irregular bleeds	Start POP. If UPSI has occurred in preceding 7 days advise IUD/IUS removal 48h after pill start

Missed pill rules for POP
- If missed traditional POP by <3 hours or desogestrel POP by <12 hours:
  - take forgotten pill and take next tablet when due.
- If missed traditional POP by >3 hours or desogestrel POP by >12 hours:
  - take last forgotten pill and next pill when due, and use condoms for 2 days.

Injectable contraception

Injectables are highly effective and have a safety record that spans 40 years. Intramuscular progestogen-only depot providing contraceptive cover for 2–3 months was one of the first long-acting hormonal preparations to be used. Progestogen-only injectables are used by ~3% of ♀ in the UK, and >20 million ♀ worldwide in over 130 countries have used it.

Two injectable contraceptive methods are available in the UK:
- Depo-Provera® (depot medroxyprogesterone acetate (DMPA)) given every 12 weeks
- Noristerat® (norethisterone oenanthate (NET-EN)) given every 8 weeks (used infrequently in the UK for short-term interim contraception).

A significant number of ♀ fail to return for their second DMPA. Prolonged/erratic bleeding is often cited as a reason for discontinuation. Pre-injection counselling, giving a realistic picture of potential side-effects in the first few injection cycles, is important.

Mechanism of action
- DMPA and NET-EN inhibit ovulation by suppressing luteinizing hormone (LH) and, to a certain extent, follicle-stimulating hormone (FSH).
- Injectables alter the cervical mucus, inhibiting spermatozoa penetration.
- Injectables prevent implantation by inducing endometrial atrophy.
- Like other progestogens, injectables modify sperm function and motility.

Advantages of progestogen-only injectables
- Very effective, reversible, and discreet method of contraception with little dependence on the user.
- Non-intercourse-related contraceptive method.
- Very safe with no reported attributable deaths.
- Safe for breastfeeding mothers.
- Helpful for ♀ with premenstrual symptoms, ovulation pain, and painful heavy periods.
- Can be used in ♀ with sickle cell disease, with evidence suggesting a ↓ in crises
- Possesses most of the non-contraceptive benefits of CHCs, including protection against PID, extra-uterine pregnancies, endometriosis, functional ovarian cysts, and fibroid formation, and a 5-fold ↓ in the risk of endometrial cancer.
- Minimal metabolic effects occur, with recent research reporting no ↑ in the risk of acute myocardial infarction, venous thrombo-embolism, or stroke.

Disadvantages of progestogen-only injectables

- Irregular prolonged vaginal bleeding/amenorrhoea. ~1/3rd experience prolonged bleeding (>10 days) after receiving their first injection, but 55% and 68% are amenorrhoeic by 1 year and 2 years, respectively.
- Intramuscular—therefore cannot be removed if side-effects occur.
- Weight gain is commonly reported (up to 2kg in the first year).
- Some may complain of progestogenic side-effects including mood changes, lassitude, loss of libido, bloating, and breast tenderness.
- Causes a short delay in the return to normal fertility with the mean time to ovulation being 5.3 months after the last injection.
- DMPA may adversely affect bone mineral density (BMD) but there are no good data suggesting that it causes osteoporosis or bone fracture. Present data suggest that BMD at the lumbar spine and femoral neck are ↓ in DMPA users compared with controls. BMD recovers to a similar level to never-users on discontinuation of DMPA (usually 3–5 years in adults and ~1 year if <18 years).
- Committee on Safety of Medicines advice:
  - In adolescents, DMPA may be used as first-line contraception but only after other methods have been discussed with the patient and considered to be unsuitable or unacceptable.
  - In all ages, careful re-evaluation of the risks and benefits of treatment should be carried out in those who wish to continue use for >2 years.
  - If significant lifestyle and/or medical risk factors for osteoporosis, other methods of contraception should be considered.
- There is no evidence that routinely giving 'add-back' oestrogen to DMPA users or additional investigations are warranted.

Starting regimens for injectable contraceptives

Circumstances	Start when?	Extra precautions for 7 days?
Quick start	At any time if it is reasonably certain that she is not pregnant	Yes
Menstruating	Up to and including day 5	No
	After day 5 of the cycle	Yes
Amenorrhoeic	Any time if it is reasonably certain that she is not pregnant	Yes
Post-abortion or miscarriage	Within 5 days	No
	After 5 days	Yes
Postpartum		
Breastfeeding or bottle-feeding	Day 21 postpartum but standard practice is to delay 1st injection until week 6 to reduce the incidence of prolonged bleeding	No
	From day 22 onwards	Yes
Switching from other hormonal methods (other than IUS)	Immediate start	No
Switching from a non-hormonal method (other than IUD)	Up to and including day 5	No
	After day 5	Yes

Circumstances	Start when?	Extra precautions for 7 days?
Switching from an IUD or IUS	Give the injection up to and including day 5 of cycle. IUD/IUS can be removed at the same time	No
	Injectables can be given at any other time, if it is reasonably certain she is not pregnant	
	If she has been sexually active	Give the injection and then remove IUD/IUS at the next period or after 7 days
	If she has not been sexually active	Give the injection and then remove IUD/IUS after 7 days or at the next period
	If she is amenorrhoeic or has irregular bleeds	Give the injection. If UPSI has occurred in preceding 7 days advise IUD/IUS removal 7 days after the injection

Contraceptive implant

A contraceptive implant offers an alternative way of delivering hormones providing long-acting low-dose reversible contraception. Norplant®, the levonorgestrel implant, was available in the UK from 1993 until 1999. It consists of 6 rods inserted subdermally ~8–10cm above the elbow on the inner aspect of the non-dominant arm. It is licensed to provide contraception over a 5-year period. UK healthcare professionals may see ♀ from sub-Saharan Africa using this multi-rod contraceptive system or the two-rod system called Jadelle®.

Implanon®, containing a single rod of 68mg etonogestrel (the active metabolite of desogestrel), was launched in 1999. It is used by 2% of ♀ in the UK and licensed to provide contraception for 3 years. It is one of the most effective contraceptives with recent method failure rates quoted as 0.01 per 100 implants. Approximately 3 million implants have been fitted worldwide.

Mechanism of action

- Etonogestrel inhibits ovulation by suppressing LH. However, up to 5% of users may ovulate in the third year.
- Implants also alter the cervical mucus, inhibiting sperm penetration and thereby preventing fertilization.
- Implants prevent implantation by inducing endometrial atrophy.
- Implants may modify sperm function and motility.

Advantages of contraceptive implants

- Long-lasting (3–5 years depending on the type of implant), effective, immediately reversible, and no effect on future fertility.
- Non-intercourse-related.
- Free from oestrogen side-effects
- High user acceptability following pre-insertion counselling, with continuation rates between 67% and 78% at 12 months.
- Requires little medical attention other than at insertion and removal.
- Can be used by those in whom synthetic oestrogen is contra-indicated.
- Implanon® does not adversely affect cardiovascular risk factors, thrombotic factors, C-reactive protein, cholesterol/HDL-cholesterol ratio, and nitrous oxide.
- Minimal effects on glucose metabolism and liver function.
- ↓ incidence in dysmenorrhoea with or without endometriosis.
- ↓ total menstrual blood loss in Norplant® and Implanon® users.
- No evidence to suggest that either Norplant® or Implanon® has an adverse effect on systemic oestrogen levels or BMD.

Disadvantages of contraceptive implants

- Unpredictable and irregular bleeding patterns are common in Implanon® users with ~10% discontinuing because of prolonged and/ or frequent bleeding. Bleeding experienced during the first 3 months is broadly predictive of future patterns. ~22% have amenorrhoea, 33% infrequent bleeding, 7% frequent bleeding, and/or 18% prolonged bleeding.
- Enlarged ovarian follicles >2.5cm may be found in 5–25% of Implanon® users. Rarely symptomatic and tend to disappear over time. ♀ with persistent follicles are more likely to complain of prolonged bleeding.
- Incidence of progestogen side-effects with Implanon® similar to that with other progestogen-only methods. Side-effects include headache, weight gain, acne, and mood changes.
- Insertion of implants requires a minor operative procedure under local anaesthetic by trained health professionals.
- Non-palpable implants have been reported in about 1 in 1000 insertions and are related to poor insertion technique. Very rarely damage to the neurovascular bundle has been reported. Referral to an 'expert' centre is advised for implant location using ultrasound scanning before removal. If non-insertion of the implant, etonogestrel assays may be required.
- Some ♀ report mild discomfort and bruising following insertion or removal of the implants.
- Infection at the insertion or removal site, migration of the implants, and scarring are rare.

Contraceptive implants may not be a suitable method for some ♀ as discontinuation is not under their control.

Starting regimens for contraceptive implants

Circumstances	Start when?	Extra precautions for 7 days?
Quick start	At any time if it is reasonably certain that she is not pregnant	Yes
Menstruating	Up to and including day 5	No
	After day 5 of the cycle	Yes
Amenorrhoeic	Any time if it is reasonably certain that she is not pregnant	Yes
Post-abortion or miscarriage	Within 5 days	No
	After 5 days	Yes
Postpartum		
Breastfeeding or bottle-feeding	Day 21 postpartum	No
	From day 22 onwards	Yes
Switching from other hormonal methods (other than IUS)	Immediate start	No
Switching from a non-hormonal method (other than IUD)	Up to and including day 5	No
	After day 5	Yes

Circumstances	Start when?	Extra precautions for 7 days?
Switching from an IUD or IUS	Insert the implant up to and including day 5 of cycle. IUD/IUS can be removed at the same time	No
	Implants can be fitted at any other time, if it is reasonably certain she is not pregnant	
	If she has been sexually active	Insert the implant and then remove IUD/IUS at the next period or after 7 days
	If she has not been sexually active	Insert the implant and then remove IUD/IUS after 7 days or at the next period
	If she is amenorrhoeic or has irregular bleeds	Insert the implant. If UPSI has occurred in preceding 7 days advise IUD/IUS removal 7 days after the implant has been inserted

Levonorgestrel intra-uterine system (IUS)

Available in the UK since May 1995 and used by ~3% of ♀. Worldwide >10 million ♀ have used it since its launch. Contains 52mg levonorgestrel in a polydimethylsiloxane reservoir on the vertical arm of a T-shaped plastic frame. Releasing ~20mcg levonorgestrel daily initially, it provides highly effective yet reversible contraception for 5 years. It is also licensed for the treatment of 1° menorrhagia and as the progestogen component of hormone replacement therapy (HRT).

Mechanism of action

- Alters cervical mucus and utero-tubal fluid, inhibiting sperm migration.
- Prevents endometrial proliferation by causing atrophic changes over time. This precludes implantation.
- May affect sperm motility and function.
- May suppress ovulation in some in the first year possibly by reducing the pre-ovulatory luteinizing hormone surge.

Advantages of IUS

- Long-acting (lasts 5 years) and independent of intercourse.
- Highly effective contraceptive (as effective as female sterilization) with an immediate return to fertility after removal. ↑ in use of LARCs such as the IUS has led to ↓ in requests for female sterilization in the UK.
- ↓ normal menstrual blood loss with 20–50% becoming amenorrhoeic.
- ↓ heavy menstrual bleeding by about 97% after 12 months use with an ↑ in haemoglobin and serum ferritin. Led to ↓ hysterectomies in the UK. Can be used in ♀ with coagulation disorders.
- Long-term use may prevent fibroid formation.
- ↓ heavy menstrual bleeding associated with fibroids and adeno-myosis.
- ↓ incidence of dysmenorrhoea.
- May be a useful medical treatment for ♀ suffering from endo-metriosis related problems with significant ↓ in severity and frequency of pain/menstrual symptoms. Good as maintenance therapy following conservative surgery for endometriosis.
- No evidence that serum oestradiol and BMD are affected.
- ↓ risk of ectopic pregnancy. Can be used in ♀ with a past history of extra-uterine pregnancies.
- ↓ incidence of PID.
- Can be used as the progestogen component of HRT.
- May protect against the development of endometrial hyperplasia. Resolves endometrial hyperplasia without atypia in 92% of cases and endometrial hyperplasia with atypia in 67%. Should not be used in early endometrial cancer.
- High user acceptance with 3 year continuation rates of 75–82%.

Disadvantages of IUS

- May cause irregular/prolonged bleeding in the first 3 months. Prolonged bleeding/spotting (>6 months following fitting) may occur in those with heavy menstrual bleeding with or without fibroids. Pre-insertion counselling should include information on menstrual disturbance.
- May be expelled or displaced in ~4–6%, particularly with intra-cavity fibroids or heavy menstrual loss.
- Fitting may be painful and seen as invasive.
- Small ↑ risk of PID within first 20 days after fitting, particularly in young ♀. Screen for STIs prior to fitting in those at risk.
- ~10% may develop functional ovarian cysts but these tend to resolve over 6 months or so and rarely require surgical intervention.
- Other rare complications, e.g. perforation of the uterus/cervix (< than 1 per 1000 devices fitted).
- Some progestogenic symptoms in the first few months, i.e. breast tenderness, bloating, or acne. These usually settle.
- Overall incidence of ectopic pregnancy is lower than in the general population, but a small risk of ectopic pregnancy in the event of IUS failure. It can be used in ♀ with a past history of ectopic pregnancy.
- Cannot be used as an emergency form of contraception.

Starting regimens for intra-uterine systems

Circumstances	Start when?	Extra precautions for 7 days?
Menstruating	Up to and including day 7 (avoiding insertion when menstrual flow is heavy thereby reducing subsequent expulsion)	No
	After day 7 of the cycle as long as it is reasonable certain that she is not pregnant	Yes
Amenorrhoeic	Any time if it is reasonably certain that she is not pregnant	Yes
Post-abortion or miscarriage	Within 5 days	No
	After 5 days	Yes
Postpartum		
Breastfeeding or bottle-feeding	After day 28 (including following a Caesarean section)	Yes
Switching from other hormonal methods (other than IUS)	Immediate start	No
Switching from a non-hormonal method (other than IUD)	Up to and including day 7	No
	After day 7	Yes
Switching from an IUD or changing an IUS	Insert the IUS up to and including day 7 of cycle	No
	After day 7, advise no sexual intercourse for 7 days prior to the IUS fitting	Yes
	If she is using an IUS and is amenorrhoeic or has irregular bleeds, advise no sexual intercourse for 7 days prior to the changing of the IUS	No

Copper intra-uterine contraceptive device (IUD)

IUDs are used by >110 million ♀ world-wide, with ~50% of these users in China. Only 4% of ♀ in the UK use IUD, possibly because of concerns and myths attached to these methods. IUDs available in the UK are small copper-containing devices in varying shapes and sizes. Most have a central frame made of polyethylene impregnated with barium, making them radio-opaque. A frameless device called GyneFix® is also available. Most devices contain >300mm^2 of copper, making them a highly effective, reversible, and inexpensive contraceptive option.

Mechanism of action

- Prevents fertilization as copper ions are toxic to sperm and ova (main mechanism).
- All IUDs ↑ the number of leucocytes in the endometrium, producing a typical 'sterile' inflammatory endometrial response which helps prevent implantation. Copper enhances this reaction.
- the increased copper content of cervico-uterine mucus inhibits sperm penetration.
▶An IUD is not an abortifacient.

Advantages of IUDs

- Long-term (up to 10 years) highly effective contraceptive with no delay in return to fertility following removal.
- Immediately effective.
- Non-intercourse related.
- Very low morbidity with a mortality rate of <1 in 500,000 users.
- No associated weight gain or hormonal side-effects.
- Very effective as an emergency contraceptive. Can be fitted up to 5 days after UPSI or 5 days after estimated time of ovulation, whichever is later.
- High acceptability and good continuation rates. Ideal for family spacing and once a family is complete.
- Inexpensive and very cost-effective.
- Risk of ectopic pregnancy is low in devices with ≥300mm^2 of copper. The incidence of ectopic pregnancy is 0.02 per 100 women-years, which is less than in those using no contraceptive method.
- May give up to 50% protection against the development of endometrial cancer.

Disadvantages of IUDs

- May cause menstrual irregularities with intermenstrual bleeding and spotting more common in the first 6 months after insertion.
- Periods may become heavier, more prolonged, and painful, especially soon after insertion. ~10% of ♀ discontinue in the first year citing menstrual bleeding ± pain as the main reason.
- ~1 in 20 IUDs are expelled; more likely within the first 3 months and similar for all types.
- Risk of PID associated with insertion, especially within the first 20 days (1.6 per 1000 women-years). May be prevented by preinsertion STI screening for those at risk.
- Rare complications such as uterine perforation may occur in up to 2 per 1000 insertions.

Starting regimens for intra-uterine devices

Circumstances	Start when?	Extra precautions for 7 days?
Menstruating	At any time in the cycle if it is reasonable certain that the ♀ is not pregnant (avoiding insertion when menstrual flow is heavy, thereby ↓ subsequent expulsion)	No
Amenorrhoeic	Any time if it is reasonably certain that she is not pregnant	No
Post-abortion or miscarriage	Immediately	No
	At any time by an experienced clinician as long as there is no concern that the pregnancy is not ongoing	No
Postpartum		
Breastfeeding or bottle-feeding	After day 28 (including following a Caesarean section) if it is reasonably certain that she is not pregnant	No
Switching from other hormonal methods	Immediate start as long as the previous method has been used correctly and consistently	No
Switching from a non-hormonal method	Immediate start as long as the previous method has been used correctly and consistently	No

Diaphragms and caps

These are often thought to be messy and difficult, and hence are used by <1% of ♀ in the UK. However the ease of use and lack of interference with intercourse often surprise ♀. Must be used correctly and consistently as typical failure rates in the first year can be high (16%). Should be fitted by a trained HCP who can advise about use of additional spermicide.

Mode of action

Physical and chemical barrier to sperm entering the upper female genital tract (when used with a spermicide). Diaphragms sit between the posterior fornix and the pubis to cover the cervix. Cervical caps fit directly over the cervix by suction and are ideal for ♀ with long cervices. Useful for ♀ with recurrent urinary tract infections (UTIs) when using diaphragms.

Advantages of diaphragms and caps

- Effective with careful consistent use (6% failure rate with perfect use).
- Can be inserted at a convenient time before sex (within 3 hours).
- May protect against human papilloma virus (HPV) transmission and development of cervical intra-epithelial neoplasia (limited evidence).
- May provide limited protection against STIs.
- No established health risks or systemic side-effects.
- Silicone alternatives available for women with latex allergies.
- User controlled.

Disadvantages of diaphragms and caps

- High failure rates in practice (16% in the first year). Therefore requires careful use on all occasions.
- Must remain in place for 6 hours after the last episode of sexual intercourse.
- May become dislodged during sex.
- May ↑ risk of cystitis or UTI
- Potential risk of toxic shock syndrome if left *in situ* longer than the recommended time specified by the manufacturer.
- Should be used with a spermicide. More spermicide should be inserted into the vagina before repeated sex occurs to ↑ efficacy.
- Spermicide is considered 'messy' by some users.
- Spermicide-induced vaginal irritation in some users.
- Needs to be fitted by a healthcare professional.

Female condom

The female condom (Femidom®) was first marketed in the UK in 1992 but very few ♀ in the UK use this method. It can be bought in pharmacies and is acceptable to some ♀ who often alternate between using male and female barrier methods.

Mode of action

The female condom is a lubricated loose-fitting, polyurethane sheath with two flexible rings. The closed end with the loose ring is inserted into the vagina and the outer ring covers the vulva. It acts as a physical barrier between sperm and ovum.

Advantages of the female condom

- No known side-effects.
- Acts as a contraceptive and may also protect against some STIs (inconsistent data).
- Theoretical benefit in helping to protect against HPV transmission and cancer of the cervix.
- Effective with careful use (5% failure rate with perfect use).
- Under direct control of the user.
- Can be inserted at any time before having sex.
- No additional spermicide required.
- Can be used with oil-based products.
- Polyurethane is stronger than latex and breakage is rare.
- No need for male erection before use.

Disadvantages of the female condom

- Has high failure rates in practice (typical failure rate 21%).
- Has a high slippage rate (about 6%).
- Requires thought before use and careful insertion to be effective.
- Can interrupt sex.
- Can be noisy and intrusive.

Spermicides

One of the oldest forms of contraception. Available in the UK as creams and pessaries. They are also the active component of vaginal sponges. Many different substances have been used in the past, but preparations available in the UK contain nonoxynol-9. Research into the viricidal potential of spermicidal substances is ongoing with the aim of developing a contraceptive which will help protect against HIV.

Advantages of spermicides
- No serious side-effects.
- Widely available in pharmacies and simple to use.
- Provide lubrication.
- Enhance efficacy of barrier methods.
- Useful during the peri-menopause (♀ >45 years with irregular cycles and some vasomotor symptoms).
- Can be used whilst breastfeeding (until menstruation returns and weaning begins).

Disadvantages of spermicides
- Must not be used as sole contraceptive in most circumstances (29% typical failure rate when used alone in fertile ♀).
- Can be messy and cause local irritation.
- Intercourse dependent.
- Waiting time of approximately 4 minutes after insertion of pessaries before they melt.
- Those available may damage the vaginal epithelium and have the potential to ↑ transmission of STIs.

Male condom

The condom or 'sheath' has been used to protect against transmission of STIs over the centuries. It is still one of the most popular contraceptive methods and is used by 24% of British couples. Readily available from a variety of outlets. Condoms must be used correctly and on all occasions when close sexual contact occurs to be effective. Typical failure rate is high (~15%).

Male condoms come in different shapes, colours, sizes, and flavours. 'Baggy' condoms may be helpful for those with erectile problems or who complain of reduced sensitivity with 'tight' latex condoms. Most are made of latex, with the only contraindication being latex allergy. The majority of reactions are type IV hypersensitivity (mild genital inflammation), although rarely anaphylaxis can occur with type I hypersensitivity. Polyurethane + deproteinized latex condoms are available as alternatives. Condoms lubricated with a non-spermicidal agent are now advised since the addition of a spermicide may cause local genital irritation and thin the vaginal mucosa in ♀, leading to possible transmission of STIs. Additional spermicide does not improve the contraceptive efficacy of male condoms. Non-oil-based lubricants are recommended, especially for anal sex, to reduce the risk of breakage (3% breakage rate compared with 21.4% when lubricant is not used), but should not be applied directly to the penis under a condom as this may cause slippage.

Users should be advised to check their condoms for safety markings (CE markings or Kitemark) and expiry date.

Mode of action
Acts as a physical barrier between sperm and ovum.

Advantages of the male condom
- No known serious side-effects.
- Acts as a contraceptive and helps to provide protection against STIs and cervical neoplasia (Box 33.1).
- Effective with careful use (~2% failure rate with perfect use).
- Latex-free condoms are available for those who have latex allergies.
- Under direct control of the user.

Disadvantages of the male condom
- High failure rates in practice.
- Transmission of STIs possible even with careful and consistent use.
- Oil-based lubricants and some vaginal preparations may affect latex condoms with ↑ risk of breakage. Aqueous-based lubricant should be used for anal sex to reduce the risk of breakage. 'Stronger' condoms result in similar breakage rates. Therefore they are not recommended.
- Requires the penis to be erect before use.
- Has a high slippage rate if lubricant is placed in the condom.
- Can interrupt sex.

Box 33.1 Male condoms and STI protection

HIV infection: condom effectiveness in preventing heterosexual transmission: 87% (range 60–96%) (meta-analysis data).

Data on other STIs is inconsistent and the degree of protection provided by male condoms is difficult to assess. However:

- Gonorrhoea and chlamydia—strong evidence that condoms reduce the risk of gonorrhoea and chlamydia in both men and women (review of 45 published studies).
- Trichomoniasis—conflicting data with no consistent evidence of benefit, but correct and regular condom use is recommended.
- Anogenital herpes—conflicting data. Evidence of protection using male condom for HSV-2 sero-discordant couples or those with >4 sex partners, but no evidence for sex workers, their clients, and GUM male heterosexual attenders. Consistent and correct use of male condoms is recommended.
- Syphilis—limited evidence available to support protective effect in higher-risk groups (e.g. Ugandan population, female and transvestite sex workers).
- Anogenital HPV—risk of cervical and vulvovaginal HPV infection reduced with consistent condom use. Regression and clearance of flat penile warts and cervical intra-epithelial neoplasia has also been reported in association with condom use.
- Hepatitis B virus—reduced core antibody rates in female sex workers who consistently use condoms.

Estimated minimum level of protection against infection provided by consistent condom use:

- HIV 85%
- *C.trachomatis* 40%
- *T.vaginalis* 60%
- *N.gonorrhoeae* 49%.

HSV infection in ♀ may be reduced but no evidence in ♂. Conflicting data on HPV infection but may ↓ incidence in ♂ and delay progression of CIN in ♀.

Natural family planning (NFP)

NFP or 'fertility awareness' has replaced the terms 'rhythm method' or using the 'safe period'. Fertility awareness relies upon the detection of ovulation. Effective if couples abstain from penetrative sex during the fertile period of the menstrual cycle or use a barrier method. Normally 3–12 months of menstrual cycle information is needed for accurate prediction of the fertile phase. Efficacy is improved if several fertility awareness methods are used concurrently, such as menstrual records, basal body temperature, and cervical mucus indicators. The failure rate is 6% with perfect use of devices such as Persona® which detect the fertile phase by measuring urinary oestriol-3-glucuronide and luteinizing hormone.

Fertility awareness is used by ~1% of couples in the UK but by many more worldwide to space their family.

Advantages of fertility awareness
- Can be used to plan pregnancy as well as prevent conception.
- No known physical side-effects.
- Non-intercourse-related method.
- No mechanical devices or hormones used.
- Acceptable to all cultures and religions.
- No follow-up is necessary once the user has learnt the method.

Disadvantages of fertility awareness
- Relatively high failure rate in practice (25%).
- Requires commitment of both partners.
- Needs to be taught in order to use successfully.
- Requires careful observation and record-keeping, which may take time to learn.
- Users must have high motivation, as long periods of abstinence from intercourse are required.
- No protection against STI transmission.

Lactational amenorrhoea method (LAM)

Breastfeeding is a natural way of spacing children since suckling suppresses LH and FSH, resulting in amenorrhoea, and stimulates prolactin, leading to lactation. LAM is very effective, offering 98% protection against pregnancy under the following conditions:

- Fully or almost fully breast-feeding (feeding with no substitutes and at regular periods on demand, day and night)
- Baby is < six months old
- Menstruation has not returned.

Coitus interruptus or 'withdrawal'

'Withdrawal' is the oldest method of birth control and is still one of the most popular natural contraceptive methods worldwide. In the UK 4% of couples use this method and it can be practised by any couple at any time.

Advantages of coitus interruptus

- Free of charge.
- Requires no prescription.
- Does not cause nausea or weight gain.
- Acceptable to many users.

Disadvantages of coitus interruptus

- High failure rate (27% in practice).
- Intercourse is incomplete.
- May be unsatisfying for both partners.
- Partial ejaculation of semen can occur.
- No protection against STI transmission.

Emergency contraception

Emergency contraception involves methods that can be used in the event of UPSI to prevent pregnancy. These methods are not abortifacients as they do not disrupt implantation of the blastocyst.

Hormonal emergency contraception

Research began in the 1960s to develop post-coital contraception. A licensed preparation that became available in the UK in the early 1980s comprised two doses of 100mcg ethinyl oestradiol and 500mcg levonorgestrel to be taken within 72 hours of UPSI. Recently, progestogen-only emergency contraception containing 1500mcg of levonorgestrel, taken in a single dose (Levonelle 1500®), has been found to be more effective with fewer side-effects. ▶♀ taking liver-enzyme-inducing drugs, such as carbamazepine or St John's wort, should take two Levonelle 1500® tablets as a single dose.

Ulipristal acetate (EllaOne®), a selective progesterone receptor modulator, has just been launched in the UK. It has a similar mode of action to progestogen-only emergency contraception but is equally effective up to 5 days after UPSI. Until further studies are published and because of its cost EllaOne® should be reserved for women who have had UPSI after day 3 and up to day 5 but decline the fitting of an IUD.

Hormonal emergency contraception is now widely available with >50% being provided by a chemist or pharmacy where it can be purchased or obtained 'free at the point of contact' through local patient group directions.

Mode of action of progestogen-only emergency contraception

The exact mode of action is unknown. Recent evidence suggests that it delays or postpones ovulation rather than preventing implantation of the blastocyst. Providers should inform users of its likely mode of action to dispel some of the myths that hormonal emergency contraception 'causes abortions', contains 'dangerous hormones', and can affect future fertility.

Advantages of progestogen-only emergency contraception

- Prevents 75% of pregnancies if taken within 72 hours of UPSI
  - 95% within 24 hours
  - 85% between 25 and 48 hours
  - 58% between 49 and 72 hours
  - 33% between 73 and 120 hours (ulipristal acetate is more effective and a copper IUD very much more effective in this situation, and should be advised).
- Easily available from GPs, nurses, community settings, pharmacies.
- Easy to take as a single dose in tablet form.
- Few side-effects and no known teratogenicity.
- Can be prescribed in advance for those using barrier methods or 'perceived to be at risk'.
- Treatment can be repeated in the same menstrual cycle if required.

Non-hormonal emergency contraception

Copper IUD is most effective, preventing almost 100% of pregnancies if fitted within 120 hours of the first episode of UPSI any time in a menstrual cycle or after multiple episodes of UPSI but no later than 5 days after the estimated time of ovulation. Copper-containing IUDs must be used rather than the levonorgestrel IUS.

Mode of action

Copper IUDs ↓ viability of the ova, ↓ sperm numbers reaching fallopian tubes, and may also prevent implantation by inducing endometrial changes.

An IUD should be offered to all ♀ requesting emergency contraception, as it is the most effective choice. However, hormonal emergency contraception should be prescribed if referral elsewhere is necessary or delay before IUD fitting is likely. This will ensure that a method of emergency contraception has been provided if IUD insertion fails or he appointment is not kept.

Advantages of using IUDs for emergency contraception

- Suitable following multiple episodes of UPSI but within 5 days after the estimated time of ovulation.
- Appropriate if vomiting follows progestogen-only emergency contraception.
- Ideal choice if an IUD is requested as a long-term contraceptive method.
- Effective contraception for rest of menstrual cycle.
- Most effective method especially if UPSI occurs close to the time of ovulation.

Disadvantages of using IUDs for emergency contraception

- Similar to copper IUDs used as a long-term contraceptive method.
- Possible pain at insertion, particularly if nulliparous.
- Not popular with those requesting emergency contraception as the fitting of an IUD is thought to be 'invasive'.
- ↑ risk of pelvic infection within the first 20 days. ►Screen for STIs prior to fitting. Some may consider antibiotic cover whilst awaiting results in high-risk groups.
- Does not protect against STI transmission.

Female sterilization

Male and female sterilization is the main method of contraception for ~18% of couples in England and Wales. Female sterilization is normally performed laparoscopically or hysteroscopically as a day-case procedure. It is regarded as permanent as reversal, which requires surgery, may not be 100% successful.

Counsel use of effective contraception prior to surgery as up to 3% of ♀ may be pregnant at the time of sterilization. Avoid routine sterilization immediately postpartum, post-abortion, or without considering other reversible options Female sterilization ↓ by ~50% over the last 15 years, with the introduction of LARC. Only 7% of couples used this method in 2007–2008.

Mode of action
Occlusion of fallopian tubes blocking the sperm and preventing fertilization.

Advantages of female sterilization
- Highly and immediately effective.
- High user satisfaction, removing fear of unplanned pregnancy.
- No weight gain or heavy periods.
- Hysteroscopic techniques requiring only local anaesthesia under development.
- May protect against breast, ovarian, and endometrial cancer, although these findings may be explained by the sterilization method employed and increasing incidence of premature menopause.

Disadvantages of female sterilization
- Normally requires a general anaesthetic.
- Reversion requires a major surgical procedure and is rarely funded by the NHS.
- Other hormonal contraceptive methods are equally effective, and are reversible with additional non-contraceptive benefits.
- Has associated complications in 0.9–1.6 per 100 cases, with clips having the lowest complication rate of 0.47 per 100 cases (Box 33.2).

Box 33.2 Complications of female sterilization

Short term

- *Anaesthetic complications* Overall mortality from anaesthetic complications is very low.
- *Operative complications* Occur in 0.5–1% of procedures.
- *Perforation* Bowel, blood vessels, bladder at the time of the procedure. The need for laparotomy as a result of a serious complication is about 1.9 per 1000 procedures and risk of death is 1 in 12,000 laparoscopies.
- *Wound infection*
- *Abdominal discomfort* and *shoulder tip pain* From intra-peritoneal gas still remaining in the abdominal cavity. This slowly improves over 24–48 hours.

Long term

- *Late re-canalization of fallopian tubes* Failure rates with Filshie clips are now quoted as 2–3 per 1000 procedures. Occurs even up to 10 years after surgery with a cumulative ectopic pregnancy rate being as high as 31.9 per 1000 procedures depending on the sterilization method used.
- *Complaints of heavy menstrual bleeding leading to hysterectomy* Women often stop hormonal methods of contraception that have controlled their menstrual loss and pain. With advancing age menstrual problems also increase and this can lead to requests for treatment. There is a 17% cumulative probability of undergoing a hysterectomy when reviewed 14 years after female sterilization.
- *Regret* Regret is not uncommon following sterilization, with 3– 10% of couples reporting this. Regret is more common when the operation has been performed in those <30 years old and within a year of the birth of a child.

Male sterilization: vasectomy

In the UK ~11% of couples rely on male sterilization as their chosen method of contraception, with ~60% of all sterilization procedures performed on ♂. This ratio is different in other parts of the world, with ♀ 10 times more likely to be sterilized than their ♂ counterparts.

Mode of action

Male sterilization techniques either occlude the vas deferens using ligation or coagulation, or use clips to block the path of the sperm and prevent fertilization. These procedures are normally performed under local anaesthetic.

Advantages of vasectomy

- Very safe and effective with a failure rate of ~1 in 2000 in a lifetime after two negative 'clearance of sperm' tests.
- Permanent method ameliorating concerns about future contraception or unplanned pregnancy.
- Minor surgical procedure, normally performed under local anaesthetic and taking 10–15 minutes.
- Can be done at a doctor's surgery or clinic.
- No evidence of an increased risk of testicular/prostate cancer following vasectomy.
- No increased risk of coronary heart disease proven.

Disadvantages of vasectomy

- Reversal is not easy and is rarely funded by the NHS.
- Couples may regret this decision especially if they are young (<30 years old).
- Not immediately effective, requiring two negative semen analyses before other methods can be abandoned
- Involves a surgical procedure with associated complications (Box 33.3).

Box 33.3 Complications of male sterilization

Short term

- *Local complications* Bruising and swelling with some discomfort or pain for a short time following the procedure. Scrotal haematoma formation occurs in 1–2% following vasectomy.
- *Wound infection* In up to 5%. May require treatment with antibiotics.
- *Failure to achieve azoospermia*. In ~0.5%. Further surgery may be required.

Long term

- *Sperm granulomata* Small tender lumps that form at the cut ends of the vas deferens caused by leakage of sperm into the tissue from the cut ends, leading to local inflammation. Can be excised.
- *Chronic scrotal pain* 0.9–5.2% complain of chronic scrotal pain following vasectomy. May be made worse by sexual arousal or ejaculation. Local scar tissue formation and induration may be the cause. Further surgery to remove the epididymis and occluded vas may be indicated in some.

HIV-positive women

Why is the discussion of contraception important?

- The vast majority of ♀ infected with HIV are of reproductive age.
- Effect of some antiretrovirals on the fetus may be severe (e.g. efavirenz resulting in anencephaly in animal studies). Long-term effects are unknown, with concerns over carcinogenesis and mitochondrial disease.
- Drug interactions with some hormonal contraceptives, antiretrovirals, and certain antibiotics (Box 33.4).
- Possible HIV transmission to the ♂ partner in an unplanned pregnancy.

Male condom

Can be recommended for use by all HIV-positive ♀ and ♂, preferably in combination with another contraceptive method if contraception is essential. If ♂ condom is unacceptable, ♀ condom should be considered.

Male/female sterilization

Both are safe in HIV infection as operative risks are no greater than in those who are HIV negative. However, if complications occur, they could be more serious in those with advanced HIV disease and so other methods may be more acceptable. Caution should also be exercised in newly diagnosed patients who may be coming to terms with their condition and could change their views with regard to future pregnancies. A longer-term reversible method may be preferable.

Combined oral contraceptives (COCs)

There are no HIV-specific contraindications in those who are well and not on any treatment. However, numerous interactions may occur in those taking antiretroviral or antibiotic treatment (Box 33.4). Therefore if a ♀ is stable on an antiretroviral regimen, it may be preferable to consider an alternative contraceptive method.

Progestogen-only pills/subdermal implants

As with COCs, there are no specific contraindications, but care needs to be taken to avoid drug interactions.

Depot medroxyprogesterone acetate (DMPA)

DMPA's efficacy is not affected by potent enzyme inducers (like rifampacin) and the injection interval does not require altering from the standard 12 weeks (Box 33.4).

Intra-uterine devices (IUDs)

- Copper IUDs are highly effective and cost-effective. No drug interactions. Risks of complications and pelvic infection following IUD insertion are similar to those in HIV-negative ♀.
- Levonorgestrel intra-uterine system (lng-ius): low failure rate (0.1–0.2/100 ♀ years) and ↓ rate of ectopic pregnancy and pelvic inflammatory disease compared with copper iuds. After 1 year, 94–97% ↓ in menstrual flow with amenorrhoea in 10–15%.

Box 33.4 Interactions and hormonal contraception

Antibiotics and COCs

- Rifampicin and rifabutin: powerful enzyme inducers. COCs not advised and alternative contraceptive measures required for 4–8 weeks following their discontinuation.
- Certain broad-spectrum antibiotics (e.g. cephalosporins, penicillin, tetracycline but not erythromicin): may ↓ COC efficacy by altering large bowel flora. Additional contraception required while taking antibiotics and for 7 days thereafter (continue next pill packet without a break if necessary). If antibiotic treatment >3 weeks, no additional precautions required as bowel flora becomes antibiotic resistant.

Antibiotics and progestogen-only contraception (POC)

- Rifampicin and rifabutin: powerful enzyme inducers, reducing efficacy of POC.
  - DMPA—not affected
  - IUS (Mirena®)—not affected
  - implant—not recommended; use additional method during and 4–8 weeks after.
  - oral—not recommended; alternative contraception required for 4–8 weeks following their cessation.
- Broad-spectrum antibiotics: not affected.

Antiretroviral drugs

- May ↑ or ↓ hormonal levels.
- All nucleoside reverse transcriptase inhibitors, including Combivir® and Truvada®, can be used safely.
- Efavirenz not compatible with oral methods, but DMPA is OK.
- Nevirapine® and Kaletra® are not compatible with any hormonal method.
- Refer to website ☍ www.hiv-druginteractions.org for interaction tables of other antiretrovirals

Cautions and contraindications

The UK Medical Eligibility Criteria for contraceptive use has adapted World Health Organization (WHO) guidance and classifies the acceptability of each contraceptive method in different conditions into one of four categories:

UKMEC definition of category

- *Category 1* A condition for which there is no restriction on the use of the contraceptive method.
- *Category 2* A condition where the advantages of using the method generally outweigh the theoretical or proven risks.
- *Category 3* A condition where the theoretical or proven risk generally outweigh the advantages of using the method. The provision of a method requires expert clinical judgement and/or referral to a specialist contraceptive provider, since use of the method is not usually recommended unless other more appropriate methods are not available or not acceptable.
- *Category 4* A condition which represents an unacceptable health risk if the contraceptive method is used.

The UKMEC guidelines are summarized in the remainder of this chapter.

	Summary sheets: common reversible methods

A **UK Category 1** indicates that there is no restriction for use. A **UK Category 2** indicates that the method can generally be used, but more careful follow-up may be required.

A contraceptive method with a **UK Category 3** can be used, however this may require expert clinical judgement and/or referral to a specialist contraceptive provider, since use of the method is not usually recommended unless other methods are not available or not acceptable. A **UK Category 4** indicates that use poses an unacceptable health risk.

UK Category	Hormonal contraception, intrauterine devices, emergency contraception and barrier methods
1	A condition for which there is **no restriction for the use** of the contraceptive method
2	A condition **where the advantages of using the method generally outweigh the theoretical or proven risks**
3	A condition where the theoretical or **proven risks generally outweigh the advantages** of using the method. The provision of a method requires expert clinical judgement and/or referral to a specialist contraceptive provider, since use of the method is not usually recommended unless other more appropriate methods are not available or not acceptable
4	A condition which represents an **unacceptable risk** if the contraceptive method is used

Initiation (I)	Starting a method of contraception by a woman with a specific medical condition.
Continuation (C)	Continuing with the method already being used by a woman who develops a new medical condition.

Fig. 33.1 UK MEC Guidelines. UK Medical Eligibility Criteria for Contraceptive use (UK MEC 2009) reproduced from the Faculty of Sexual and Reproductive Health Care of the Royal College of Obstetricians and Gynaecologists, with permission.

COMMON REVERSIBLE METHODS SUMMARY TABLE						
CONDITION	**CHC**	**POP**	**DMPA/ NET-EN**	**IMP**	**Cu-IUD**	**LNG-IUD**
I = Initiation, C = Continuation						
PERSONAL CHARACTERISTICS AND REPRODUCTIVE HISTORY						
PREGNANCY	NA	NA	NA	NA	NA	NA
AGE	Menarche to <40=1 ≥40=2	Menarche to >45=1	Menarche to <18=2 18-45=1 >45=2	Menarche to >45=1	Menarche to <20=2 >20=1	Menarche to <20=2 >20=1
PARITY						
a) Nulliparous	1	1	1	1	1	1
b) Parous	1	1	1	1	1	1
BREASTFEEDING						
a) <6 weeks postpartum	4	1	2	1		
b) ≥6 weeks to <6 months (fully or almost fully breastfeeding)	3	1	1	1		
c) ≥6 weeks to <6 months postpartum (partial breastfeeding medium to minimal)	2	1	1	1		
d) ≥6 months postpartum	1	1	1	1		
POSTPARTUM (in non-breast-feeding women)						
a) <21 days	3	1	1	1		
b) ≥21 days	1	1	1	1		
POSTPARTUM (breastfeeding or non-breastfeeding, including post-caesarean section)						
a) 48 hours to <4 weeks					3	3
b) ≥4 weeks					1	1
c) Puerperal sepsis					4	4
POST-ABORTION						
a) First trimester	1	1	1	1	1	1
b) Second trimester	1	1	1	1	2	2
c) Immediate post-septic abortion	1	1	1	1	4	4
PAST ECTOPIC PREGNANCY	1	1	1	1	1	1
HISTORY OF PELVIC SURGERY	1	1	1	1	1	1
SMOKING						
a) Age <35 years	2	1	1	1	1	1
b) Age ≥35 years						
(i) <15 cigarettes/day	3	1	1	1	1	1
(ii) ≥15 cigarettes/day	4	1	1	1	1	1
(iii) Stopped smoking <1 year ago	3	1	1	1	1	1
(iv) Stopped smoking ≥1 year ago	2	1	1	1	1	1
OBESITY						
a) ≥30–34 kg/m^2 body mass index	2	1	1	1	1	1
b) ≥35 kg/m^2 body mass index	3	1	1	1	1	1
CARDIOVASCULAR DISEASE						
MULTIPLE RISK FACTORS FOR CARDIOVASCULAR DISEASE (such as old age smoking diabetes hypertention and obesity)	3/4	2	3	2	1	2

UKMEC	DEFINITION OF CATEGORY
CATEGORY 1	A condition for which there is no restriction for the use of the contraceptive method.
CATEGORY 2	A condition where the advantages of using the method generally outweigh the theoretical or proven risks.
CATEGORY 3	A condition where the theoretical or proven risks generally outweigh the advantages of using the method. The provision of a method requires expert clinical judgement and/or referral to a specialist contraceptive provider, since use of the method is not usually recommended unless other more appropriate methods are not available or not acceptable.
CATEGORY 4	A condition which represents an unacceptable health risk if the contraceptive method is used.

Fig. 33.1 (Continued).

COMMON REVERSIBLE METHODS SUMMARY TABLE						
CONDITION	CHC	POP	DMPA/ NET-EN	IMP	Cu-IUD	LNG-IUD
I = Initiation, C = Continuation						
HYPERTENSION						
a) Adequately controlled hypertension	3	1	2	1	1	1
b) Consistently elevated blood pressure levels (properly taken measurements)						
(i) systolic >140 to 159mmHg or diastolic >90 to 94mmHg	3	1	1	1	1	1
(ii) systolic ≥160mmHg or diastolic ≤95mmHg	4	1	2	1	1	1
c) Vascular disease	4	2	3	2	1	2
HISTORY OF HIGH BLOOD PRESSURE DURING PREGNANCY (where current blood pressure normal)	2	1	1	1	1	1
VENOUS THROMBOEMBOLISM (VTE)						
a) History of VTE	4	2	2	2	1	2
b) Current VTE (on anticoagulants)	4	2	2	2	1	2
c) Family history of VTE						
(i) First-degree relative age <45 years	3	1	1	1	1	1
(ii) First-degree relative age ≥45 years	2	1	1	1	1	1
d) Major surgery						
(i) With prolonged immobilisation	4	2	2	2	1	2
(ii) Without prolonged immobilisation	2	1	1	1	1	1
e) Minor surgery without immobilisation	1	1	1	1	1	1
f) Immobility (unrelated to surgery) e.g.- wheelchair use, debilitating illness	3	1	1	1	1	1
KNOWN THROMBOGENIC MUTATIONS (e.g. Factor V Leiden, Prothrombin mutation, Protein S, Protein C, and Antithrombin deficiencies)	4	2	2	2	1	2
SUPERFICIAL VENOUS THROMBOSIS						
a) varicose veins	1	1	1	1	1	1
b) superficial thrombophlebitis	2	1	1	1	1	1

UKMEC	DEFINITION OF CATEGORY
CATEGORY 1	A condition for which there is no restriction for the use of the contraceptive method
CATEGORY 2	A condition where the advantages of using the method generally outweigh the theoretical or proven risks
CATEGORY 3	A condition where the theoretical or proven risks generally outweigh the advantages of using the method. The provision of a method requires expert clinical judgement and/or referral to a specialist contraceptive provider, since use of the method is not usually recommended unless other more appropriate methods are not available or not acceptable.
CATEGORY 4	A condition which represents an unacceptable health risk if the contraceptive method is used

Fig. 33.1 (Continued)

COMMON REVERSIBLE METHODS SUMMARY TABLE

CONDITION	CHC	POP	DMPA/ NET-EN	IMP	Cu-IUD	LNG-IUD
I = Initiation, C = Continuation						
CURRENT AND HISTORY OF ISCHAEMIC HEART DISEASE	4	I 2 / C 3	3	I 2 / C 3	1	I 2 / C 3
STROKE (history of cerebrovascular accident, including TIA)	4	I 2 / C 3	3	I 2 / C 3	1	I 2 / C 3
KNOWN HYPERLIPIDAEMIAS	2/3	2	2	2	1	2
VALVULAR AND CONGENITAL HEART DISEASE						
a) Uncomplicated	2	1	1	1	1	1
b) Complicated (eg. With pulmonary hypertension, atrial fibrillation, history of subacute bacterial endocarditis)	4	1	1	1	2	2
NEUROLOGIC CONDITIONS						
HEADACHES	I / C					
a) Non-migrainous (mild or severe)	I 1 / C 2	1	1	1	1	1
b) Migraine without aura, at any age	I 2 / C 3	I 1 / C 2	2	2	1	2
c) Migraine with aura, at any age	4	2	2	2	1	2
d) Past history (≥5 years ago) of migraine with aura, any age	3	2	2	2	1	2
EPILEPSY	1	1	1	1	1	1
DEPRESSIVE DISORDERS						
DEPRESSIVE DISORDERS	1	1	1	1	1	1
BREAST AND REPRODUCTIVE TRACT CONDITIONS						
VAGINAL BLEEDING PATTERNS						
a) Irregular pattern without heavy bleeding	1	2	2	2	1	1
b) Heavy or prolonged bleeding (includes regular and irregular patterns)	1	2	2	2	2	I 1 / C 2
UNEXPLAINED VAGINAL BLEEDING (suspicious for serious condition) Before evaluation	2	2	3	3	I 4 / C 2	I 4 / C 2
ENDOMETRIOSIS	1	1	1	1	2	1
BENIGN OVARIAN TUMOURS (including cysts)	1	1	1	1	1	1
SEVERE DYSMENORRHOEA	1	1	1	1	2	1

UKMEC	DEFINITION OF CATEGORY
CATEGORY 1	A condition for which there is no restriction for the use of the contraceptive method
CATEGORY 2	A condition where the advantages of using the method generally outweigh the theoretical or proven risks
CATEGORY 3	A condition where the theoretical or proven risks generally outweigh the advantages of using the method. The provision of a method requires expert clinical judgement and/or referral to a specialist contraceptive provider, since use of the method is not usually recommended unless other more appropriate methods are not available or not acceptable.
CATEGORY 4	A condition which represents an unacceptable health risk if the contraceptive method is used

Fig. 33.1 (*Continued*)

COMMON REVERSIBLE METHODS SUMMARY TABLE								
CONDITION	CHC	POP	DMPA/ NET-EN	IMP	Cu-IUD		LNG-IUD	
I = Initiation, C = Continuation								
GESTATIONAL TROPHOBLASTIC DISEASE (GTD)* (includes hydatidiform mole, invasive mole, and placental tumour)								
a) Decreasing or undetectable β-hCG levels	1	1	1	1	1		1	
b) Persistently elevated β-hCG levels or malignant disease	1	1	1	1	4		4	
CERVICAL ECTROPION	1	1	1	1	1		1	
CERVICAL INTRAEPITHELIAL NEOPLASIA	2	1	2	1	1		2	
CERVICAL CANCER (awaiting treatment)					I	C	I	C
	2	1	2	2	4	2	4	2
BREAST DISEASE								
a) Undiagnosed mass	I	C	2	2	2	1		2
	3	2						
b) Benign breast disease	1	1	1	1	1		1	
c) Family history of cancer	1	1	1	1	1		1	
d) Carriers of known gene mutations associated with breast cancer (eg.BRCA1)	3	2	2	2	1		2	
e) Breast cancer								
(i) Current	4	4	4	4	1		4	
(ii) Past and no evidence of current disease for 5 years	3	3	3	3	1		3	
ENDOMETRIAL CANCER					I	C	I	C
	1	1	1	1	4	2	4	2
OVARIAN CANCER					I	C	I	C
	1	1	1	1	3	2	3	2
UTERINE FIBROIDS								
a) Without distortion of the uterine avity	1	1	1	1	1		1	
b) With distortion of the uterine cavity	1	1	1	1	3		3	
ANATOMICAL ABNORMALITIES								
a) Distorted uterine cavity (any congenital or acquired uterine abnormality distorting the uterine cavity in a manner that is incompatible with IUD insertion)					3		3	
b) Other abnormalities (including cervical stenosis or cervical lacerations) not distorting the uterine cavity or interfering with IUD insertion					2		2	
PELVIC INFLAMMATORY DISEASE (PID)								
a) Past PID (assuming no current risk factors of STIs)	1	1	1	1	1		1	
b) Current PID					I	C	I	C
	1	1	1	1	4	2	4	2

* Advice should be sought from the specialist managing a woman's gestational trop-hoblastic disease as clinical guidelines can vary within the UK.

UKMEC	DEFINITION OF CATEGORY
CATEGORY 1	A condition for which there is no restriction for the use of the contraceptive method
CATEGORY 2	A condition where the advantages of using the method generally outweigh the theoretical or proven risks
CATEGORY 3	A condition where the theoretical or proven risks generally outweigh the advantages of using the method. The provision of a method requires expert clinical judgement and/or referral to a specialist contraceptive provider, since use of the method is not usually recommended unless other more appropriate methods are not available or not acceptable.
CATEGORY 4	A condition which represents an unacceptable health risk if the contraceptive method is used

Fig. 33.1 (Continued)

COMMON REVERSIBLE METHODS SUMMARY TABLE								
CONDITION	**CHC**	**POP**	**DMPA/ NET-EN**	**IMP**	**Cu-IUD**		**LNG-IUD**	
I = Initiation, C = Continuation								
SEXUALLY TRANSMITTED INFECTIONS (STIs)								
a) Chlamydial infection					**I**	**C**	**I**	**C**
i) Symptomatic	1	1	1	1	4	2	4	2
ii) Asymptomatic	1	1	1	1	4	2	4	2
b) Current purulent cervicitis or gonorrhoea	1	1	1	1	4	2	4	2
c) Other STIs (excluding HIV and hepatitis)	1	1	1	1	2		2	
d) Vaginitis (including *Trichomonas vaginalis* and bacterial vaginosis)	1	1	1	1	2		2	
e) Increased risk of STIs	1	1	1	1	2		2	
HIV / AIDS								
HIGH RISK OF HIV	1	1	1	1	2		2	
HIV INFECTED								
a) Not using anti-retroviral therapy	1	1	1	1	2		2	
b) Using anti-retroviral therapy (see drug interactions section)	1-3	1-3	1-2	1-2	2-2/3		2-2/3	
AIDS	2	2	2	2	2		2	
OTHER INFECTIONS								
SCHISTOSOMIASIS								
a) Uncomplicated	1	1	1	1	1		1	
b) Fibrosis of liver (if severe see cirrhosis)	1	1	1	1	1		1	
TUBERCULOSIS								
a) Non-pelvic	1	1	1	1	1		1	
b) Known pelvic	1	1	1	1	**I**	**C**	**I**	**C**
					4	3	4	3
MALARIA	1	1	1	1	1		1	
ENDOCRINE CONDITIONS								
DIABETES								
a) History of gestational diabetes	1	1	1	1	1		1	
b) Non-vascular disease								
(i) non-insulin dependent	2	2	2	2	1		2	
(ii) insulin dependent	2	2	2	2	1		2	
c) Nephropathy/retinopathy/ neuropathy	3/4	2	3	2	1		2	
d) Other vascular disease	3/4	2	3	2	1		2	
THYROID DISORDERS								
a) Simple goitre	1	1	1	1	1		1	
b) Hyperthyroid	1	1	1	1	1		1	
c) Hypothyroid	1	1	1	1	1		1	

UKMEC	DEFINITION OF CATEGORY
CATEGORY 1	A condition for which there is no restriction for the use of the contraceptive method
CATEGORY 2	A condition where the advantages of using the method generally outweigh the theoretical or proven risks
CATEGORY 3	A condition where the theoretical or proven risks generally outweigh the advantages of using the method. The provision of a method requires expert clinical judgement and/or referral to a specialist contraceptive provider, since use of the method is not usually recommended unless other more appropriate methods are not available or not acceptable.
CATEGORY 4	A condition which represents an unacceptable health risk if the contraceptive method is used

Fig. 33.1 (*Continued*)

COMMON REVERSIBLE METHODS SUMMARY TABLE						
CONDITION	CHC	POP	DMPA/NET-EN	IMP	Cu-IUD	LNG-IUD
I = Initiation, C = Continuation						
GASTROINTESTINAL CONDITIONS						
GALL BLADDER DISEASE						
a) Symptomatic						
(i) treated by cholecystectomy	2	2	2	2	1	2
(ii) medically treated	3	2	2	2	1	2
(iii) current	3	2	2	2	1	2
b) Asymptomatic	2	2	2	2	1	2
HISTORY OF CHOLESTASIS						
a) Pregnancy related	2	1	1	1	1	1
b) Past COC related	3	2	2	2	1	2
VIRAL HEPATITIS	I C					
a) Acute or flare	3/4 2	1	1	1	1	1
b) Carrier	1	1	1	1	1	1
c) Chronic	1	1	1	1	1	1
CIRRHOSIS						
a) Mild (compensated without complications)	1	1	1	1	1	1
b) Severe (decompensated)	4	3	3	3	1	3
LIVER TUMOURS						
a) Benign						
i) Focular nodular hyperplasia	2	2	2	2	1	2
ii) Hepatocellular (adenoma)	4	3	3	3	1	3
b) Malignant (hepatoma)	4	3	3	3	1	3
INFLAMMATORY BOWEL DISEASE (includes Crohn's Disease and ulcerative colitis)	2	2	1	1	1	1
ANAEMIAS						
THALASSAEMIA	1	1	1	1	2	1
SICKLE CELL DISEASE	2	1	1	1	2	1
IRON DEFICIENCY ANAEMIA	1	1	1	1	2	1
RAYNAUD'S DISEASE						
a) Primary	1	1	1	1	1	1
b) Secondary						
(i) without lupus anticoagulant	2	2	1	1	1	1
(ii) with lupus anticoagulant	4	2	2	2	1	2
RHEUMATIC DISEASES						
SYSTEMIC LUPUS ERYTHEMATOSUS (SLE) People with SLE are at an increased risk of ischaemic heart disease, stroke, and venous thromboembolism and this is reflected in the categories given.						
a) Positive (or unknown) antiphospholipid antibodies	4	3	3	3	3	3
b) Severe thrombocytopenia	2	2	I 3 C 2	2	I 3 C 2	2
c) Immunosuppressive	2	2	2	2	I 2 C 1	2
d) None of the above	2	2	2	2	1	2

UKMEC	DEFINITION OF CATEGORY
CATEGORY 1	A condition for which there is no restriction for the use of the contraceptive method
CATEGORY 2	A condition where the advantages of using the method generally outweigh the theoretical or proven risks
CATEGORY 3	A condition where the theoretical or proven risks generally outweigh the advantages of using the method. The provision of a method requires expert clinical judgement and/or referral to a specialist contraceptive provider, since use of the method is not usually recommended unless other more appropriate methods are not available or not acceptable.
CATEGORY 4	A condition which represents an unacceptable health risk if the contraceptive method is used

Fig. 33.1 (Continued)

COMMON REVERSIBLE METHODS SUMMARY TABLE						
CONDITION	CHC	POP	DMPA/ NET-EN	IMP	Cu-IUD	LNG-IUD
I = Initiation, C = Continuation						

DRUG INTERACTIONS

ANTIRETROVIRAL THERAPY
This section relates to the SAFETY of contraception use in women using these antiretrovirals. EFFECTIVENESS may be reduced and pregnancy itself may have a negative impact on health for some women with certain medical conditions.

Antiretroviral therapy and hormonal contraception: Antiretroviral drugs have the potential to either decrease or increase the bioavailability of steroid hormones in hormonal contraceptives. Limited data suggest potential drug interactions between many antiretroviral drugs (particularly some non-nucleoside reverse transcriptase inhibitors and ritonavir-boosted protease inhibitors) and hormonal contraceptives. These interactions may alter the safety and effectiveness of both the hormonal contraceptive and the antiretroviral drug. Thus, **if a woman on antiretroviral treatment decides to initiate or continue hormonal contraceptive use, THE CONSISTENT USE OF CONDOMS IS RECOMMENDED**. This is for both preventing HIV transmission and to compensate for any possible reduction in the effectiveness of the hormonal contraceptive. When a COC is chosen, a preparation containing a minimum of 30mcgs EE should be used.

Antiretroviral therapy and IUDs: There is no known interaction between antiretroviral therapy and IUD use. However, AIDS as a condition is classified as Category 3 for insertion and Category 2 for continuation unless the woman is clinically well on antiretroviral therapy, in which case both insertion and continuations are classified as Category 2. (See AIDS condition).

					I	C	I	C
a) Nucleoside reverse transcriptase inhibitors	1	1	DMPA=1 NET-EN=2	1	2/3	2	2/3	2
b) Non-nucleoside reverse transcriptase inhibitors	2	2	DMPA=1 NET-EN=2	2	2/3	2	2/3	2
c) Ritonavir-boosted protease inhibitors	3	3	DMPA=1 NET-EN=2	2	2/3	2	2/3	2

ANTICONVULSANT THERAPY
This section relates to the SAFETY of using methods of contraception in women using these medications. EFFECTIVENESS may be reduced and pregnancy itself may have a negative impact on health for some women with certain medical conditions.

Certain anticonvulsants and combined oral contraception: When a COC is chosen, a preparation containing a minimum of 30mcgs EE should be used. **THE CONSISTENT USE OF CONDOMS IS RECOMMENDED***.

Certain anticonvulsants and progestogen-only contraception: Although the interaction of certain anticonvulsants with POPs, NET-EN and implants is not harmful to women, it is likely to reduce the effectiveness of POPs, NET-EN and implants. Whether increasing the hormone dose of POPs alleviates this concern remains unclear.

If a woman on certain anticonvulsants decides to use CHC, POP or implant **THE CONSISTENT USE OF CONDOMS IS RECOMMENDED***. Use of other contraceptives should be encouraged for women who are long-term users of any of these anticonvulsant drugs. Use of DMPA is a Category 1 because its effectiveness is NOT decreased by the use of certain anticonvulsants.

Lamotrigine: When a COC is chosen, a preparation containing a minimum of 30mcgs EE should be used. Anticonvulsant treatment regimens that combine lamotrigine and non-enzyme inducting antiepileptic drugs (such as sodium valproate) do not interact with COCs.

a) Certain anticonvulsants (phenytoin, carbamazepine, barbiturates, primidone, topiramate, oxcarbazepine)	3*	3*	DMPA=1 NET-EN=2	2*	1	1
b) Lamotrigine	3	1	1	1	1	1

UKMEC	DEFINITION OF CATEGORY
CATEGORY 1	A condition for which there is no restriction for the use of the contraceptive method
CATEGORY 2	A condition where the advantages of using the method generally outweigh the theoretical or proven risks
CATEGORY 3	A condition where the theoretical or proven risks generally outweigh the advantages of using the method. The provision of a method requires expert clinical judgement and/or referral to a specialist contraceptive provider, since use of the method is not usually recommended unless other more appropriate methods are not available or not acceptable.
CATEGORY 4	A condition which represents an unacceptable health risk if the contraceptive method is used

Fig. 33.1 (Continued)

COMMON REVERSIBLE METHODS SUMMARY TABLE						
CONDITION	**CHC**	**POP**	**DMPA/ NET-EN**	**IMP**	**Cu-IUD**	**LNG-IUD**
I = Initiation, C = Continuation						

DRUG INTERACTIONS

ANTIMICROBIAL THERAPY
This section relates to the **SAFETY** of contraceptive use in women using these antimicrobials.
EFFECTIVENESS may be reduced and pregnancy itself may have a negative impact on health for
some women with certain medical conditions.

There is intermediate level evidence that the contraceptive effectiveness of COC is not affected by co-administration of most broad-spectrum antibiotics. **Rifampicin or rifabutin therapy and combined oral contraception:** When a COC is chosen, a preparation containing a minimum of 30mcgs EE should be used. **THE CONSISTENT USE OF CONDOMS IS RECOMMENDED*.** Rifampicin or rifabutin therapy and progestogen-only contraception: Although the interaction of rifampicin or rifabutin with POPs, NET-EN and implants is not harmful to women, it is likely to reduce the effectiveness of POPs, NET-EN and implants. Whether increasing the hormone does of POPs alleviates this concern remains unclear. If a woman on rifampicin or rifabutin decides to use CHC, POP or implant **THE CONSISTENT USE OF CONDOMS IS RECOMMENDED*.** Use of other contraceptives should be encouraged for women who are long-term users of rifampicin or rifabutin. Use of DMPA is a Category 1 because its effectiveness is unlikely to be decreased by the use of rifampicin or rifabutin.						
a) Broad spectrum antibiotics	1*	1	1	1	1	1
b) Antifungals	1	1	1	1	1	1
c) Antiparasitics	1	1	1	1	1	1
d) Rifampicin or rifabutin therapy	3*	3*	DMPA=1 NET-EN=2*	2*	1	1

UKMEC	DEFINITION OF CATEGORY
CATEGORY 1	A condition for which there is no restriction for the use of the contraceptive method
CATEGORY 2	A condition where the advantages of using the method generally outweigh the theoretical or proven risks
CATEGORY 3	A condition where the theoretical or proven risks generally outweigh the advantages of using the method. The provision of a method requires expert clinical judgement and/or referral to a specialist contraceptive provider, since use of the method is not usually recommended unless other more appropriate methods are not available or not acceptable.
CATEGORY 4	A condition which represents an unacceptable health risk if the contraceptive method is used

Fig. 33.1 (Continued)

Psychological aspects and sexual dysfunction

Psychological aspects

Personality types

In those attending clinics for STIs:
- extroversion—associated with ↑ sexual partners, varied sexual behaviour, and ↑ STIs.
- psychoticism—related to ↑ sexual curiosity, promiscuity, and hostility.
- neuroticism—associated with ↓ sexual satisfaction but ↑ sexual guilt, inhibition, and exaggerated concerns about STIs.

Clinic patients

20–40% of new patients attending clinics for STIs have been classified as 'psychiatric cases' based on general health questionnaire scores showing high levels of anxiety. It is important to recognize and manage this during the consultation to help address the presenting problem as well as improve subsequent attendance. The origins of anxiety at presentation are multi-factorial, although stigma and shame are prominent. New diagnoses of HIV infection, anogenital herpes, and syphilis generate the greatest anxiety and are also the most common STIs associated with phobias.

The greatest psychological reaction usually arises from a diagnosis of HIV infection. It does not necessarily relate to the stage of the disease and may exhibit a 'bereavement'-type reaction—disbelief, denial, anxiety, and depression. There may also be suicidal tendencies. In addition, such feelings may be complicated by guilt, resentment, and stigmatization. Regular support is important, ensuring that information is given at and over a time best suited to the individual. Referral for specialist advice/treatment may also be required.

Certain procedures (e.g. colposcopy for abnormal cervical cytology) are associated with very high levels of anxiety. Stress and depression are common features of chronic conditions, e.g. HIV infection, vulval vestibulitis, chronic pelvic pain, prostatitis, and persistent anogenital warts. They are also reported with conditions that may recur (e.g. anogenital herpes, warts, and vaginal candidiasis). Patients need sufficient time to express their anxiety and a careful explanation of the condition (with written information) is important. Therapeutic intervention (e.g. antiretroviral treatment for HIV and suppressive treatment for frequent recurrences of herpes) may ↓ psychological morbidity. Stigma and shame, associated especially with chronic STIs, fuel anxiety and may hinder disclosure to sexual partners.

Neuroses associated with STIs

Over-reaction and hypochondriasis

Examples include:
- inappropriate reaction to the condition diagnosed
- undue vigorous penile squeezing to produce a urethral discharge
- obsessional attention to genital marks and irregularities.

May be a symptom of some other underlying problem (e.g. rumours about a sexual partner). Managed by exploring the patient's anxieties and correcting misinformation.

Phobias

Excessive and inappropriate anxiety reactions triggered by specific situations or objects, despite having an insight into the lack of reason or appropriateness. Often triggered by stress and media publicity. Likely to be prompted by underlying guilt or a sexual concern which should be addressed when formulating management strategies.

Factitious illness and Munchausen's syndrome

In GUM often related to HIV infection with imagined positive test result. Reasons and motivation are often unclear, but may be used to gain sympathy, hospital care, or social benefits. Psychiatric referral is often required.

Sexual dysfunction

Classification by the American Psychiatric Association

- Sexual desire disorders:
  - hypoactive
  - sexual aversion
- Sexual arousal disorder
- Orgasmic disorder
- Sexual pain disorders:
  - dyspareunia
  - vaginismus

After organic problems have been identified and treated the management of sexual dysfunctions requires the cooperation and support of both partners. Emotional issues which may also underlie or complicate the presenting problem should be explored and addressed through counselling. Simple counselling, provided to an individual or couple, is often brief:

- it provides basic information and corrects false ideas
- it makes suggestions, e.g. positions during intercourse
- it provides permission and reassures—often linked with a new suggestion (e.g. the use of vibrators and other sex aids)
- it facilitates communication between partners in particular to develop self-assertiveness and self-protection.

This may lead to behavioural psychotherapy for individuals, couples, or sometimes groups. The framework consists of the following:

- setting behavioural tasks (i.e. 'homework').
- analysis of the patient's or couple's success, identifying obstacles or difficulties
- provision of help, support, and advice to address the obstacles and problems
- review of the new situation with new tasks set or revised.

More common problems seen in women presenting to GUM

Low sexual desire/arousal (sexual anhedonia) and orgasmic dysfunction
Heterogeneous condition
Causal factors include:

- partner conflict and disharmony
- ignorance
- psychological causes (e.g. anxiety, depression, body dysmorphism)
- physical causes—local (e.g. endometriosis, cystitis), systemic (e.g. diabetes mellitus, multiple sclerosis), drugs (e.g. oral contraceptives, hypotensives, tranquillizers), surgery affecting body image (e.g. hysterectomy, mastectomy)
- post-menopause— ~15% significant decline in arousal.

Management

- Definition and management of any underlying problem. In post-menopausal ♀ hormone replacement treatment with androgenic activity (e.g. tibolone).
- Testosterone transdermal patch (Intrinsa®)—licensed for female hypoactive sexual desire disorder in bilaterally oopherectomized and hysterectomized (i.e. surgically induced menopause) ♀ receiving concomitant oestrogen therapy, although only recommended up to the age of 60 years. Statistically significant improvement in sexual desire demonstrated in 6 month duration clinical trials although ↑ adverse effects, mainly hirsutism and acne, also demonstrated.
- Sensate focus (of benefit despite level of inhibition)—a three-stage programme in which the couple progresses stepwise from non-genital pleasuring through genital pleasuring to non-demanding coitus under the control of the ♀.
- Insufficient data on drugs but apomorphine may benefit some with arousal and hypoactive sexual disorders. Phosphodiesterase-5 inhibitors appear to be disappointing.

Dyspareunia

Genital pain just before, during, or after sexual intercourse. More common in ♀ and liable to be exacerbated by vaginismus (involuntary bulbo-cavernosus muscle spasm) and psychological factors especially anxiety and marital/partner adjustment.

Vulvovaginal problems

- Congenital—e.g. rigid hymen
- Physiological—inadequate lubrication (e.g. oestrogen deficiency)
- Traumatic—e.g. episiotomy, radiation therapy
- Inflammatory:
  - infective—e.g. candidosis, trichomoniasis
  - ulcerative—e.g. genital herpes, syphilis, aphthosis, Behçet's disease
  - dermatological—e.g. irritant dermatitis, lichen sclerosis or planus
  - degenerative—atrophic vulvovaginitis
  - vulvar vestibulitis
- Neoplastic—e.g. squamous cell carcinoma
- Bartholin gland—abscess, cyst

Uterine/pelvic problems

Retroverted uterus, pelvic congestion, cervicitis, endometritis, pelvic inflammatory disease, pelvic adhesions, endometriosis, fibroids, adnexal pathology (e.g. ovarian cysts, tumours).

Anal/intestinal problems

Anal fissure/fistula, irritable bowel, inflammatory bowel disease.

Urinary problems

Urethritis, urethral caruncle, cystitis.

Vaginismus

A learned response, often secondary to dyspareunia (e.g. from vestibulitis, atrophic vaginitis, trauma), leading to recurrent or persistent involuntary contraction of the musculature of the outer third of the vagina, interfering with coitus and causing distress. Other causes/factors include fear of pregnancy, loss of control, association of intercourse with violence, previous sexual abuse, relationship difficulties, and religious/cultural taboos. Tampons are usually avoided, and external towels are used for menstruation. Involuntary perineal spasms may occur while preparing for/conducting a pelvic examination which is often evaded.

Management

Management is in stages—problem-oriented therapy with behavioural and desensitization exercises.

- Exclude or manage physical causes and psychological factors. Inform and correct misunderstanding of sexual functioning, ideally with the partner's involvement if agreeable.
- Encourage ♀ to become comfortable touching her genitalia and inserting a finger into the vagina.
- Proceed to more fingers and/or the use of lubricated graded dilators.
- Advise Kegel's exercise—perineal contraction (against inserted finger(s) or dilators) followed by relaxation, to help muscle control.
- Suggest partner involvement—gentle introduction of a finger into the vagina, slowly escalating to more fingers or dilators.
- When comfortable, proceed to penetrative sexual intercourse with the ♀ adopting a position (e.g. superior) to maintain control.

More common problems seen in men presenting to GUM

Erectile dysfunction (ED) (Table 34.1)

Common, affecting over 50% aged 40–70 years (although only 10% fail to achieve nocturnal erections): 60% organic, 15% psychogenic, 25% mixed.

Main causes

- Lifestyle factors: obesity, smoking (×1.5), alcohol, recreational drugs.
- Trauma and iatrogenic, e.g. prolonged bicycle riding, prostatic/pelvic surgery, pelvic fracture, and local radiation treatment.
- Drugs, e.g. antidepressants (most), antipsychotics (many), hypotensives (most), androgen inhibitors (e.g. finasteride for benign prostatic hypertrophy).
- Vascular: responsible for nearly 50% of cases in those aged >50 years, e.g. ischaemic heart disease (IHD), hypertension, peripheral vascular disease. Coexisting IHD (up to 40%) manifests a mean of ~38 months after ED (penile arteries 1–2mm, coronary 3–4mm).
- Endocrine: diabetes mellitus (~50% have ED), neurogenic and vascular factors; hyper/hypothyroidism; hypogonadism, both physiological and pathological; hyperprolactinaemia.
- Neurological: multiple sclerosis; Parkinson's disease.
- Psychogenic (depression, anxiety): ↑ sympathetic tone. Performance anxiety may become self-perpetuating.

Table 34.1 International index of erectile function-5 (IIEF-5) scoring system

Over the past 6 months	Score				
	1	**2**	**3**	**4**	**5**
Confidence in getting and keeping an erection	Very low	Low	Moderate	High	Very high
Erections on sexual stimulation hard enough for penetration	Never/ almost never	<50% of the time	~50% of the time	>50% of the time	Always/ almost always
Maintaining erection afterpenetration	Never/ almost never	<50% of the time	~50% of the time	>50% of the time	Always/ almost always
Maintaining erection to completion of intercourse	Extremely difficult	Very difficult	Difficult	Slightly difficult	Not difficult
Satisfactory intercourse	Never/ almost never	<50% of the time	~50% of the time	>50% of the time	Always/ almost always

IIEF-5 score ≤21 correlates with ED (98% sensitive and 88% specific)

Basic assessment
- History: for risk factors; libido, shaving (need and frequency).
- Examination: genital abnormalities including hypogonadism, facial/body hair, neurological (S2–S4 dermatomes), blood pressure/peripheral pulses.
- Investigations: exclude diabetes (urinalysis/blood glucose); consider serum testosterone, prolactin + other endocrine tests (thyroid, pituitary function). Ultrasonography and angiography rarely required.

First-line management
- Psychosexual therapy (alone or in combination).
- Phosphodiesterase-5 inhibitors:
  - Sildenafil: recommended dose 50mg (range 25–100mg) 1 hour before intercourse. Advise 1 dose in 24 hours (100mg maximum). 29% ↓ in plasma concentration with food. Half-life, 4–5 hours.
  - Vardenafil: recommended dose 10mg (range 2.5–20mg) 25–60 minutes before intercourse. Advise 1 dose in 24 hours (20mg maximum). 20% ↓ in plasma concentration with food. Half-life, 4.8–6 hours.
  - Tadalafil: recommended dose 10mg (range 10–20mg) 30 minutes–12 hours before intercourse. Maximum dose over 24 hours, 20mg. No ↓ in plasma concentration with food. Half-life, 17.5–21 hours.

Success rates (erection suitable for intercourse) of phosphodiesterase-5 inhibitors up to 75%, but high placebo rates (22–38%). Contraindicated in patients taking nitrates (both therapeutic and recreational) and those with hypotension, unstable angina, recent cerebrovascular accident, or myocardial infarction.

Alternative management methods
- Central dopamine agonist: apomorphine. Recommended dose 2mg (up to 3mg) sublingually 20 minutes before intercourse. Minimum of 8 hours between doses. Success rate ~50% (32% with placebo). Contraindications include hypotension, severe unstable angina, severe heart failure, or recent myocardial infarction. With the exception of Parkinson's disease, $\male$ with neurological disease do not respond.
- Synthetic prostaglandin E_1 agent (e.g. alprostadil): available as intra-urethral pellets (usual starting dose 250mcg up to 1mg) or as an intra-cavernosal injection (usual dose range 5–20mcg). Up to 90% response rate with injection and 40–60% with pellets.
- Testosterone (IM or transdermal): should only be considered when ED is related to hypogonadism, otherwise no evidence of benefit. Hepatotoxic.
- Pelvic floor exercises with biofeedback (including perineal muscle electrical stimulation). Only if ED related to venous leakage or occlusion (success rate ~50%).
- Mechanical aids:
  - Vacuum devices: suck venous blood into the penis, causing an erection maintained by a firm constricting band. Lacks spontaneity, may cause bruising and produces a venous (cold/blue) erection.
  - Implants: e.g. inflatable devices, malleable rods.

Premature ejaculation
Most common sexual dysfunction in $\male$ under 40 years, reported in ~40%. Difficult to define as dependent on sexual partner and may indicate delayed $\female$ orgasm, but generally indicative of ejaculation with minimal sexual satisfaction occurring before the person wishes. Generally considered to be a psychological problem; rarely reported with chronic prostatitis.
- *Primary* Patient has always ejaculated prematurely. Often considered to be a conditioned response from teenage masturbatory practices but may reflect deep sexual anxiety from childhood traumatic experiences including sexual assault and/or familial conflict. Current research suggests genetic susceptibility and ↓ central serotonin (5-hydroxy tryptamine (5-HT)) mediated neurotransmission are also important factors.
- *Secondary* Previous ejaculatory control. Probably largely related to performance anxiety.

Management
If associated with erectile dysfunction treat this first.
- Stop/start: manual stimulation (initially) by partner or patient until ejaculation is imminent. Then cease for 30 seconds before resuming. The sequence is repeated until ejaculation is required.
- Squeeze technique: similar approach but firm pressure is applied across the penis at the frenum, aborting imminent ejaculation.

Over time these methods progress to vulval contact and then vaginal penetration (♀ superior), stopping for 30 seconds or withdrawing and squeezing as ejaculation approaches. Success rate 65–90% with active participation of partner.

- Ejaculation 1–2 hours before coitus: young ♂—longer latent period for coital ejaculation. (Older ♂ may have problems attaining erection even after 2 hours.)
- Reduce sensation:
  - local anaesthetic gel/ointment, e.g. lidocaine (provided that there is no allergy)
  - use of less sensitive condoms.
- Drug treatment (not licensed): selective serotonin re-uptake inhibitors (SSRIs) and clomipramine delay ejaculation by their effect on central 5-HT receptors. SSRIs take at least 3 weeks to produce the effect but clomipramine is effective after a single dose. Regimens shown to be effective:
  - daily—clomipramine 10–40mg or SSRI (paroxetine 20–40mg, sertraline 50–100mg, or fluoxetine 20mg).
  - 'On-demand'—clomipramine 10–50mg 5–6 hours before coitus.
- Pelvic floor (Kegel) exercises.

Retarded ejaculation

Difficulty, delay, or absence of orgasm following sufficient sexual stimulation which causes personal distress.

Aetiology

- Physiological: ↓ sensitivity, inadequate stimulation
- Congenital: Wolffian and Mullerian duct malformations
- Benign prostatic hypertrophy, prostatic carcinoma
- ↑ age: neuronal degeneration, ↓ sensitivity associated with ↓ testosterone
- Pelvic surgery: e.g. prostatectomy (transurethral/radical), bladder neck surgery, proctocolectomy
- Neurological: e.g. multiple sclerosis, spinal cord damage
- Endocrine: diabetes mellitus (neuropathy), hypogonadism
- Drugs: e.g. alcohol, most anti-depressants and drugs for treating obsessive–compulsive disorders, α- and β-blockers, anticholinergic agents
- Psychological: e.g. fear of being seen, pregnancy, infection.

Management

Treat underlying cause, when relevant. If associated erectile dysfunction, this should be managed first. If drug related, consider altering medication or adding pharmacological adjuvants, e.g. amantadine (100–400mg for 2 days prior to coitus), bupropion (75–150mg), buspirone (15–60mg), cyproheptadine (4–12mg), or yohimbine (5–10mg), all as needed, if SSRI induced (⚠ outwith product licences).

- Psychological approach.
- Explore and resolve any underlying anxieties.
- Establish extra-genital ejaculation, with suitable stimulation (mechanical, visual, etc. as required), gradually introducing vaginal contact and insertion into the programme.
- Male superior position—facilitates ejaculation.

Dyspareunia
Genital
- Congenital/post-traumatic: e.g. phimosis, tight frenum
- Inflammatory: urethritis, genital herpes, syphilis, candidosis, dermatological (e.g. lichen sclerosis), aphthosis, Behçet's disease
- Peyronie's disease
- Iatrogenic (e.g. intracorporeal and transurethral alprostadil; rarely priapism following phosphodiesterase type-5 inhibitor use)
- Testicular lesions: e.g. epididymitis, torsion
- Neoplastic: e.g. squamous cell carcinoma

Ejaculatory pain
- Seminal vesicle disorders: calculi, cystic malformations, metastatic cancer
- Other pelvic causes: chronic prostatitis, benign prostatic hypertrophy and prostatic carcinoma, urethral stricture, pelvic arteriovenous malformation, hernia repair
- Drugs: antidepressants, neuroleptics
- Mercury poisoning
- Psychogenic: e.g. fear of being seen

Anal
Anal dyspareunia during receptive anal intercourse may be due to psychogenic factors or intestinal tract diseases including anal fissures, inflammatory disease, and irritable bowel disease.

HIV infection

- Bereavement reaction with new HIV-positive result
- Extreme anxiety and phobia generated by HIV
- May be associated with reduced testosterone levels due to hypogonadism (or possibly related to the aromatization of testosterone to oestrogen) leading to a ↓ in libido and ED
- Effect of lipodystrophy for those on antiretroviral treatment on self-image and self-esteem
- Retarded ejaculation associated with peripheral neuropathy related directly to either HIV infection or drug toxicity
- Recreational and illicit drugs used by some HIV-infected men who have sex with men may ↑ unsafe sex and contribute to poor therapeutic adherence

HIV: introduction and epidemiology

History

In 1981 an epidemic of a previously unknown acquired immune deficiency syndrome (AIDS) was described in the USA. A lentivirus (subfamily of retroviruses) was subsequently identified. Lentus (from the Latin for slow) denotes the long latent phase between infection and the development of symptoms. Retroviruses use the enzyme reverse transcriptase (RT) to generate proviral DNA from RNA (reverse of the usual direction of genetic transcription). The term human immunodeficiency virus (HIV) was accepted in 1986. In the same year a related virus (HIV-2), endemic in West Africa and sharing common features including the induction of immune deficiency, was identified.

Origin of HIV

There are structural and genomic organizational similarities between HIV and simian immune deficiency virus (SIV). Phylogenetically, HIV-1 and HIV-2 cluster with chimpanzee (*Pan troglodytes*) (SIVcpz) and sooty mangabey (SIVsm) simian retroviruses, respectively. SIVcpz is almost identical to HIV-1.

The structural differences between HIV-1 and HIV-2 may explain the differences in natural history, pathogenicity, and susceptibility to antiretroviral drugs.

Evidence that the virus existed for some time before its effects became clinically apparent in 1981 is supported by the following.

- HIV detected in a blood sample taken in 1959 from an adult male living in the former Zaire. A different subtype was detected in a lymph node biopsy taken in 1960 from an adult female from the same country. Phylogenetic analysis of these two samples suggests that HIV may have crossed species some 35–75 years previously.
- HIV found in tissue samples from an African American teenager who died in St Louis, USA, in 1969.
- HIV found in tissue samples from a Norwegian sailor who died around 1976.

Prevalence

Worldwide (Table 35.1)

33 million people (15 million women and 2.5 million children under 15 years) were estimated living with HIV in 2007. Two-thirds of them are in sub-Saharan Africa. The estimated proportion of population infected with HIV has stabilized since 2001, mainly because of changes in high-risk behaviour and maturity of the pandemic in sub-Saharan Africa.

In the developed countries the number of people living with HIV is likely to   because of migration, continuing transmission, and availability of life-prolonging drugs. Infection rates are likely to stay high in countries with poverty, inadequate healthcare, and limited resources for prevention. The socio-economic impact is greater in developing countries.

UK (Fig. 35.1)

Cumulative total of 93,000 reported cases of HIV in the UK by the end of 2007, with an estimated 73,000 living with HIV of whom one-third are unaware of their infection.

New infections have accelerated among ♂ who have sex with ♂ (MSM) since 1999, and by end of 2006 40% of people living with HIV were MSM.

Heterosexually acquired infections have been ↑ since the early years of the epidemic and outnumber those acquired through sex between ♂ since 1999. Over the past 10 years the migration of people into the UK from areas in the world with high HIV prevalence has contributed significantly to the increase in heterosexually transmitted infection.Injecting drug use plays a small role in the UK epidemic. The age at diagnosis of this group has risen, suggesting that new diagnoses are being made on a population mostly infected in the mid-1980s before widespread needle exchange programmes where introduced.

Screening blood donations and heat treatment of blood products to inactivate HIV was introduced in the UK in 1985. Since then there have been no recorded transmissions of HIV through contaminated clotting factors given to haemophilia patients. However, there have been five cases where HIV infection could have been acquired through blood transfusion. Current estimated blood transfusion risk in the UK is <1 in 1 million units.

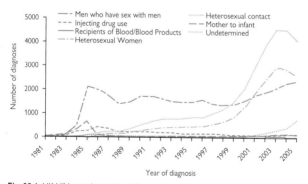

Fig. 35.1 UK HIV prevalence by risk factor. *Source:* From the Health Protection Agency ♪ www.hpa.org.uk

Table 35.1 HIV seroprevalence rates in adults aged 15–49 years (based on 2007 UNAIDS data)

Heterosexuals	
UK	
North America, Western and Central Europe	0.1–<1.0%
Eastern Europe	0.1–2%
South America and Caribbean	0.1–3%
South, Eastern, Southeast Asia	<0.1–2%
Oceania	<0.1–2%
Middle East	<0.1–3%
Africa	
Southern	20–28
Central and Eastern	5–<15
Northern	<0.1–<0.5
Western	1–<5
MSM	
London	15%
Rest of UK	2–3%
Injecting drug users	
London	4.7%
Rest of UK	0.2%

The viruses and their epidemiology

HIV-1 and HIV-2

HIV-1 and HIV-2 differ in several aspects.

- HIV-1: found worldwide, a rapidly mutating virus eventually producing divergent quasi-species. More virulent and rapidly progressive than HIV-2.
- HIV-2: predominantly found in West Africa but also reported in Portugal and France and increasingly in India and South America. Predominantly heterosexually transmitted. Lower viral loads (VLs) than HIV-1 independent of the duration of infection. Rate of vertical transmission ↓ than HIV-1.

HIV-1 and 2 are classified into groups according to their genetic diversity.

HIV-1

- Group M (main group—90% of infection). Further divided into subtypes or clades with at least 11 genetically distinct subtypes: A1, A2, B, C, D, (E now considered a circulating recombinant form, RF01_AE), F1, F2, G, H, J, and K (I now classified as a CRF complex). Some variants are termed U category, i.e. uncertain or unclassifiable, and may represent new subtypes or recombinant forms. More than 40 circulating recombinant forms have been described so far and are likely to increase, as is their proportion in the pandemic.
- Group O (outlier group).
- Group N (new group).

HIV-2

Divided into groups: non-recombinant (A–G) and recombinant (AB).

Geographical distribution of HIV groups and subtypes

Group M is the most common group worldwide. The majority of its subtypes are found in Africa, while certain subtypes predominate in other regions.

Groups N and O are rare and remain confined to Western and Central Africa. Population movement and international travel will erode the geographical boundaries of subtype location.

Predominant subtype distribution

- B—America, Europe, Australia, and Japan; Thailand and Southeast Asia (IV drug users). At least 25% of infections in Europe now are non-B subtypes.
- A and D—sub-Saharan Africa.
- C—Southern and Eastern Africa and India. Responsible for almost half of the infections worldwide.
- E (CRF01_AE)—Thailand and Southeast Asia.
- F—Brazil (also in Romania).
- H—localized to Central Africa.
- J—Central America.

Biological implications of HIV subtypes
- Mode of transmission of HIV-1 subtypes:
  - subtype B is mainly found in MSM.
  - subtypes E (CRF01_AE) and C are more commonly seen in heterosexuals. They replicate more easily than subtype B in Langerhans' cells (normally found in the vagina, cervix, and prepuce, but not in the rectum).
- Infectivity: subtype E (CRF01_AE) is transmitted more easily than subtype B.
- Natural history: subtype D causes more progressive disease than subtype A.
- Response to therapy:
  - implications of subtype diversity need continuous assessment as they may influence the response to treatment
  - HIV-2 is intrinsically resistant to non-nucleoside RT inhibitors.
- Vaccine production: unclear whether a vaccine provides subtype cross-protection. Genetic variations may be important and necessitate periodic vaccine modification (as with influenza vaccine).
- Diagnosis and screening strategies: diagnostic tests must reliably detect the various strains, subtypes, and circulating recombinant forms. Modifications of tests can be made to ensure that all those with HIV infection are detected. This is also important for ensuring safety of the blood supply.

Phenotypic classification

HIV can also be classified on its ability to form a syncytium with CD4 cells *in vitro*. This ability is not directly related to the genotypic characteristic of the virus. Therefore, within each HIV subtype, there are isolates that are syncytium-inducing (SI) and non-syncytium-inducing (NSI). Most 1° HIV strains are NSI, while SI strains tend to appear with disease progression. This switch depends on cellular tropism for macrophages or T cells and on the chemokine co-receptor used to gain entry into the CD4 cell. Most NSI strains use CCR5 co-receptors and most SI strains use CXCR4 co-receptors.

Risk factors (Table 35.2) and routes of transmission

HIV is exclusively transmitted through body fluids . Routes of transmission include:

- Sexual intercourse: between ♂ and ♀, ♂ and ♂, and rarely ♀ and ♀. Although sex between ♂ and ♂ characterized the initial HIV epidemic seen in the USA, Western Europe, and Australasia, elsewhere it is typically spread heterosexually. The relative risk of infection depends on the local prevalence and also the type of sexual practice.
- Sharing infected needles and syringes among drug users.
- Transfusion of blood and blood products: now very rare in countries where blood is screened for HIV. Transmission may still occur in the developing world through re-use of contaminated surgical equipment and needles.
- Vertically from an infected mother to baby: antepartum, intrapartum, and postpartum (breastfeeding).
- Occupational exposure: to healthcare professionals (HCP). Only one documented case of an HCP transmitting HIV to patients.

Table 35.2 HIV transmission risk following a single exposure to HIV infection*

Sexual intercourse	
Anal: receptive	0.1–3%
Anal: insertive	0.06%
Vaginal: receptive	0.1–0.2%
Vaginal: insertive	0.03–0.09%
Oral (fellatio): receptive	Up to 0.04%
Oral: cunnilingus and insertive fellatio	No data but estimated to be at least half receptive rate
Sharing injecting equipment	0.7%
Single unit of blood	90–100%
Occupational	
Needlestick injury	0.3%
Mucous membrane contact	0.1%

*Influenced by plasma and genital VLs, breaks in mucosal surfaces (e.g. trauma, genital ulcer disease).

Frequently asked questions

What is HIV?

HIV (human immunodeficiency virus) is a virus which damages the body's immune system. HIV destroys a type of white blood cell called the CD4 cell. This cell spearheads/leads the body's defence against infection. When a person's CD4 count becomes low he/she is more susceptible to certain infections.

What is AIDS?

AIDS (acquired immune deficiency syndrome) is the final stage of HIV infection. When the CD4 cells drop to a very low level (usually <200 cells/μL), the ability to resist certain infections is seriously impaired. Certain opportunistic conditions (AIDS-defining illnesses) can develop, e.g. *Pneumocystis jiroveci* (*carinii*) pneumonia (PCP), Kaposi's sarcoma.

How is HIV transmitted?

- Having unprotected sex with an infected person.
- Sharing a needle/equipment to take drugs.
- Receiving a blood transfusion from an infected person (unlikely in the UK where blood has been tested for HIV since 1985).
- Transmission from a positive mother to her baby during pregnancy or delivery, and by breastfeeding.

Can it be passed on by kissing?

There is no evidence of transmission by kissing, and viral levels in saliva are very low. Body fluids which contain high levels of HIV correlating with infection are blood, seminal fluid, vaginal/menstrual fluid, and breast milk.

Can it be passed on by oral sex?

Yes, especially with receptive fellatio.

Does HIV have symptoms?

Some people have flu-like symptoms 4–8 weeks after infection. They usually settle within 1–2 weeks. A person can have HIV for many years before developing symptoms (and may never do so).

Does a negative HIV antibody test mean I have not contracted HIV?

This depends on when your last risk activity was. An antibody test can be negative in the first few weeks after transmission. A further negative test at 3 months should confirm that transmission has not occurred

Delay between infection and a positive HIV antibody test

Although most infected people test positive within 2–6 weeks, it can take up to 3 months for enough antibodies to be produced to give a positive HIV antibody test. During this time the person is often very infectious with a high viral load.

Pathogenesis of HIV infection

HIV structure

HIV-1 and HIV-2 are structurally similar (icosahedral) with the following components (Fig. 36.1).

- **Envelope**: a lipid bilayer formed from host cell lipids and viral proteins. Embedded in the envelope is a complex protein (env) containing the viral surface glycoprotein (gp120) and a transmembrane glycoprotein (gp41). Both are derived from a precursor (gp160).
- **Matrix**: encapsulated by the envelope and made up of viral protein p17.
- **Core**: comprises
  - RNA dimer—two identical copies of single-stranded RNA linked together, each containing ~9500 nucleotides. Associated with nucleocapsid (p7 and p6).
  - Capsid protein p24 encapsulates the ribonucleoprotein core which contains three enzymes—reverse transcriptase (p66/51), integrase (p31), and protease (p15).

Genetic organization of HIV

- Genetic information is stored as RNA.
- Gene maps for HIV-1 and HIV-2 are similar except that HIV-2 has *vpx* instead of *vpu*.
- Both sides of the HIV provirus are flanked by a repeated sequence known as the long-terminal repeat.

HIV genes and their major functions

Major structural proteins	*gag*	Encodes for capsid, matrix, and nucleocapsid
	pol	Encodes for viral enzymes
	env	Encodes for envelope glycoproteins
Regulatory proteins	*tat*	Regulates HIV transcription
	rev	Induces transition from early to late genes
Accessory proteins	*vpu*	Enhances virus particle release
	vpr	Facilitates import of preintegration complex and cell growth arrest
	vif	Maintains replication of HIV in lymphocytes and macrophages
	nef	Downregulates CD4 receptors andstimulates HIV infectivity

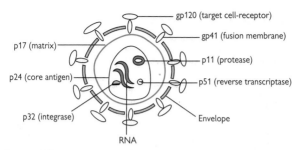

Fig. 36.1 HIV structure: gp and p refer to glycoprotein and protein, respectively, and the numerical values ($\times 10^3$) indicate molecular weight.

HIV replicative cycle

Replication occurs in the following sequence: binding → fusion and entry → reverse transcription → integration → proviral transcription → cytoplasmic expression → assembly → budding and maturation.

Binding/attachment

Glycoprotein120 binds to the extracellular component of the CD4 receptor (expressed in helper T-cells, macrophages, monocytes, and microglial, dendritic, and Langerhans' cells). A chemokine co-receptor (CCR5 or CXCR4) is also required for infection of helper T-cells or macrophages.

Fusion

Binding of gp120, CD4, and co-receptors produces a conformational change in gp41, leading to virion and cell membrane fusion and release of the viral core into the cell.

Reverse transcription

Viral reverse transcription complex includes viral RNA, transfer RNA (tRNA^{Lys}), viral reverse transcriptase, integrase, matrix and nucleocapsid proteins, viral protein R (*vpr*), and various host proteins. Reverse transcription yields HIV pre-integration complex, composed of double-stranded viral cDNA, integrase, matrix, *vpr*, reverse transcriptase, and the high-mobility group DNA-binding cellular protein HMGI (Y). Pre-integration complex travels towards the nucleus using microtubules. Reverse transcription is error prone, producing a mistake every cycle and generating multiple mutations instrumental in both the development of drug resistance and escape from immune surveillance.

Integration

Integrase mediates the integration of the viral DNA into the host cell chromosome. It also removes terminal nucleotides from the proviral DNA, correcting the ragged ends generated by the terminal activity of reverse transcriptase.

Proviral transcription

Transcription is controlled by host factors. NF-κ B induced by T-cell receptor stimulation, IL-1, and TNF-α binds (NF-κ B) to DNA binding sites to activate transcription. Host factors regulate transcription of provirus. Transcription generates different multiple spliced HIV-specific transcripts, which are transported rapidly into the cytoplasm and encode *nef, tat, and rev*. Single-spliced or unspliced viral transcripts remain in the nucleus and encode the structural, enzymatic, and accessory proteins that are needed for the assembly of fully infectious virions.

rev-independent and *rev*-dependent cytoplasmic expression

During early HIV synthesis only multiple spliced mRNA transcripts are available for translation. Later on unspliced and singly spliced mRNAs diffuse into the cytoplasm where translation to structural protein synthesis starts.

Virion assembly

The HIV particles generated assemble at the host cell surface.

- *env* proteins are synthesized in the endoplasmic reticulum and transported to the cell surface where gp41 anchors gp120 to the plasma membrane.
- *gag* and *gag–pol* proteins are cleaved by viral proteases during budding to produce mature products.

Mature virions are released ready to infect new cells and begin the replication cycle once again. The entire process is extremely active, with 10^8–10^{10} viral particles produced each day.

HIV and its receptors

- CD4 antigen is the principal receptor, and is mainly expressed on the surface of helper T lymphocytes. It is expressed to a lesser degree in CD4 dendritic cells, including Langerhans' cells, CD4 monocytes, macrophages, and microglial cells.
- Co-receptors: several chemokine receptors have been described, but CCR5 and CXCR4 are the most important co-receptors for HIV attachment in vivo. CCR5 is the co-receptor for NSI strains and CXCR4 is the co-receptor for SI strains.
- gp120: contains hypervariable regions (V1–V5) which vary from one HIV isolate to another. V3 loop is not involved in CD4 binding but is important for HIV tropism for macrophages or T-lymphoid cell lines. It is also the target for neutralizing antibodies that block HIV-1 infectivity.

Factors influencing HIV disease progression

Host factors

- Age: ↑ age is associated with ↑ progression.
- Co-infection: may affect immune system resulting in ↑ progression (e.g. tuberculosis and hepatitis C). Cytomegalovirus is associated with ↑ progression in haemophiliacs.
- Gender: ♀ appear to have higher viral loads at any CD4 level and may progress more rapidly.
- Psychosocial factors: depression, impaired intellectual functioning, drug use, and social deprivation may be associated with ↑progression.
- Genetic susceptibility:
  - Up to 20% of individuals of northern European descent have a deletion in the CCR5 gene resulting in a mutant (CCR5Δ32). Homo-zygous individuals (1–2% of the Caucasian population) are almost resistant to HIV infection and heterozygotes are slow progressors. CCR2 (a minor co-receptor) deletion (CCR-V641) is widespread in all ethnic groups and results in slower progression to aids.
  - Certain HLA types are associated with ↓ or ↑ progression.
  - Possession or lack of certain genes: e.g. low copy number of CCL3L1 associated with ↑ susceptibility to HIV acquisition and progression.
- Nutrition: poor premorbid state associated with ↑ progression.
- Pharmacological variability: individual drug metabolism and elimination modifies response to therapy.

Viral factors

Changes in the phenotype and genotype of the virus enable it to 'escape' control by the immune system. In late HIV infection switching from CCR5 to CXCR4 (i.e. from NSI to SI) leads to infection of both active and resting immune cells, resulting in ↑ disease progression. Mutations may alter viral 'fitness' influencing pathogenicity. Gene mutation involving *nef* is associated with progression, and some drug-resistant mutations (e.g. M184V which induces lamivudine resistance) may ↓ viral fitness.

Drug susceptibility depends largely on HIV genotypic and phenotypic characteristics with genotype mutations rendering some drugs ineffective. Other factors such as efflux pumps may also be involved.

Staging, classification, and natural history of HIV disease

Clinical staging

Early in the epidemic, before HIV was discovered, diagnosis of AIDS was largely based on finding *Pneumocystis jiroveci* (previously *P.carinii*) pneumonia (PCP) or Kaposi's sarcoma. HIV antibody testing led to patients being identified as having asymptomatic infection, AIDS-related complex, or AIDS. The Centers for Disease Control and Prevention (CDC) devised a classification system, revised in 1993, based on clinical features, AIDS-defining illnesses, and CD4 counts (Table 37.1). The CD4 count is a useful predictor for the development of opportunistic infections (OIs) and malignancies, but it should be recognized that this may be influenced by other factors such as inter-current infection.

This system was originally designed as a categorization tool for public health purposes and was not intended for staging.

Category A
- Asymptomatic HIV infection
- Persistent generalized lymphadenopathy
- Acute retroviral syndrome

Category B
- Bacillary angiomatosis
- Candidiasis:
  - oral
  - recurrent vaginal
- Cervical dysplasia/carcinoma *in situ*
- Constitutional symptoms
- Oral hairy leukoplakia
- Herpes zoster
- Idiopathic thrombocytopenic purpura
- Listeriosis
- Pelvic inflammatory disease
- Peripheral neuropathy

Category C (AIDS-defining conditions)
- CD4 count <200cells/μL
- Candidiasis:
  - pulmonary
  - oesophageal
- Cerebral toxoplasmosis
- Cervical cancer
- Coccidioidomycosis
- Cryptosporidiosis
- Cytomegalovirus
- Herpes simplex:
  - chronic (>1 month)
  - oesophageal
- HIV encephalopathy
- Histoplasmosis (extrapulmonary)
- Isosporiasis
- Lymphoma
- *Mycobacterium avium* complex
- *Mycobacterium tuberculosis*
- *Pneumocystis jiroveci*
- Pneumonia (recurrent)
- Progressive multifocal leucoencephalopathy
- Salmonella (septicaemia, recurrent)
- Wasting syndrome due to HIV

Table 37.1 Revised classification of HIV disease (CDC, January 1993)*

CD4 (counts/μL)	A	B	C
>500	A1	B1	C1
200–500	A2	B2	C2
<200	A3	B3	C3

*Those in categories A3, B3, C1, C2, and C3 have AIDS under the 1993 surveillance case definition.

Natural history of untreated HIV infection

Characterized by progressive loss of immune function allowing the development of some virulent bacterial infections, certain opportunistic infections, and malignancies that define AIDS (Fig. 37.1). Progression rate varies depending on interactions between host, viral, and environmental factors. The average time between HIV acquisition and AIDS is ~10 years if untreated.

The course of the disease can be divided into five continuous stages: 1° infection followed by early, middle, advanced, and late stages. There is significant individual variation between patients in the same clinical stage.

- 1° HIV infection: disseminates widely in the body at seroconversion, usually with a very high VL and a rapid CD4 cell ↓ which is spontaneously but not fully reversible.
- Early stage: CD4 count >500cells/µL. After 1° stage viraemia ↓ (rarely becoming undetectable). Usually asymptomatic apart from generalized lymphadenopathy and certain skin disorders (e.g. seborrhoeic dermatitis, aphthous ulcers, eosinophilic dermatitis, and psoriasis) which may deteriorate or appear for the first time.
- Middle stage: CD4 count 200–500cells/µL. Mostly asymptomatic/mildly symptomatic. Skin disorders of early stage may worsen. Recurrent herpes simplex infection, varicella zoster, diarrhoea, weight loss, and intermittent fever may develop. Lung infections caused by community-acquired organisms such as *Streptococcus pneumoniae, Haemophilus influenzae*, and *Mycobacterium tuberculosis* become more common.
- Advanced stage: CD4 count 50–200cells/µL. ↑ VL with classical manifestations of AIDS, especially PCP, Kaposi's sarcoma, lymphomas, and *Mycobacterium avium* complex (MAC) infection.
- Late stage: CD4 count <50cells/µL. Very high levels of viraemia. Further development of conditions associated with severe immune deficiency, e.g. CMV retinitis, disseminated MAC. Neurological manifestations ↑ due to 1° brain lymphoma, multifocal leukoencephalo-pathy, and dementia. HIV wasting disease is commonly seen at this stage.

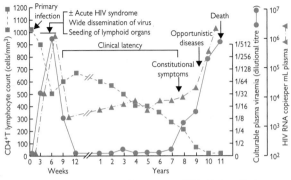

Fig. 37.1 Schematic representation of progression of HIV infection with time. Reproduced with permission of Professor Giuseppe Pantaleo, Centre Hospitalier Universitaire Vaudois.

HIV: diagnosis and assessment

HIV pre-test discussion

UK surveillance data show that ~1/3rd of HIV infections in adults remain undiagnosed and that ~25% of newly diagnosed individuals have a CD4 count <200cells/μL and even with treatment have a significantly higher mortality than those diagnosed when CD4 count >200cells/μL. HIV testing has been largely confined to individuals requesting the test. There is a need to increase the offer and uptake of testing, necessitating a shift from in-depth counselling to a brief discussion with normalization of testing.

Testing should routinely be offered to the following patients:
- GUM/sexual health clinic attendees
- women antenatally and those seeking terminations
- IV drug users
- those with TB, HCV, or HBV
- men and women who have high risk sexual contact
- those undergoing transplantation or dialysis, or blood donors
- patients presenting with an AIDS-defining illness.

Testing should also be considered in those with indicator disease (e.g pneumonia, oral candidiasis, Hodgkin's lymphoma) and in areas of high–prevalence acute admissions and patients registering with a GP (Table 38.1).

HIV infection is usually diagnosed by detecting antibodies in a serum sample. Fourth generation testing should be standard and include p24 antigen with increased sensitivity and a false–positive rate of ~0.2%. However, in suspected 1° infections or 2–4 weeks after a specific high-risk incident (e.g. needlestick injury) plasma should be tested for HIV RNA by a nucleic acid amplification technique (e.g. PCR). Testing should always be done with informed consent and assurance about the confidential nature of the process. Point-of-care testing by fingerprick or mouth swab provides results within a few minutes and may be considered in community settings.

Pretest discussion should cover the following
- Risk assessment: e.g. sexual practices, travel, drug use, occupation, blood/blood products prior to 1985 (in the UK).
  - Very high risk:
    – unprotected sexual contact with an HIV-infected partner
    – receipt of infected blood/ blood products
    – sharing injecting equipment with HIV-infected person.
- If risk within 72 hours consider post-exposure prophylaxis (📖 Chapter 53, Post-exposure prophylaxis, p. 599)
  - High risk:
    – ♂ to ♂ unprotected anal sex (especially receptive)
    – sex or sharing injecting equipment with people from countries with a high HIV prevalence.
- Assess patient knowledge: ensure that the individual understands the nature and transmission of HIV. Advise on risk reduction.

- Standard antibody test—serum (saliva and finger-prick tests available if venepuncture impossible/refused):
  - Detects antibodies to HIV-1 and HIV-2, does not diagnose AIDS.
  - Seroconversion often within 4–6 weeks but may take up to 12 weeks 'window period'; therefore repeat testing may be required. Repeat saliva testing advised 14 weeks after risk. Therefore it is important to determine the date of the last risk.
  - Positive standard screening tests need to be validated by different method(s) which may incur delays. Rarely indeterminate results are obtained, requiring repeat sampling.
  - If the patient lacks capacity they may only be tested if the test is in the patient's best interest. The patient's attorney may need to be contacted and any advanced directives must be considered. Discussion of reason for refusal should take place to ensure that it is not based on misconceptions.
- Implications of testing
  - Early diagnosis allows monitoring with pre-symptomatic highly active antiretroviral therapy (HAART), if appropriate, and development of strategies to avoid transmission including post-exposure prophylaxis
  - If pregnant, allows informed choices about the management of pregnancy, especially the use of antiretroviral treatment (both mother and infant) and avoidance of breastfeeding to ↓ vertical transmission. Arrangements for early monitoring of the infant's health.
  - If negative, elimination of needless anxiety and no consequence on life insurance or mortgage application.
  - If positive:
    –psychological impact of result
    –social and work implications (e.g. surgeon); may affect travel to or work in certain countries
    –life insurance restrictions/weightings; a positive result (or awaiting a test result) must be declared on application forms
- Arrangements for giving results
  - How/when the result will be provided (especially in high-risk situations)
  - If positive, who will he/she tell? How will the individual cope? What support is available?
- Document that information has been provided on:
  - positive, negative, and indeterminate results
  - how, when, and where results will be given and whether written confirmation is required
  - follow-up and the possible need for repeat testing to confirm positive results or cover the window period.
- Obtain and document informed consent.

Table 38.1 Suggested HIV pre-test checklist

Risk assessment	Yes	No	Further information
Prior HIV test			When
Blood transfusion/products			When Where
Injecting drug user (shared equipment)			Last time:
Sex with people from countries with high HIV prevalence			Where: Last time:
MSM or sex with MSM*			Last time:

Contact with HIV
  Low risk
  Higher risk
			Last time:

Information provided			
Benefits of early identification and treatment explained Implication of positive result (especially if high risk) 3-month window explained Insurance explained Result giving explained			
Consent to test obtained			
HIV test taken			
Repeat test required			When:

*MSM, ♂ who has sex with ♂.

Post-test counselling

The content and timing of the discussion will depend on the patient's reaction to a positive or negative result.

Aims of post-test counselling

- Address the immediate concerns and provide support for those who are positive and also negative (especially the very anxious).
- Provide information on the prevention of HIV transmission.
- Ensure patient is aware of need for confirmatory/repeat testing if appropriate.
- Discuss modifiable risk factors.

If HIV positive

- Address immediate reactions and assess need for psychological intervention.
- Provide further basic information about the natural history of HIV, reinforcing the difference between HIV and AIDS and the efficacy of treatment.
- Construct a management plan which meets the needs of the patient.
- Give details of support services.
- Offer follow-up appointments and ongoing support which may include addressing issues concerned with employment, travel, legal matters, and support for carers and partners.
- Discuss measures needed to prevent transmission and possibility of PEPSI for partners
- Provide information on what further investigations will be required.

Seronegative HIV infection

Negative HIV antibody test with HIV infection (after excluding specimen-handling errors) is well recognized during the window period. It is otherwise very rare and identified only when clinical presentation suggests HIV/AIDS with a negative HIV antibody test but positive PCR for HIV RNA/DNA (or viral culture). Possible causes:

- profound hypogammaglobulinaemia
- seroreversion—extremely rare
- HIV group O infection
- unknown.

Medical situations in which to consider HIV infection
- Reticulo-endothelial abnormalities:
  - impaired immunity
  - unexplained lymphadenopathy
  - blood dyscrasia
- Infections:
  - tuberculosis or atypical mycobacterial infection
  - *Pneumocystis jiroveci (carinii)* pneumonia
  - cerebral toxoplasmosis
  - oral or oesophageal candidiasis
  - herpes zoster (in younger people)
  - cytomegalovirus retinitis
  - aseptic meningitis
  - transverse myelitis
  - peripheral neuropathy
- Tumours:
  - non-Hodgkin's lymphoma/Hodgkin's lymphoma
  - cerebral lymphoma
  - cervical cancer
  - lung cancer
  - head and neck cancer
  - anal cancer
- Dermatological conditions
  - Seborrhoeic dermatitis
  - Recalcitrant psoriasis
- General:
  - symptoms suggesting seroconversion illness, especially if associated with another STI
  - oral hairy leukoplakia
  - unexplained weight loss
  - unexplained diarrhoea
  - night sweats
  - pyrexia of unknown origin

Assessment of an HIV-positive patient

Initial assessment

Objectives
- Reinforce the patient's understanding of HIV infection and how to avoid further transmission.
- Identify medical, socio-economic, and legal problems.
- Establish stage of disease.
- Establish a rapport with patient (essential to ensure efficient follow-up).
- Full history, medical examination, and baseline investigations to plan future management and drug therapy. Further tests depend on the circumstances and stage of disease.

History
- Sexual history including sexual partners/practices, condom use, and contraception.
- Current and previous medical history (especially tuberculosis, STIs, or hepatitis) and surgical, gynaecological, and obstetric history.
- Extensive systemic enquiry covering GI, neurological, visual, respiratory, and cardiovascular systems.
- Current medication and allergies.
- Drug, substance, and alcohol use.

Clinical examination
- General: weight, temperature, pulse, blood pressure, respiratory rate, pallor, and jaundice.
- Lymph glands: lymphadenopathy—site, size, symmetry, tenderness, and consistency.
- Mouth and throat: gum and tooth disease, oral ulceration, hairy leukoplakia, candidiasis, and enlarged pharyngeal lymphoid tissue.
- Cardiovascular: routine examination.
- Respiratory: routine examination.
- Abdomen: routine examination.
- Neurological: routine examination. Specifically assess eyes, checking visual acuity, visual fields, pupil size, pupil reactivity, and extra-ocular movements. Examine retinae, ideally with pupils dilated; if CD4 <50cells/µL slit-lamp examination by ophthalmology.
- Genital/pelvic examination: discharges, ulcers, condylomata, testicular enlargement or atrophy, cervical abnormalities, pelvic masses, and STI screening.
- Cervical cytology: annual review with close follow-up if abnormal.
- Perianal and rectal examination: anal/rectal discharge, condylomata, ulcers, prostate assessment, and tests for STIs as appropriate.
- Skin: general skin examination specifically checking for seborrhoeic dermatitis, fungal nail infection, warts, Kaposi's sarcoma, molluscum contagiosum, and abnormal pigmentation.

Laboratory investigations

- Full blood count, urea, electrolytes and liver function tests, glucose, triglycerides, and cholesterol.
- Serological tests: hepatitis A, hepatitis B (surface antigen and core antibody), hepatitis C, CMV IgG, toxoplasma, varicella zoster virus (VZV) IgG, and syphilis.
- Viral load (VL)—informs on likely rate of disease progression and monitors response to therapy:
  - undetectable VL indicates level <20–50copies/mL (depending upon test used)
  - <5000copies/mL generally suggests low rate of progression in the coming 5 years
  - >55,000copies/mL is associated with ↑ rate of progression.
- CD4 count—usually measured as part of lymphocyte subsets:
  - main indicator of risk of opportunistic infection and possible need for prophylactic treatment in the asymptomatic patient
  - individual results may be influenced by other factors, e.g. inter-current infections
  - repeat if unexpectedly low or high count.
  - trend is more useful than single readings.
- Plasma samples for viral resistance testing.

Frequently asked question

Do I have to tell people that I am HIV positive?

When you are diagnosed you will speak to a health adviser who will discuss this and similar issues with you. You should be careful who you tell, as once it's done, there's no going back. Although safety precautions are taken, you should inform anyone who could come into contact with infected body fluids (e.g. dentists, surgeons) and your doctor, especially if you develop unusual symptoms which may be related to or altered by the HIV infection. If you are a healthcare professional (HCP) you should seek appropriate counselling, as certain invasive procedures cannot be performed by HIV-positive HCPs.

It is important to act responsibly where others are concerned, especially sexual (or drug-sharing) partners. There are court cases where HIV-positive individuals have been prosecuted for infecting partners without informing them that they are HIV positive.

Further investigations and follow-up
- Chest X-ray.
- Estimate stage of HIV infection from initial assessment and baseline investigations.
- Assess disease progression: HIV-related infections and malignancies, response to therapy, and signs of drug toxicity.
- Monitor VL and CD4 count at regular intervals; frequency depends on the patient's clinical status. Asymptomatic patients with stable disease may have their VL and CD4 count measured every 3–6 months but shorter intervals may be necessary for those with more advanced disease.

Drug prophylaxis
- *Pneumocystis jiroveci (carinii)* pneumonia (PCP): when CD4 count <200cells/μL, first choice is trimethoprim/sulfamethoxazole (co-trimoxazole) orally 960mg 3 times a week. If allergic consider desensitization (Table 38.2). Alternatives are: dapsone 50–100mg daily, dapsone 50mg plus pyrimethamine 50mg 3 times a week, atovaquone 750mg 3 times a week, or nebulized pentamidine 300mg once a month. Azithromycin 500mg 3 times a week may be effective as 1° prophylaxis.
- Tuberculosis (TB): prior BCG vaccination provides unreliable protection. A negative tuberculin test may be due to anergy and does not exclude TB. Chemoprophylaxis is recommended for close contacts of smear-positive pulmonary TB. Six months of isoniazid 300mg daily or 3 months of isoniazid 300mg daily plus rifampicin 600mg daily is effective.
- Toxoplasmosis: if CD4 count <100cells/μL and toxoplasma IgG positive. Co-trimoxazole (as for PCP prophylaxis).
- VZV: varicella zoster immunoglobulin (5 vials IM) if seronegative for VZV antibodies within 72 hours of significant exposure.
- *Mycobacterium avium* complex: prophylaxis may be considered with CD4 counts <50 cells/μL (📖 Chapter 46, *Mycobacterium avium* complex p. 532).

Vaccination
Inactivated rather than live vaccines should be used (e.g. polio). If travelling abroad additional vaccination may be required (📖 Chapter 55, Vaccination p. 612). Those who are immunodeficient may not mount a good response to vaccination. Vaccination can be delayed until immune reconstitution ensues, although unnecessary delay should be avoided if there is a specific infection risk.
- Influenza vaccination: can be given to all patients.
- Hepatitis A: if immuno-naive.
- Hepatitis B: if immuno-naive.
- Pneumovax: controversial, but safer if given to those whose HIV infection is suppressed by antiviral therapy with CD4 >200cells/μL.

Table 38.2 Suggested desensitization schedule for trimethoprim–sulfamethoxazole (TS)

Day	Dose	TS
1	1mL of 1:20 paediatric suspension	0.4mg/2mg
2	2mL of 1:20 paediatric suspension	0.8mg/4mg
3	4mL of 1:20 paediatric suspension	1.6mg/8mg
4	8mL of 1:20 paediatric suspension	3.2mg/16mg
5	1mL of paediatric suspension	8mg/40mg
6	2mL of paediatric suspension	16mg/80mg
7	4mL of paediatric suspension	32mg/160mg
8	8mL of paediatric suspension	64mg/320mg
9	1 tablet	80mg/400mg
10	1 double-strength tablet	160mg/800mg

Thereafter 1 double strength tablet 3 days a week until CD4 count is >200cells/µL for at least 3 months.

Reprinted from Absar, N. Daneshvar, H., Beall, G. (1994). *J Allergy Clin Immunol*, **93**, 1001–5. © 1994 with permission from Elsevier.

HIV: primary infection

Definitions

Primary HIV infection (PHI)

The period of time from the onset of infection until the immune system establishes a balance with viral replication. Characterized by rapidly increasing viraemia with transient immune suppression. Usually takes weeks–months to stabilize.

Acute seroconversion illness—acute retroviral syndrome (ARS)

The symptomatic development of HIV-specific antibodies.

Prevalence of acute seroconversion illness

Difficult to determine because of the wide spectrum of clinical presentations which may be mild and non-specific (Table 39.1). These explain the wide range of reported prevalence of 30–93% in those recently infected. Clinician awareness, experience, and high index of suspicion ↑ diagnostic rate. It is unclear what determines the severity of symptoms. The inoculum size, HIV strain virulence, and patient's immune status may be factors. Almost all reports of ARS are in adults with HIV-1, but it may occur in children or those with HIV-2 infection.

Clinical features of acute seroconversion illness

Symptoms usually begin 2–6 weeks after infection, typically lasting 5–10 days and rarely >14 days. Subjective symptoms such as fatigue may continue for several weeks or even months, but eventually almost all patients enter an asymptomatic phase that may last for years. Within 2–4 weeks of infection very high levels of free HIV and p24 antigen can be detected in the peripheral blood. Symptoms coincide with peak levels of plasma viraemia.

Usual clinical features

Fever followed by lymphadenopathy, pharyngitis, and skin rash.

Others

- Dermatological manifestations (involving face, neck, and trunk > limbs):
  - maculopapular skin rashes
  - mucosal ulceration of genitals, mouth, and oesophagus
  - additional skin lesions include pustules, urticaria, erythema multiforme, and alopecia
- Infectious mononucleosis like illness:
  - fever, pharyngitis, myalgia, arthralgia, and lymphadenopathy
  - oral ulceration (highly suggestive of acute seroconversion illness)
  - no prominent tonsillar involvement (unlike infectious mono-nucleosis).

Table 39.1 Acute retroviral syndrome—frequency of clinical features

Fever	80–97%
Lymphadenopathy	40–77%
Pharyngitis	44–73%
Skin rashes	51–70%
Myalgia or arthralgia	49–70%
Thrombocytopenia	45–51%
Leucopenia	35–40%
Diarrhoea	32–33%
Headache	30–70%
↑ serum transaminases	21–23%
Nausea and vomiting	20–60%
Hepatosplenomegaly	14–17%
Weight loss	13–32%
Oral candidiasis	10–12%
Encephalopathy	8%
Neuropathy	8%

- Evidence of immune deficiency:
  - oral and oesophageal candidiasis
  - *Pneumocystis jiroveci* (*carinii*) pneumonia.
- Neurological manifestation:
  - meningitis, peripheral neuropathy, brachial neuritis, Bell's palsy, myelopathy, encephalitis, Guillain–Barré syndrome.

Severe and prolonged illness, especially with neurological manifestations, is associated with a poorer prognosis. Resolution of symptoms coincides with ↓ in plasma viraemia and the development of a CD8 cell-specific immune response with the later emergence of HIV-specific antibodies (usually within 4–6 weeks of infection but may be up to 3 months).

Immune responses in primary HIV infection

Cellular response

More important than humoral immunity in containing HIV infection and develops earlier. HIV-specific immune responses, particularly cytotoxic CD8 cells, influence the natural history of HIV infection.

1° infection is characterized by active viral replication and very high levels of plasma viraemia. The virus disseminates throughout the body, particularly to the lymphoid system where its replication is never completely suppressed. During the first few days of infection both CD4 and CD8 cells are suppressed, resulting in lymphopenia approaching levels seen in patients with advanced disease. This is followed by relative lymphocytosis, predominantly CD8 cells, that declines when acute seroconversion is complete. However, the CD4 count, although increasing, does not return to baseline values. These changes result in reversal of the CD4/CD8 ratio to <1. One feature of acute HIV infection is the rapid depletion of CD4 cells in the gut lymphoid tissue which persists despite immune reconstitution with HAART.

HIV viraemia ↓ with HIV-specific immune responses, gradually stabilizing within 6–12 months to reach a 'viral set-point'. Higher set-points indicate ↑ risk of disease progression.

Humoral response

Antibody response usually becomes detectable within 10–21 days of the onset of symptoms but may take up to 3 months from infection. Anti-bodies to gp160 and p24 develop first, followed by anti-gp120 and anti-gp41. Anti-p24 diminishes with time and may disappear with advanced disease. However, anti-gp120 and anti-gp41 persist for life. Poor prognosis if inadequate HIV antibody response. Neutralizing antibodies are usually detected 4–8 weeks after resolution of the viraemic peak. Non-neutralizing antibodies to envelope and p24 antigens develop much earlier, coinciding with seroconversion.

Diagnosis

PHI usually presents before the development of antibodies and therefore is diagnosed by finding p24 antigen or HIV RNA in the appropriate clinical setting. Fourth-generation HIV antibody tests also detect p24 antigen, and can test positive at the later stages of PHI but can be falsely negative. HIV RNA levels are usually extremely high, often $>10^6$copies/mL.

Atypical lymphocytes are commonly seen in the peripheral blood with levels up to 30%. Anaemia, thrombocytopenia, abnormal liver function tests, or ↑ inflammatory markers may also be found (see Box 39.1 for differential diagnoses).

Box 39.1 Main differential diagnoses of acute seroconversion illness

- Epstein–Barr virus (infectious mononucleosis)
- Cytomegalovirus infection
- Toxoplasmosis
- Viral hepatitis
- 2° syphilis
- Rubella
- 1° herpes simplex virus infection
- Drug reaction
- Aseptic meningitis
- Streptococcal pharyngitis

Management of primary HIV infection

PHI is the time of highest infectivity in HIV infection. The plasma level of HIV RNA strongly predicts the progression rate. Early intervention has theoretical advantages as the virus is likely to be homogenous and the immune system intact. Antiretroviral treatment may ↓ the number of infected cells, preserve HIV-specific immune responses, and possibly ↓ the viral set-point. However, the long-term benefit of therapy has not been demonstrated.

It is unusual for PHI to be identified unless patients present with symptoms (ARS), the nature and severity of which may influence the decision to treat. If treatment is considered it is common practice to be offered entry into controlled clinical trials. Failing this, standard HAART may be given when CD4 is persistently low, or there is severe CNS disease or development of an AIDS-defining illness. Possible benefits of treatment should be weighed against drug toxicity, adherence, and potential for drug resistance in discussion with the patient. The optimum duration of treatment is not yet established. Benefit from structured treatment interruptions in stimulating host immune response has not been conclusively demonstrated. The role of drugs that inhibit activation of latently infected CD4 cells (e.g. hydroxycarbamide and ciclosporin A), with subsequent inability of virus production, is not known.

Other possible benefits of diagnosing PHI:
- early identification of partners most at risk
- advice on reduction/prevention of infection
- if treated ↓ viral load may ↓ infectivity
- minimizing late HIV diagnosis when immune system already damaged.

HIV: gastrointestinal disorders

Introduction

The gut harbours the largest lymphoid tissue in the body and contains 70–80% of immune cells which are depleted within a few weeks after infection and are not replenished even after immune reconstitution with HAART. HIV directly infects the gut mucosal cells, and interaction between gp120 and certain mucosal proteins results in efficient cell–cell spread of HIV. Alteration in gut permeability and microbial translocation is thought to play a role in immune activation and disease progression.

Oral disease

Oral disease is very common in HIV infection and may indicate the diagnosis. Detailed oral examination should be part of the assessment of the newly diagnosed HIV +ve individual. Various lesions of ulcerative, raised, white, or pigmented appearance may be encountered (Boxes 40.1 and 40.2). Advice from an oral or maxillofacial surgeon should be obtained when necessary.

Viral infections

Herpes simplex virus (HSV)

HSV infection is very common, with seropositivity rates approaching 80% in HIV +ve MSM. Oral HSV, like herpes infection elsewhere, is characterized by latency (in the trigeminal ganglia).

- *1° episodes*: vesicles normally appear on lips, gingiva, hard palate, or rarely the dorsal aspect of the tongue. Unlike herpes zoster, primary HSV infection is not associated with viraemia. Lesions are initially vesicular, followed by ulcers, crusting, and then healing. It may take up to 3 weeks for 1° HSV lesions to heal. The duration is longer in the severely immunocompromised.
- *Recurrent HSV*: tends to localize to the vermilion border of the lips. Some patients experience pain or tingling sensation before the appearance of the lesions. It may take 7–10 days for oral HSV lesions to heal. Recurrent HSV infection may be more common in patients with symptomatic HIV disease, and severely immunocompromised patients tend to have more frequent and more severe attacks.
- *Complications*:
  - ocular keratitis occurs with the same frequency as in HIV –ve individuals.
  - herpes oesophagitis, usually with severe odynophagia, occurs more frequently in patients with late HIV disease but not necessarily associated with concomitant oral herpes,
  - HSV meningitis is more likely to be 2° to 1° genital herpes but can occur in acute oral herpes.
- *Management*: Labial herpes can be treated with topical aciclovir 4–6 times daily. Systemic treatment, see 📖 Anal disease p. 470.

Box 40.1 Differential diagnosis of white lesions in the oral cavity

- Candidiasis
- Oral hairy leukoplakia
- Frictional keratosis
- Tobacco-induced leukoplakia
- Lichen planus
- White sponge naevus
- Geographical tongue
- Primary syphilis and syphilitic mucous patches
- Squamous cell carcinoma

Box 40.2 Differential diagnosis of oro-pharyngeal ulcers

Viral
- Herpes simplex virus
- Cytomegalovirus
- Herpes zoster virus

Bacterial
- Necrotizing ulcerative periodontitis
- Necrotizing stomatitis
- *Mycobacterium tuberculosis*
- *Mycobacterium avium* complex
- *Treponema pallidum*

Fungal
- Histoplasmosis

Tumours
- Lymphoma
- Kaposi's sarcoma

Other causes
- Aphthous ulcers
- Behçet's disease

Cytomegalovirus (CMV)

Seroprevalence rates rise with age. >90% prevalence rates have been found in HIV +ve MSM.

- *CMV oral ulcers:*
  - mucosal, intra-oral, typically solitary, deep, necrotic ulcers with a red margin and a white halo; difficult to differentiate from those of other aetiology
  - arise when CD4 count <50cells/μL
  - usually occur as part of disseminated CMV disease and attempts must be made to exclude infection of other organs such as the retina
  - diagnosis is established by the biopsy finding of typical owl's eye inclusions; CMV PCR on tissue sample may help.
- *Management:* 📖 Chapter 44, Opportunistic infections p. 514

Varicella zoster virus (VZV)

Reactivation of VZV causes herpes zoster (HZ)/shingles in the immuno-compromised host, including HIV infection at any stage. Rarely found as a 1° infection in those without previous exposure to the virus. People with HIV infection are 15 times more likely to have HZ than age-matched controls. Oral HZ is latent in the trigeminal nerve. Mandibular branch involvement results in lesions in the lower lip and lateral border of the tongue, and maxillary branch involvement results in lesions on the hard palate. Oral vesicles only last for a few hours and are followed by painful ulcers, while the concomitant skin lesions may last for 2–4 weeks.

Diagnosis and management: 📖 see pp. 518–9.

Oral hairy leukoplakia (OHL)

White adherent vertically corrugated lesion seen only in the mouth, most commonly on the lateral aspect of the tongue (Plate 15). The affected area may fluctuate in size.

Caused by Epstein–Barr virus (EBV). Demonstrated by finding EBV DNA, RNA, and proteins in biopsies of OHL. Usually asymptomatic but a few patients may complain of pain and altered taste. Reported in all risk groups but more common in adults, ♂, and smokers. It is not pathognomonic and occurs in HIV −ve immunocompromised individuals such as bone marrow and renal transplant recipients. Incidence and persistence increase with advancing HIV disease and declining CD4 counts. Its occurrence is associated with faster progression towards AIDS even after adjustment for CD4 count. It is not pre-malignant and does not need specific treatment but regresses with improved immune function associated with HAART.

Human papilloma virus (HPV)

HPV types 7, 13, 18, and 32 are the most commonly identified causes of oral warts in HIV +ve individuals. Mutant strains are frequently reported. Oral warts are more common in HIV +ve individuals than in the general population but there is no association with the stage of infection. HPV16 has been associated with oral squamous cell carcinoma in HIV-infected ♂. Although mostly localized to the oral cavity, laryngeal warts may occur and may be solitary or multiple, pedunculated, or sessile with small papilliferous or cauliflower-like projections.

Management: Surgical excision, laser, or cryotherapy.

Bacterial diseases

Periodontal disease

Dental hygiene is very important in HIV infection because of the high incidence of gum and periodontal disease. Periodontal disease should be managed in consultation with a maxillofacial or dental surgeon. Mild gingivitis and dental abscesses are common at all stages of infection. Linear gingival erythema (LGE), necrotizing ulcerative periodontitis (NUP), and necrotizing stomatitis (NS) occur more frequently in HIV infection. They are characterized by rapid onset, increased severity, and poor response to conventional treatment.

- *Linear gingival erythema* Patients present with spontaneous painless gum bleeding. Examination reveals an oedematous erythematous band parallel to the free gingival margin, which may be a precursor of NUP. Commonly isolated organisms include *Bacteroides gingivalis*, *Fusobacterium nucleatum*, and Actinobacilli. The response to treatment is poor but attention to oral hygiene and chlorhexidine mouthwash is helpful. Systemic metronidazole may be required.
- *Necrotizing ulcerative periodontitis* An acute onset severe and rapidly progressive condition, usually seen in patients with advanced HIV disease. Tends to occur in clean mouths with little plaque. A few teeth may be affected, but in severe cases all may be involved. Severe gum pain precedes the appearance of signs which include soft tissue necrosis with destruction of periodontal ligament and bone. NUP may resemble intra-oral lymphoma.
- *Necrotizing stomatitis* Also called necrotizing ulcerative stomatitis. Very difficult to differentiate from NUP although usually localized and less severe. It is a rapidly progressive process involving the gingiva, alveolar bone, and palate, causing severe deep pain. Bone sequestration may occur and management includes oral hygiene, chlorhexidine mouthwashes, and systemic antibiotics such as metronidazole and amoxicillin together with gentle debridement.

Tuberculosis

The most common oral manifestation is irregular ulceration of the tongue or palate. Culture has been shown to be insensitive in its detection from this site (2–17%), so polymerase chain reaction should also be considered.

Fungal disease

Oral and pharyngeal candidiasis

Probably the most common opportunistic infection (OI) in HIV disease. >90% will have oro-pharyngeal candidiasis at some stage. Commonly caused by *Candida albicans*, but other species such as *Candida glabrata* and *Candida tropicalis* are implicated. Although oro-pharyngeal candidiasis may occur at acute seroconversion, it becomes more frequent as the CD4 count ↓.

Clinical features

- *Pseudomembranous candidiasis* The pseudomembranous appearance results from overgrowth of candidal hyphae mixed with desquamated epithelium and inflammatory cells. Appears as white plaques at any site of the mouth or pharynx and leaves an erythematous raw bleeding mucosa on scraping. Patient may complain of soreness and altered taste (Plate 16).
- *Erythematous candidiasis* Appears as flat red patches of varying morphology that can be difficult to recognize and therefore diagnosis may be delayed. The most common sites are the palate and the dorsal surface of the tongue. Usually asymptomatic, but soreness and burning sensation may be reported.
- *Angular cheilitis* Appears solely or in conjunction with other forms of oro-pharyngeal candidiasis, resulting in redness, ulcers, and fissuring of one or both corners of the mouth.
- *Hyperplastic candidiasis* This the rarest form of candidiasis in HIV +ve individuals. Lesions appear as white and hyperplastic but are more easily removed than in the pseudomembranous form.

Diagnosis

Can be made on the clinical appearance. Candidal hyphae can be demonstrated on Gram or periodic acid–Schiff staining of smears from the lesions. Culture may be used, particularly in recalcitrant infection, to identify the candidal type, which may guide treatment. Sensitivities may be difficult to interpret. It does not help in making the diagnosis, as candida is a commensal of the oropharynx.

Management

- Systemic antifungal (standard mode of therapy):
  - fluconazole: 50–100mg once daily for 7–14 days
  - itraconazole solution: 100–200mg once daily for 7–14 days.
- ⚠ Avoid terfenadine as risk of arrhythmias.
- Topical antifungal (consider in mild cases):
  - nystatin (as pastilles or as suspension): 100,000–500,000 units 4 times daily after food for 7 days or continue for 48 hours after lesions have resolved.
  - amphotericin (lozenges and suspension): dissolve 1 lozenge (10mg) slowly 4 times a day after food for 10–15 days or continue for 48 hours after lesions have resolved.
  - miconazole oral gel: 5–10mL after food and retained near lesions 4 times daily; continue treatment for 48 hours after lesions have resolved.

Topical treatment must be retained in the mouth in contact with lesions for sufficient time.

Prognosis

Relapses are common and may be the result of poor compliance rather than resistance to antifungals. Consider prophylactic therapy (fluconazole 50mg daily) when recurrences are common but risk of resistance ⚠.

Neoplasia

Kaposi's sarcoma (KS) (📖 Chapter 52, Kaposi's sarcoma p. 567)

Oral KS was among the first recognized features early in the AIDS epidemic. More common in MSM. Usually presents as a blue, purple, or red lesion that may be flat, papular, nodular, or rarely a large tumour (Plate 17). Large nodular lesions may ulcerate and be secondarily infected. Occasionally the adjacent mucosa is stained yellow (by haemosiderin). Most common site is the hard palate but may be seen on the gingiva, tongue, soft palate, and buccal mucosa. Local pain may be a feature in secondarily infected ulcerative KS lesions. Mucosal lesions may indicate more extensive visceral involvement requiring good systemic enquiry and radiological investigation with CXR and possibly computed tomography (CT) scanning.
Management: 📖 Chapter 52, Kaposi's sarcoma, Management, p. 569.

- Immune reconstitution achieved by HAART may result in KS resolution, improves survival and response to therapy.
- Small lesions respond to local therapy such as surgical excision (⚠ may bleed excessively), laser excision, and intralesional chemotherapy.
- Larger lesions may be treated with radiation therapy, which may be complicated by mucositis.

Oral lymphoma

Caused by Epstein–Barr virus. The vast majority are B-cell non-Hodgkin's lymphomas. Oral lymphoma may precede the development of lymphomas at other sites. Presents as a rapidly growing tumour at any site in the mouth (Plate 18). May be diffuse or discrete nodules or may present as ulcers of variable morphology. Diagnosis must be confirmed by tissue biopsy.

Management

Once the diagnosis is established, lymphoma must be staged by appropriate imaging. Systemic chemotherapy and local radiation are the mainstay of therapy in collaboration with the maxillofacial surgeons to minimize oral side-effects.

Idiopathic aphthous ulcers

Recurrent oral ulceration resembling aphthous ulcers is a common phenomenon in HIV +ve individuals. Usually well circumscribed, superficial, and varying in size.

- Herpetiform: appear as clusters of 1–2mm ulcers, usually in the mouth and soft palate.
- Minor: usually solitary, 0.5–1.0cm in diameter.
- major: 2–4cm in size and necrotic. Usually found on the tonsils and tongue base and rarely the pharynx and nasopharynx. Typically very painful, persisting for several weeks.

Management
- Topical steroids: clobetasol in Orabase© 3–4 times daily is usually effective.
- Systemic steroids may be used if associated with oesophageal ulcers: 40–60mg daily for 7–10 days. Infective aetiology must be excluded.
- Thalidomide (50–200mg/day) produces an excellent response in resistant cases. Prescribing thalidomide needs fulfilment of special requirements, especially the avoidance of pregnancy ⚠.

Salivary gland disease
In HIV infection the salivary glands may become infiltrated with lymphocytes, predominantly CD8 cells, resulting in enlargement especially affecting the parotids. Xerostomia may be caused by drugs such as didanosine, antihistamines, and antidepressants, but also as a manifestation of HIV infection where the precise aetiology is unclear. Salivary amylase levels may be raised in drug-related cases.

Management
- Salivary stimulants such as sugarless sweets and chewing gum for symptomatic relief.
- Artificial saliva as necessary.
- Careful dental hygiene.

Parotid gland enlargement
- Diffuse infiltrating lymphocytosis syndrome (DISL) due to CD8 expansion, may also involve the cervical lymph nodes and lungs. Presents with dry mouth and parotid gland enlargement.
- Benign lympho-epithelial cysts: usually painless and soft, may be single or multiple and may enlarge gradually to involve the superficial lobes of both glands.

Imaging techniques and fine-needle aspiration help to confirm diagnosis. Parotidectomy rarely needed other than for cosmetic reasons.

Oesophageal disease

Dysphagia ± odynophagia are the main symptoms of oesophageal disease. Symptoms and signs are not discriminative enough to establish the underlying aetiology (Box 40.3). Assessment of the nutritional status and hydration is essential in managing such patients.

Dysphagia investigations

- Endoscopy and biopsy are required to establish a definitive diagnosis.
- Double-contrast barium swallow may differentiate between infection and neoplasm but is rarely diagnostic.
- More than one pathology may coexist and therefore multiple biopsies (>6) from different sites are advisable.
- Generally culture of oesophageal specimens is not helpful as it does not differentiate between colonization and actual tissue invasion, but it may be useful in identifying viral and mycobacterial pathogens.

Candidal oesophagitis

Most common cause of oesophagitis in HIV infection. A patient with oral candidiasis and odynophagia can be treated empirically for oesophageal candidiasis and investigated if it fails to respond. It usually occurs when the CD4 count <200cells/μL and is rarely asymptomatic. Candidal exudate can be seen during upper GI endoscopy.

Management

- Fluconazole 100–200mg or itraconazole 200mg once daily for 7–14 days.
- Itraconazole suspension 200mg twice daily (the suspension formulation of itraconazole has a better bioavailability than the capsular form). This is especially useful in fluconazole-resistant candidiasis (rare and seen in those with very low CD4 count who have had repeated courses of fluconazole).
- Liposomal amphotericin B (e.g. AmBisome®) or voriconazole in refractory cases.

CMV oesophagitis

CMV causes large distal oesophageal ulcers. Biopsy required to confirm diagnosis and to exclude other or concomitant causes of oesophagitis.

Management

CMV disease is treated with ganciclovir, cidofivir, or foscarnet until clinical improvement. Patients may be given maintenance oral valganciclovir to prevent CMV retinitis (🕮 Chapter 44, Opportunistic infections p. 514).

Box 40.3 Causes of oesophagitis

Infections
- *Candida* spp
- Cytomegalovirus
- Herpes simplex virus
- *Mycobacterium avium* complex

Malignancies
- Kaposi's sarcoma
- Lymphoma

Idiopathic oesophageal ulceration (non-HIV related)
- Reflux oesophagitis
- Pill-induced oesophagitis (e.g. zidovudine)

Enteric disease

Diarrhoea is an extremely common symptom in HIV infection (Box 40.4). It may be debilitating and require extensive and invasive investigation. In patients with CD4 >200cells/μL it is usually caused by virulent organisms and managed as in the immunocompetent. When CD4 <200cells/μL it is usually more severe, more likely to be caused by OIs, more difficult to diagnose, and less responsive to treatment. Large bowel diarrhoea is typically of small volume, may be bloodstained, and is associated with lower abdominal pain and tenesmus. Small bowel diarrhoea is characteristically of large volume, offensive, and of pale colour. Diarrhoea is described as being chronic when it persists >1 month.

Although infection with *Campylobacter*, *Shigella*, and other enteric pathogens occurs (📖 Chapter 19, Infections not usually sexually transmitted p. 250), particularly important organisms are *Cryptosporidium*, *Microsporidium*, *Isosopora*, and *Salmonella*.

Cryptosporidiosis

Cryptosporidium parvum (4–6μm intracellular protozoon) has a complete life-cycle (with a sexual and an asexual stage) in the intestinal mucosa of a single host. The oocyst can survive in the environment for >3 months. As it is small, it may bypass water filtration systems and standard home and hospital disinfectants are ineffective in its killing. The infectious dose for human is around 130 oocysts. Infection is self-limiting and usually asymptomatic in the immunocompetent host, but can cause debilitating symptoms in patients with advanced HIV disease. Human disease is limited to the jejunum but may involve all the gastrointestinal and respiratory epithelium in the immunocompromised.

Important factors in transmission
- Zoonotic infection (e.g. rural communities)
- Contaminated water (occurs occasionally in UK domestic water supply) and food
- Travellers to countries with poor sanitation systems
- Human-to-human transmission which may include sexual
- Oocysts may be excreted for 2 weeks after recovery.

Postulated mechanism of diarrhoea in cryptosporidiosis
- Osmotic
- Cholera-like cryptosporidial toxin production resulting in cyclic adenosine production
- Villous atrophy resulting in malabsorption.
- Substance P (SP), a neuropeptide and pain transmitter, is upregulated in the inflamed bowel during *Cryptosporidium* infection with ↑ chloride and glucose secretion.

Clinical features

- HIV +ve with preserved immune function—similar to HIV −ve immunocompetent.
- In advanced HIV disease—persistent watery diarrhoea of variable frequency and volume (1–15L/day). Commonly associated with nausea, abdominal cramps, malabsorption, weight loss, and electrolyte disturbances. Sclerosing cholangitis, interstitial lung disease, chronic sinusitis, and otitis media are rare features.

Diagnosis

The parasite can easily be missed on routine stool analysis- inform lab that diagnosis is being considered. Special staining techniques such as phenol auramine (fluorescent stain) are required. Intestinal mucosal biopsies may identify the organism.

Management

Attention to fluid and nutrition is important. No proven effective regimens, although paromomycin, azithromycin, and other antibiotics are used with variable degrees of success.

- Best response is achieved by improving the immune function with specific treatment of HIV itself by HAART.
- Antidiarrhoeal agents:
  - loperamide
  - opiates
  - diphenoxylate.
- Octreotide (somatostatin analogue)—effective in secretory diarrhoea.

Prevention

- Raising awareness of modes of transmission.
- If CD4 <50cells/µL boil water for minimum of 10 minutes.
- Use of fine filters to the mains water supplies.

Microsporidiosis

Caused by small (1–7μm) obligate intracellular protozoa. Several hundred species identified but only a few cause disease in humans, rarely in immunocompetent. The most common *Microsporidia* causing disease in patients with advanced HIV infection are as follows.

- *Encephalitazoon intestinalis*: accounts for 80% of microsporidial diarrhoea. Infects the small intestinal epithelium and biliary tract and presents with chronic watery diarrhoea (usually less severe than that of cryptosporidiosis), cramps, weight loss, and cholangiopathy. May infect macrophages, leading to dissemination with pulmonary, sinus, renal, and conjunctival disease.
- *Enterocytozoon bieneusi*: accounts for most of remainder of microsporidial diarrhoea. Infects enterocytes (jejunum) and causes abdominal symptoms, as above, but does not disseminate.

Diagnosis

Identification of the organism in the stools with immunofluorescent stains or modified trichrome stain. Transmission electron microscopy of intestinal biopsies considered as gold standard if available. Various staining methods are used to visualize the organism in tissue biopsies. Serological tests are unreliable and PCR of limited use.

Management

- Albendazole 400mg twice daily for 4 weeks produces best results for *Encephalitazoon* infection.
- Some relief of symptoms has been described with metronidazole, co-trimoxazole, erythromycin, and octreotide but all fail to eradicate the organism.
- Significant symptom improvement has been achieved with HAART.

Isospora belli

A common cause of epidemic diarrhoea in tropical countries and travellers. Infection is caused by ingestion of the 25μm oocysts contaminating food and water. Infection is usually confined to the small intestine but may cause acalculous cholecystitis and may disseminate in patients with advanced HIV disease.

Clinical features

- Crampy abdominal pain, watery diarrhoea, and weight loss similar to cryptosporidiosis
- Steatorrhoea (involvement of the pancreatic and biliary tracts)
- Eosinophilia
- Rarely involves the spleen, liver, and abdominal lymph nodes

Diagnosis

Oocysts are visualized in the stools by using a modified Kinyoun stain (an acid fast stain) or in duodenal aspirate or biopsy.

Management

- Co-trimoxazole 960mg 2–4 times daily for 2–4 weeks gives good results.
- 2° prophylaxis recommended because relapses are common, e.g. co-trimoxazole as for PCP.
- HAART results in significant improvement of symptoms.

Management of chronic diarrhoea in HIV infection

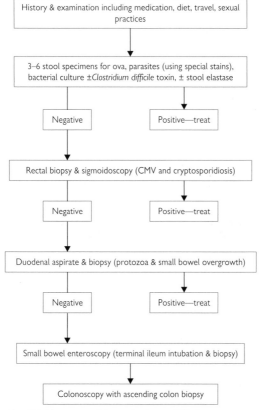

Algorithm 40.1 Management of chronic diarrhoea in HIV infection

Salmonellosis

Salmonellae are Gram-negative non-spore-forming rods belonging to the Enterobacteriaceae family. Non-typhoidal *Salmonella* infections occur with ↑ frequency in HIV infection, particularly with *Salmonella typhimurium*. Major sources are poultry and eggs. *Salmonella* multiplies in the intestinal epithelium, and if not contained it invades the mesenteric lymph nodes and disseminates. Cellular immune responses are important defence mechanisms.

Clinical features

In HIV infection *Salmonella* tends to cause more systemic symptoms. A common feature is severe gastroenteritis and fever. Localized extra-intestinal focal infection may occur. Bacteraemia is common in patients with advanced HIV disease, may be recurrent, and may not be accompanied by GI symptoms.

Diagnosis

- Isolation of the organism is necessary for a definitive diagnosis
- *Salmonella* may be isolated in the blood before stools become positive
- Diagnosis should be considered in all HIV +ve patients with fever ± diarrhoea, and blood and stool cultures taken.

Management

Salmonella requires prompt treatment in HIV +ve individuals because of severity, high relapse rates, and higher risk of dissemination:
- fluid and electrolyte replacement
- oral ciprofloxacin 750mg twice daily (the drug of choice)
- ceftriaxone 1–2g daily
- amoxicillin, but bacterial resistance is ↑.

Prevention

- Risk reduction by avoiding eating undercooked food, with particular care during travel.
- Long-term suppressive antibiotic therapy may be required if recurrent episodes. It may be possible to stop such therapy if there is significant immune reconstitution with HAART. Ciprofloxacin is the drug of choice although co-trimoxazole has some effect.
- AIDS patients have ↑ rates of carriage, which has implications in those working in the food industry.

HIV enteropathy

HIV has been found in gut-associated lymphoid tissue, macrophages of the lamina propria, and enterochromaffin cells. HIV can also affect local humoral immunity and gut motility because of autonomic dysfunction. Villous atrophy with variable degrees of compensatory crypt hyperplasia is a common finding. This leads to rapid cell turnover and functional immaturity of intestinal epithelium with a resultant reduction in enzyme production, leading to impaired absorption of sugars and peptides. Evidence of malabsorption such as abnormal D-xylose test, low vitamin B_{12} levels, and impaired triolein breath tests are described in patients with advanced HIV disease.

These abnormalities may occur in the absence of intestinal disease. HIV enteropathy is a diagnosis only entertained after exclusion of other pathogens.

Management

There are no agreed criteria for the diagnosis of HIV-related enteropathy. Every attempt should be made to find an underling cause, especially infection. Principles of therapy are attention to nutrition and symptomatic control of diarrhoea. Improves with HAART.

Factors contributing to diarrhoea such as alcoholism and drugs must be addressed.

Box 40.4 Causes of diarrhoea in HIV

Infections
- Bacterial
  - *Samonella, Shigella, Campylobacter, Escherichia coli, Clostridium difficile*
  - CD4 < 50 cells/µL—MAC
- Parasitic
  - *Giardia, Cryptosporidium, Microsporidum, Isospora, Entamoeba.*
  - CD4 < 50 cells/µL—*Cryptosporidium, Microsporidium*
- Viral
  - Enteroviruses, HIV enteropathy
  - CD4 < 50 cells/µL—CMV, HSV

Other causes
- Drugs—most anti-retrovirals
- Chronic pancreatitis
- Lymphoma
- Bowel cancer

Anal disease

Anal complaints and anal lesions are frequent presentations in those with HIV infection, especially MSM. Anal pain, pruritus, discharge, and bleeding should be assessed by enquiring about sexual practices, followed by anal and rectal examination by proctoscopy. Gonorrhoea, chlamydia, syphilis, and anogenital warts are common and must be excluded.

Anal HSV infection

Although HSV-2 causes the majority of infection, HSV-1 is increasing in frequency. Patients with advanced HIV disease tend to have more recurrences and prolonged episodes that are less likely to resolve spontaneously.

Typical painful vesicles and ulcers occur in the anal and peri-anal region. Severe disease may result in diffuse peri-anal ulceration. The distal rectum may be involved, resulting in anal discharge, painful defecation, rectal bleeding, and tenesmus. Fever and painful inguinal adenopathy occur more commonly in primary attacks.

Diagnosis 📖 Chapter 21, Diagnosis p. 266.

Management

Prompt treatment with specific antiviral drugs reduces the duration of symptoms and viral shedding. Chronic episodes (>4 weeks) occur more frequently in patients with advanced HIV disease. Aciclovir-resistant HSV has been reported, usually in association with HIV infection. Valaciclovir and famciclovir have better bioavailability.

Recommended initial treatment in the immunocompromised:
- aciclovir 400mg 4 times daily for 10 days
- famciclovir 500mg twice daily for 7 days
- valaciclovir 500mg twice daily for 5 days (up to 10 days if severe)—similar regimen to immunocompetent.

Suppressive treatment (interrupted and reviewed every 6–12 months):
- aciclovir 200mg 4 times daily (or 400mg twice daily)
- valaciclovir 500mg twice daily
- famciclovir 500mg twice daily.

Human papilloma virus (HPV) infection

Anal warts are common in HIV +ve individuals, especially in MSM. HPV6 and 11 are the most frequently found types but others, including HPV16, 18, 31, and 33, have been detected. Patients with advanced HIV disease may have exuberant plaques in the peri-anal region as well as flexural areas. Extensive anal and peri-anal warts may present with rectal bleeding and constipation.

Management: 📖 Chapter 21, Management p. 266.

No treatment ensures HPV eradication. Treatment is similar to those who are HIV –ve, although persistence and recurrences are more common but may improve with immune reconstitution produced by HAART.

Anal intra-epithelial neoplasia (AIN)

The epithelium of the transitional zone between the anus and the colonic mucosa has the same embryonic origin as the cervix and is susceptible to intra-epithelial neoplasia and invasive cancer similar to those seen in the cervix. AIN1–3 precedes the development of anal cancer similar to cervical cancer. HPV16 and 18 infection, receptive anal intercourse, and HIV infection are cofactors associated with the development of these changes.

Anal carcinoma may be prevented by the early detection and treatment of AIN3. Anal cytology can be used to detect dyskaryosis, although this is not routine clinical practice. In the absence of anal cytology, annual digital rectal examination is recommended to detect early lesions. It is anticipated that the incidence of AIN and anal carcinoma will increase as life expectancy rises with the introduction of HAART (which does not appear to be protective).

Low-grade AIN lesions can be treated conservatively by regular monitoring and high-grade lesions (AIN3) by ablative surgical techniques.

Pancreatic disease

Pancreatic involvement in HIV infection is common but is usually asymptomatic. Drugs, alcohol, and OIs are the usual causes. Pancreatic disease tends to occur in conjunction with hepatic and hepatobiliary disease.

Clinical presentation may be with acute or chronic pancreatitis, though elevation of serum amylase or lipase may predate the development of symptoms.

Acute pancreatitis

Patients are usually severely ill, in shock, with acute abdominal pain, nausea, and vomiting. It is associated with OIs including:
- CMV—most common infective cause
- cryptococcus and toxoplasmosis
- cryptosporidiosis, HSV, non-Hodgkin's lymphoma and KS (less common).

Drugs such as didanosine, zalcitabine, co-trimoxazole, and pentamidine are probably the most common cause of acute pancreatitis. Very high levels of triglycerides associated with protease inhibitors may also cause pancreatitis. Serum amylase is elevated and CT scanning demonstrates an oedematous enlarged pancreas with surrounding fluid. Admission to a high dependency unit for cardiovascular and electrolyte support is usually required.

Chronic pancreatitis

Typically presents with pancreatic exocrine deficiency. Chronic diarrhoea and malabsorption are the usual presenting features. As with HIV –ve patients, the discontinuation of any offending drugs and alcohol may result in symptomatic improvement. Associated HIV-related cholangiopathy is a recognized underlying cause.

Diagnosis

Chronic abdominal pain (especially if there is history of acute pancreatitis) is suggestive of chronic pancreatitis. This may be accompanied by pancreatic insufficiency symptoms, e.g. steatorrhoea, weight loss, and other evidence of malabsorption. Screen by measuring faecal elastase and triolein breath tests (serum amylase and lipase are usually normal). The best diagnostic test is endoscopic retrograde cholangiopancreatography (ERCP).

Management
- Pain control
- Pancreatic enzyme supplement

Hepatic and biliary tract disease

HIV itself has been found in Kupffer cells, hepatic macrophages, and hepatocytes. The liver in those with HIV infections is a target of specific viral, bacterial, fungal, and protozoal infections. Infection with hepatitis B or C viruses may predate HIV infection. With improved life expectancy and the effect of drugs, more liver-related problems are being identified.

Hepatic disease

>80% of those with HIV infection are estimated to have abnormal liver function tests (LFTs) at some time during the course of their infection. This does not necessarily indicate the presence of liver disease. Important causes of abnormal LFTs and liver disease are as follows (Box 40.5).

- Viral co-infections: HCV, HBV, HDV, CMV, EBV.
- Drugs
  - Antiretrovirals—all may cause raised ALT, more common in hepatitis co-infection. Grade 3/4 ALT occurs in ~12% patients on any HAART. Atazanavir causes clinically insignificant raised bilirubin 2° to uridine–glucuronosyl transferase inhibition.
  - Many of the drugs used in prophylaxis and treatment of OI lead to liver toxicity.
  - NRTIs, particularly D4T, DDI, and AZT, may cause mitochondrial toxicity leading to hepatic steatosis.
- Alcohol.
- Bacterial, fungal, and protozoal infections and neoplasms occur much less frequently. The pattern of LFTs and the clinical stage of HIV infection may help to narrow the diagnostic options.

Liver damage may lead to the following:

- Hepatic steatosis is more common in HIV infection because of NRTI-induced mitochondrial toxicity, as part of the metabolic syndrome associated with protease inhibitor (PI) and HCV co-infection. May lead to steatohepatitis and cirrhosis.
- Cirrhoisis is a common cause of morbidity and mortality. Point prevalence ~8%. Generally associated with viral hepatitis. However, ~10% of cirrhotics do not have co-infection and may have developed cirrhosis 2° to drugs.
- Nodular regenerative hyperplasia is a cause of portal hypertension and variceal bleed in the absence of fibrosis and may be caused by HIV ± antiretrovirals.

History

Prior infection with viral hepatitis, alcohol intake, prescribed and recreational drug use, antiretroviral history, and recent travel.

Examination

Fever, hypotension, signs of chronic liver disease and nutritional status (obesity and malnutrition).

Abnormal LFTs

Mixed hepatitic and obstructive liver enzyme abnormalities are common but rarely diagnostic in isolation.

- Predominant ↑ of serum transaminases usually indicate hepatitis but lacks sensitivity and specificity. A new hepatitis viral infection or reactivation of hepatitis B and/or C infection with immune reconstitution should be excluded. Consider drug hepatotoxicity and investigate for other infections.
- Predominant ↑ of serum alkaline phosphatase usually indicates biliary obstruction. Initial assessment is by ultrasound scan or CT of the liver and abdomen. Lesion identified can be targeted by image-guided biopsy. ERCP must be considered if imaging techniques reveal intra- and/or extra-hepatic duct dilatation.

Biliary tract disease

Presents with right upper quadrant abdominal pain and weight loss. Investigations to exclude common biliary conditions such as cholelithiasis should proceed before attributing to HIV infection.

HIV-associated cholangiopathy

Similar to sclerosing cholangitis presenting with right upper abdominal pain associated with nausea, vomiting, fever, and marked elevation of serum alkaline phosphatase. Ultrasound shows dilated intra- and/or extra-hepatic bile ducts. ERCP provides further structural delineation. Some cases are associated with cryptosporidial and CMV infections.

Acalculous cholecystitis

Presents with similar symptoms to HIV-associated cholangiopathy. Ultrasound of the abdomen normally shows thickened dilated gall bladder but may be normal. Can be complicated by recurrent cholangitis. Associated with CMV, *Cryptosporidium parvum*, microsporidia, and MAC infection but no cause in >50%. Diagnosis by ultrasound or technetium scintigraphy. Treatment is cholecystectomy.

Box 40.5 Main causes of liver disease in HIV patients

Viral
- Hepatitis B virus
- Hepatitis C virus
- Cytomegalovirus

Alcohol

Drugs
- Recreational
- Therapeutic (e.g. antiretroviral and antituberculous)

Other infections
- Mycobacteriosis

Neoplasia
- Lymphoma
- Kaposi's sarcoma

HIV: hepatitis virus co-infection

Introduction

Since the introduction of HAART, deaths from HIV, in particular those resulting from opportunistic infection (OI) have markedly ↓. Conversely, liver-related mortality has ↑. Hepatitis B, hepatitis C, and HIV can all be transmitted via blood and sexual contact, and consequently co-infection is common. Assessment of co-infection requires a multidisciplinary approach with attention to ongoing drug and alcohol use, psychiatric illness, progressive liver disease, and degree of HIV immune suppression. Alcohol should be strongly discouraged. Injecting drug users (IDUs) should enter a maintenance programme.

If immuno-naive, hepatitis A/B vaccination should be provided.

HIV–hepatitis B virus (HBV) co-infection

Epidemiology

In high endemic areas of sub-Saharan Africa, Eastern Europe, South and Southeast Asia co-infection rates of 10–15% are found. In the UK, HBV-associated HIV infection is 5–8% with co-infection more common in haemophiliacs, IDUs, and those from high prevalence areas. Co-infection rates vary regionally within the UK.

Natural history and clinical features

Co-infection is usually associated with a higher HBV viraemia and a more rapid progression to cirrhosis. Although HBV does not appear to influence the natural history of HIV, there is ↑ rate of hepatotoxicity in relation to antiretroviral therapy. HBV reactivation can occur in those who appear to have cleared their HBV infection. This can lead to transient HB surface antigenaemia or chronic HBV infection and may occur more frequently when CD4 counts are ↓. In addition the natural clearance of HBe antigen is ↓ but spontaneous recovery from chronic HBV infection may occur in those whose CD4 count ↑.

Diagnosis and investigations

- As for HBV and HIV (📖 Chapter 24, HBV infection p. 294, Chapter 38, HIV pre-test discussion p. 436). However, if ALT is raised persistently, HBV DNA must be measured to exclude HBV disease.
- It is important to repeat HBV serology regularly in immuno-naive patients with HIV infection. Other factors causing liver disease/ infection require exclusion.
- AFP and liver ultrasound should be performed in all at diagnosis and 6 monthly if cirrhotic. Six-monthly screening should be considered in Asian patients >40 years, African patients >20 years, family history of hepatocellular carcinoma (HCC), and if HBV VL high and ALT abnormal.
- If ALT raised, screen for other causes of liver disease.
- Liver biopsy is important when active HBV replication (high HBV–DNA, abnormal liver function, or advanced liver disease). HBV genotyping may be considered. Testing for resistance (e.g. YMDD

motif codon substitution in lamivudine resistance) should be done if previous treatment or suppression of HBV DNA is not achieved by 6 months.
- Fibroscan® has not been validated in HBV infection.
- Increased monitoring of liver function on HAART (due to enhanced hepatotoxicity of most antiretroviral drugs).

Management (Box 41.1)

In chronic HBV–HIV co-infection the aim of HBV treatment is to suppress viral replication. Only rarely is it curative (loss of surface antigen). Available treatment options include lamivudine, tenofovir, adefovir, pegylated interferon, emtricitabine, and most recently entecavir.

HBe-antigen –ve patients with normal liver function and low viral load 2000 IU/mL (<10^4copies/mL) do not require treatment. In these patients, monitor LFTs and HBV VL annually. If started on HAART, avoid lamivudine as only HBV drug. Patients with HBV–DNA >10^5copies/mL and/or abnormal liver function should have a liver biopsy. Ishak score for fibrosis should be measured: mild disease ≤2; moderate ≥2 to <6; cirrhosis >6.

The optimum time to initiate treatment is unknown. Early intervention may be aided by higher CD4 counts but the risk of emergence of HIV drug resistance must be considered.

⚠ Interferon must not be used in HBV-infected cirrhotic patients.

Treatment prior to HAART
- Mild liver disease: if HBV VL ≥10^4 copies/mL, eAg +ve or –ve, and raised ALT, consider treatment with pegylated interferon or adefovir.
- Moderate liver disease: if VL ≥10^4 copies/mL, eAg +ve or –ve, consider treatment with adefovir or pegylated interferon (if ALT raised).
- Cirrhosis: if VL ≥10^3 copies/mL, eAg +ve or –ve, treat with adefovir.

Treatment regime
Co-infected patients requiring HAART should be treated with a regime containing tenofovir and emtricitabine or lamivudine. Lamivudine, tenofovir or emtricitabine should only be used as part of HAART. If HAART regimens containing lamivudine or tenofovir achieve good HBV response, but need to be changed, these agents should be maintained in addition to the new HAART combination. The dose for lamivudine in co-infected patients should be 150mg twice daily or 300mg daily not 100mg daily as in HBV mono-infection.

Assessment for liver transplantation if cirrhosis develops should not be denied.

Box 41.1 HIV–HBV co-infection management

- Initial investigations: CD 4, LFT, hepatitis B viral load
- Stage liver fibrosis: ideally by liver biopsy
- Decision to treat based on LFTs, liver histology, CD4 and HBV DNA
- CD4 >500:
  - minimal fibrosis, normal ALT and HBV DNA <2000IU/L →
    monitor 3–6 monthly
  - minimal fibrosis in Hep eAg +ve +↑ALT, HBV DNA >2000IU/L →
    pegylated interferon for 12 months.
  - significant fibrosis → HBV exclusively active agent
- CD4 <350 → HAART including agents active against HBV.

CD4 350–500 +significant fibrosis → consider HAART containing agents active against HBV.

HIV–hepatitis C virus (HCV) co-infection

Epidemiology

HCV infection is a major risk for end-stage liver disease (ESLD) in HIV infection. HCV prevalence is much higher in HIV-infected individuals than in the rest of the population (in the UK 5–15% compared with 0.4%). Higher rates are found in HIV-positive haemophiliacs, IDUs, MSM, and those from Southern or Eastern Europe.

Heterosexual HCV transmission is infrequent but may be more likely with anal sex or coexisting STIs.

Natural history and clinical features

Co-infection with HCV accelerates the progression of HIV and results in a poorer CD4 increase with HAART.

HCV-infected individuals co-infected with HIV have a faster progression to cirrhosis if untreated (median time decreases from 32 to 23 years with ~50% cirrhotic at 30 years post-HCV infection) with death from ESLD more common. Vertical transmission of HCV ↑ to 14–17%.

Otherwise clinical features as for mono-infection (📖 Chapter 24, HCV infection p. 298).

Diagnosis and investigations

- As for HCV and HIV (📖 Chapter 24, HBV infection p. 294, Chapter 38, HIV pre-test discussion p. 436) including HCV genotype testing. HIV patients with low CD4 may have occult HCV and HCV VL should be measured if ALT persistently raised and HCV Ab –ve.
- Liver biopsy currently recommended except if bleeding disorder present.
- Fibroscan® may be helpful, but some evidence suggests overestimation of fibrosis in co-infection if standard cut-off of 12kpa used for cirrhosis.
- Monitoring of progression of liver disease with α-fetoprotein, abdominal ultrasound, and Doppler scan of portal vein yearly, and if severe liver disease/cirrhosis 6 monthly. Monitoring should continue if severe liver disease after successful treatment.
- Increased monitoring of liver function on HAART (because of enhanced hepatotoxicity of most antiretroviral drugs).

Management (Box 41.2)

Treatment should be considered in all patients but can be difficult with ↑ side-effects in the co-infected. Pre-treatment investigations as above with TSH, FBC, U+Es, LFTs, and CD4 count.

Pre-treatment

- Consider the following:
- HAART should be started if CD4 <350cells/µL and HCV treatment should be delayed until CD4 has increased >200cells/µL (treatment success improves with ↑ CD4 percentage >25%). A temporary CD4 drop of up to 150cells/µL occurs on interferon; percentage is normally preserved.
- Didanosine and Zidovudine should be avoided in combination with ribavirin (increased SE). Abacavir may lead to ↓ response.

Treatment regime (Box 41.2)

- Non-cirrhotic: pegylated interferon 2α (180mcg/week) or pegylated interferon 2β (1.5mcg/kg/week) + ribavirin (<75kg 600mg + 400mg; >75kg 600mg bd).
- Cirrhosis: increased side-effects. Seek specialist advice—escalating dose regime may be necessary.
- Ophthalmology review if hypertension or diabetic—increased retinal disease with interferon

Treatment should be monitored with 2 weekly and then monthly FBC, LFTs, 3 monthly TFTs and CD4, and HCV viral load at 4, 12, 24, and 48 weeks. Responders are HCV RNA –ve at 12 weeks post-treatment. Further RNA should be checked to confirm.

Side-effects ↑ in co-infection, particularly haematological disturbance. Consider erythropoietin to maintain ribavirin dose particularly in early stages up to week 12 of treatment.

Treatment length

- Genotypes 2 and 3:
  - 48 weeks if HCV RNA –ve at week 4: consider 24 weeks treatment particularly if poor tolerance
- Genotype 1
  - HCV RNA –ve at week 4: 48 weeks treatment
  - HCV RNA +ve week 4, >2log drop week 12 and –ve week 24: consider 72 weeks treatment.
- Acute HCV (new HCV Ab +ve when previously –ve): treat within 6 months of infection with HCV.
  - 24 weeks with VL at 12 weeks.

⚠ Interferon should be stopped if HCV RNA +ve at week 12 in all genotypes as sustained virological response <1% at end of treatment.

Patients with genotypes 2 and 3 and mild/moderate liver disease have a sustained viral response of ~60%. Patients with genotype 1 have a sustained viral response of ~30% at best (48 week regimen). Patients must be warned that virological response does not lead to immunity to HCV and transmission may recur with resumption of high-risk activity.

Those with stable HIV disease requiring liver transplantation should not be denied assessment although current experience is small.

Box 41.2 HIV–HCV co-infection management

- Baseline tests+ LFTs, HCV genotype, HCV RNA, CD4.
- Liver fibrosis assessment: ideally liver biopsy (not required for genotype 2 and 3) if available fibroscan or fibrosis biomarkers.
- CD4 >350 → treat as for HCV mono-infection.
- CD4 <350 → HAART + pegylated interferon + ribavarin (consider drug interactions and toxicity).
- During treatment measure HCV RNA at 4, 12, 24 and 48 weeks.
- Duration of treatment:
  - 24 weeks for genotypes 2 and 3 if rapid virological response achieved, otherwise 48 weeks if RNA –ve at 24 weeks
  - 48 weeks for genotypes 1 and 4 but extend to 72 weeks if >2log RNA drop at 12 weeks and RNA –ve at 24 weeks.

HIV: respiratory disorders

Introduction

Respiratory symptoms with a wide disease spectrum are common in HIV infection (Box 42.1). They include processes not directly related to HIV, e.g. bronchogenic carcinoma, smokers' bronchitis, or IV drug use associated pulmonary vascular disease.

In HIV infection

- HIV itself, without pulmonary opportunistic infection (OI), leads to ↓ lung function.
- Respiratory disease ↑ in frequency with falling CD4 counts and ↑ duration of HIV infection.
- Risks of OI ↑ by other factors, e.g. cigarette smoking (further damages lung defences).
- The advent of HAART (where available) has significantly ↓ the burden of HIV-associated respiratory disease.

Pathology varies with:

- Age, e.g. lymphocytic interstitial pneumonitis (LIP) occurs predominantly in children
- Exposure (travel to or residence in areas endemic for specificpathogens), e.g. histoplasma
- Level of immune function
- Specific immune defects, e.g. failure to produce antibodies against pneumococcal capsular antigen (independent of CD4 count)
- HIV infection by modifying typical clinical presentations and influencing results of investigations, e.g. ↓ rate of sputum smear positivity in pulmonary TB.

Considerable overlap of symptoms and signs in different conditions and dual infections may occur. Uncommon for a particular constellation of symptoms, clinical findings, and radiological abnormalities to be absolutely diagnostic—a full investigation is always required. However, radiological appearances may suggest different groups of conditions.

Chest X-ray appearances

Interstitial	*Pneumocystis jiroveci (carinii)* pneumonia (PCP), Cryptococcosis (rare) LIP (in children), rarely CMV
Lobar	Bacterial infection
Nodular	Kaposi's sarcoma (KS), septic emboli, fungal infection, non-Hodgkin's lymphoma
Miliary	Tuberculosis (TB)
Pneumatocele	PCP, staphylococcal pneumonia
Pleural effusion	KS, TB, lymphoma
Mediastinal and/or hilar lymphadenopathy	Mycobacteriosis, lymphoma, fungal infection

As deterioration can sometimes be rapid it is important that 'best guess' therapy is initiated while awaiting the results of microbiology.

Box 42.1 Spectrum of respiratory illnesses in HIV-infected patients

Infections (organisms identified most commonly)
- Bacteria
  - *Streptococcus pneumoniae*
  - *Haemophilus influenzae*
  - Gram-negative bacilli (*Pseudomonas aeruginosa, Klebsiella pneumoniae*)
  - *Staphylococcus aureus*
  - *Mycobacterium tuberculosis*
  - Atypical mycobacteria (*Mycobacterium kansasii, Mycobacterium avium* complex)
  - *Rhodococcus equi*
- Fungi
  - *Pneumocystis jiroveci (carinii)*
  - *Cryptococcus neoformans*
  - *Histoplasma capsulatum*
  - *Aspergillus* spp
  - *Candida* spp
  - *Coccidioides immitis*
- Viruses
  - Cytomegalovirus
  - Herpes simplex virus
- Parasites
  - *Strongyloides stercoralis*
  - *Toxoplasma gondii*
- Neoplasia
  - Kaposi's sarcoma
  - Non-Hodgkin's lymphoma
  - Bronchogenic carcinoma
- Other respiratory illnesses
  - Upper respiratory tract infection (sinusitis, pharyngitis)
  - Lymphocytic interstitial pneumonitis
  - Non-specific interstitial pneumonitis
  - Acute bronchitis
  - Obstructive lung disease (asthma, chronic bronchitis)
  - Bronchiectasis
  - Emphysema
  - Pulmonary vascular disease
  - Illicit-drug-induced lung disease
  - Medication-induced lung disease
  - 1° pulmonary hypertension
  - Bronchiolitis obliterans organizing pneumonia

Bacterial pneumonia

Before HAART bacterial pneumonia was the most frequent pulmonary complication of HIV, occurring in up to 42% in autopsy studies. An episode of bacterial pneumonia is associated with subsequent ↑ morbidity and ↓ survival time.

Aetiology

Most common pathogens are *Streptococcus pneumoniae*, *Haemophilus influenzae*, and *Staphylococcus aureus* which occur more frequently in the general population as a cause of pneumonia. In pneumococcal infection rate of bacteraemia is ↑ and there may be ↑ incidence of penicillin-resistant isolates. Intravenous drug use further ↑ the risk of bacterial pneumonia. Less common causes include *Rhodococcus equi* which produces a cavitatory pneumonia of insidious onset.

Clinical and diagnostic features

Most bacterial pneumonias present acutely with symptoms and radiological patterns similar to that seen in HIV −ve patients (lobar or broncho-pneumonic consolidation). However, the radiological presentation may be indistinguishable from other OIs, and *H.influenzae* has been reported to present with diffuse opacities mimicking PCP (Table 42.1). As immunodeficiency becomes more advanced, pneumonias due to *Staph.aureus* and *Ps.aeruginosa* become more important and may produce cavitation.

Management

In patients presenting with a clinical diagnosis of bacterial pneumonia:
- Assess and correct hypoxia, volume depletion, and hypotension.
- Gauge severity by presence of confusion, ↑ blood urea, ↑ respiratory rate, ↓ blood pressure, older age group, and co-pathologies.
- Obtain sputum and blood cultures and baseline atypical pneumonia serology. Consider urine testing for legionella antigen.
- Check inflammatory markers and white cell count, although white cell response may be ↓ if there is HIV-induced marrow suppression.
- Commence IV antibiotic therapy with:
  - either cefuroxime 1.5g three times daily plus a macrolide (e.g. clarithromycin 500mg twice daily)
  - or amoxicillin 1g three times daily plus a macrolide.
- consider modification of these combinations if there are features to suggest involvement with *Staph.aureus, Ps.aeruginosa*, or atypical organisms such as *R.equi*.
- if recurrent and evidence of ↓ antibody production consider IV immunoglobulin therapy or prophylactic antibiotics.

For outpatient and less severe pneumonia oral amoxicillin may suffice and a macrolide may be added if no improvement.

Table 42.1 Comparison of bacterial pneumonia and PCP

	PCP	Bacterial pneumonia
CD4 cell count	<200cells/µL	Any
Symptoms	Non-productivecough	Productive cough (purulent sputum)
Duration	Typically weeks	Typically 3–5 days
Signs	50%—clear lungs	Focal lung abnormalities common
Laboratory tests		
White blood count	Varies	Frequently ↑
Serum lactic dehydro-genase	↑	Varies
Chest radiograph		
Distribution	Diffuse > local	Focal > diffuse
Location	Bilateral	Unilateral, segmental/lobular
Pattern	Reticular, granular	Alveolar
Cysts	15–20%	Rarely
Pleural effusions	Very rarely	25–30%

Pneumocystis jiroveci (carinii) pneumonia (PCP)

The AIDS indicator disease in ~65% of patients before the initiation of 1° prophylaxis programmes and effective antiretroviral therapy. Initially thought to be protozoan, but genetic analysis indicates that the organism is a unicellular fungus. Infection usually occurs when CD4 counts <200cells/µL or CD4 percentage <15%. Although natural colonization/infection occurs frequently in early life it is thought that clinical pneumonitis represents new infection rather than reactivation of latent organisms.

PCP is almost completely preventable using 1° prophylaxis. The gold standard is co-trimoxazole. Dapsone, dapsone and pyrimethamine, atovaquone, and pentamidine are alternatives (📖 Chapter 38, p. 442). Cutaneous hypersensitivity reactions to co-trimoxazole are common, but 80% of HIV +ve patients can be desensitized by the use of gradually ↑ doses (📖 Chapter 38, Table 38.2).

Clinical features

Usually presents sub-acutely with symptoms ↑ over weeks with night sweats, systemic symptoms and weight loss, dry cough, progressive dyspnoea initially on exertion and eventually at rest, occasionally with a spontaneous pneumothorax. Abnormalities on respiratory examination often minimal or absent and significant ↓ of pulmonary function may occur despite minimal chest X-ray changes.

Diagnosis

Radiology

- High-resolution computed tomography shows ground glass appearance of interstitial pathology.
- Chest X-ray may be normal in early and mild disease but in severe PCP the typical pattern is bi-basal perihilar interstitial infiltrates (Plate 19). Less commonly unilateral infiltrates and pneumatoceles, and rarely pneumothorax or pleural effusion.
- Atypical upper lobe involvement may be seen if the patient has been on nebulized pentamidine prophylaxis. They may also develop extra-pulmonary involvement of various organs including eyes, spleen, and skin (due to lack of systemic effect).
- Gallium-67 scanning is highly sensitive but less specific. Its high cost and 2 day time delay in getting results limits its use to those with suspected relapse.

Oximetry

If history is suspicious but normal resting oxygen saturations, exercise oximetry showing ↓ in oxygen saturation by 5% or to <90% is highly suggestive of PCP.

Respiratory secretions/lung tissue

Specific diagnosis requires demonstration of *Pneumocystis jiroveci* cysts in respiratory secretions or lung tissue. Patients with borderline lung function may require sputum induction and bronchoscopy.

- Sputum should be induced by 3% saline using an ultrasonic nebulizer. When stained with fluorescene, linked monoclonal antibodies— sensitivity up to 77%, negative predicted value up to 64%.
- Fibreoptic bronchoscopic alveolar lavage (BAL)—sensitivity ~90%.
- Transbronchial biopsy with histology of fixed tissue—sensitivity up to 98%.

Management

Prior to initiating investigations in those presenting with a history suggestive of PCP, it is essential to assess pulmonary impairment and the need for oxygen supplements by pulse oximetry and arterial blood gases.

▶If there is pulmonary impairment, delays in initiating PCP therapy should be kept to a minimum. HAART should be started within 2 weeks of treatment of PCP. Delaying HAART is associated with ↑ AIDS progression and death.

Gold standard antibiotic therapy is co-trimoxazole 120mg/kg in four divided doses daily for 21 days. Haematology, liver function tests, and the skin must be monitored carefully for evidence of toxicity or developing hypersensitivity. Folinic acid supplements may be considered if there is evidence of impaired marrow function. For non-responders or hypersensitive patients alternative regimens include clindamycin (600mg four times daily) and primaquine (15–30mg/day), dapsone (100mg/day) and trimethoprim (5mg/kg every 4–6 hours), atovaquone (750mg three times daily), IV pentamidine (600mg/day), and trimetrexate (45mg/m^2/day IV plus folinic acid). Caspofungin (70mg/day) in addition to co-trimoxazole has been used successfully in some patients not responding.

In patients with arterial oxygen pressures <9.3kPa steroid therapy is recommended as it ↓ risk of respiratory failure and mortality. Conventional regimen is prednisolone (or equivalent) 40mg twice daily for 5 days, 40mg once daily for 5 days, followed by 20mg daily for 5–10 days. There is no significant ↑ in risk of other OIs except *Candida* spp and local herpes simplex virus.

Patients with severe PCP may progress to respiratory failure requiring ventilatory support with constant positive airways pressure (CPAP) or intubation and ventilation. Pneumothorax may require chest drain insertion. Adverse prognostic indicators include ↑ serum lactic dehydrogenase (LDH) levels, need for high ventilatory pressures, and prolonged stay in intensive therapy unit (ITU).

Maintenance and withdrawal of 2° prophylaxis

Following successful treatment, 2° prophylaxis, with the same regimens as for 1° presentation, should be continued.

- For patients receiving 1° or 2° PCP prophylaxis discontinue when the CD4 count has been >200 cells/μL for at least 3 months (rate of OIs does not ↓ until after 2 months of HAART).

Tuberculosis (TB)

On a worldwide scale TB is the most important HIV-associated OI, and as a result the prevalence of TB in the developed world has ↑. In sub-Saharan Africa up to ~65% of patients with extra-pulmonary TB have HIV infection. Patients presenting primarily with TB should have their risk profile for HIV infection assessed and be offered HIV testing as appropriate. Those with known HIV infection and pulmonary disease should have TB excluded. Proven or suspected TB should be notified and contact tracing with assessment initiated.

Clinical features

TB can occur at any stage of HIV infection. Classic presentation of pulmonary TB is night sweats/fever, cough, pleuritic chest pain, haemoptysis, and weight loss. Atypical presentations occur as CD4 count ↓. Lobar distribution of pulmonary infection may mimic community-acquired pneumonia. Disseminated and extra-pulmonary diseases are more common with ↓ CD4 count. Although most cases are caused by reactivation of latent infection, 1° infection with rapid progression to active TB can occur when CD4 counts are <100cells/μL. TB has an additional immunosuppressive effect in HIV infection.

Diagnosis

- Radiology: in patients with preserved immune function typical upper lobe cavitatory changes occur. In those with lower CD4 counts appearances may be more extensive, mimicking other infections.
- Examination of at least three sputum samples by microscopy of Ziehl–Neelsen or auramine stained samples and culture. Induced sputum or BAL samples if patients cannot produce sputum or if sputum AFB −ve. Smear positivity ↓ if advanced immunodeficiency.
- If extra-pulmonary findings (e.g. lymphadenopathy, bone marrow abnormalities) tissue cultures may be diagnostic.
- Molecular methods, e.g. interferon γ production from peripheral blood mononuclear cells in response to antigenic stimulation (e.g. Quantiferon Gold® or T SPOT™), have an undefined role in diagnosis and may be −ve in active disease. Rifampicin mutation gene probe should be considered in AFB +ve specimens if the patient is from a high-risk area for multidrug-resistant TB (MDRTB) or has had previous TB diagnosis. If +ve treat as MDRTB.

Management

Drug therapy of TB-co-infected HIV +ve patients is complex because of ↑ drug toxicities, drug interactions, and paradoxical reactions. If TB is strongly suspected, empirical therapy with four drugs should be initiated immediately after cultures sent. Even if cultures are negative, a full course may be required if there is clinical response despite negative cultures. Treatment of active TB may lead to ↑ in CD4 counts.

A 6 month short course of anti-TB therapy is sufficient for respiratory disease and most extra-pulmonary TB with fully sensitive organisms.

TB meningitis requires 12 months treatment. Treatment should preferably start with quadruple therapy using isoniazid (300mg daily), rifampicin (600mg daily), pyrazinamide (1.5–2g daily), and ethambutol (15mg/kg/day) with standard monitoring precautions until mycobacterial drug sensitivities are known. After 2 months switch to rifampicin and isoniazid for a further 4 months.

⚠ If MDRTB suspected seek expert advice on initial regime.

►Check visual acuities prior to starting ethambutol. Monitor visual symptoms and liver function tests regularly.

►There are very important drug–drug interactions between anti-TB and anti-HIV therapies because of their varying enzyme-inducing and enzyme-inhibiting effects (📖 Table 53.1). Joint management involving physicians experienced in TB and HIV therapy is important. Rifampicin produces across-the-board ↓ in HAART levels. When used in conjunction with rifampicin, efavirenz should be increased to 800mg/day in Caucasians. Evidence suggests that 600mg/day is sufficient in Black Africans or Caucasians <50kg. Protease inhibitors should not be used with rifampicin; rifabutin may be used at a lower dose, i.e. 150mg every other day.

Drug interactions may be minimized as follows.

- Defer HAART until after completion of anti-TB drugs, particularly if CD4 count ↑ on anti-TB medication.
- If CD4 count 100–200/μL, defer HAART until anti-TB medication is reduced to dual therapy.
- Make careful choice of HAART and anti-TB drugs to reduce interactions. This may reduce anti-TB efficacy.
- Consider monitoring efavirenz and/or rifampicin levels.

TB treatment regimens with declining evidence of efficacy

- Standard short course of rifampicin-containing regimen for 6 months.
- Standard short course of induction with rifabutin/rifampicin substitution at 2 months.
- Rifabutin/rifampicin substitution throughout 6 month course.
- Standard induction followed by non-rifamycin continuation—total duration of 8 months.
- 8 month non-rifamycin regimen.

► If CD4 counts <100/μL there is significant risk of developing additional OIs and the initiation of HAART should not be deferred.

Where there is no suspicion of resistant organism the patient would be regarded as no longer an infection risk after 2 weeks of therapy.

Immune reconstitution syndrome (📖 Chapter 53, Immune reconstitution p. 592)

A further complication of anti-TB with HAART is the development of an immune reconstitution syndrome with high fevers and malaise as a result of improved immune function directed at mycobacteria. This may require steroids for its control or interruption of HAART until the TB is better controlled.

Opportunist mycobacterial infections

Mycobacterium avium complex infections occur in HIV-infected individuals in CD4 counts of <100/μL and characteristically produce generalized bacter-aemic disease. Colonization of the respiratory tract can occur without evi-dent morbidity, but this presages the occurrence of disseminated disease. During immune reconstitution as a result of HAART, previously subclinical infection in the lungs may become apparent as an inflammatory response develops, leading to pulmonary inflammation and X-ray changes.

Other fungal infections

Pulmonary cryptococcosis

Pulmonary disease is diagnosed less frequently than meningitis in patients with AIDS although the lung is the most likely portal of entry. Pulmonary involvement can be asymptomatic, but precedes the onset of disseminated disease in the majority of patients. Pulmonary involvement can produce cough, fever, malaise, shortness of breath, and pleuritic pain.

Diagnosis

- Chest X-rays show focal or diffuse infiltrates that may mimic PCP. Less commonly, mass lesions, hilar and mediastinal adenopathy, and pleural effusions occur.
- Organisms are more likely to be isolated from BAL samples than from sputum.

Management

Treating the pulmonary lesion can prevent disseminated disease. Consists of amphotericin B combined with flucytosine as induction therapy, followed by fluconazole or itraconazole.

Pulmonary aspergillosis

Aspergillus infections in advanced HIV disease are uncommon and occur in conjunction with other OIs. Invasive disease occurs predominantly in patients with severe neutropenia. In HIV disease the lung is the most important site of invasive aspergillosis. Symptoms include fever, dyspnoea, cough, chest pain, and haemoptysis. ~20% have unilateral or bilateral diffuse or nodular infiltrates.

Diagnosis

- Chest X-ray
  - ~30% have thick-walled upper lobe cavities
  - ~20% have unilateral or bilateral diffuse or nodular infiltrates.
- CT of chest may show 'halo' sign.
- Microbiology
  - Sputum, BAL, blood, bone marrow, and tissue biopsies should be examined by microscopy and cultured for fungi. Only 10–30% have positive findings on sputum culture. BAL has a higher yield.
  - Culture is required as microscopy alone cannot distinguish Aspergillus from other fungal species.
  - PCR and/or galactomannan ELISA may be helpful, but need careful interpretation in suspected disease.

Management

- Amphotericin B 1mg/kg/day or higher doses in liposomal form
- Itraconazole or voriconazole
- Caspofungin 70mg stat then 50mg/day

In patients with severe neutropenia granulocyte macrophage colony stimulating factor may have an adjunctive role.

Other conditions

Cytomegalovirus (CMV) pneumonitis

Patients with PCP often have CMV isolated from bronchial washings or lung biopsy. In most cases this represents viral replication without pneumonitis and the patient responds to PCP therapy alone. Active pneumonitis occurs much less frequently than in patients taking immunosuppressive therapy post transplant. Hypoxia is usual.

Diagnosis
- Chest X-ray shows diffuse interstitial infiltrates
- Identification of CMV in lung tissue

Management

Patients with interstitial pneumonia and positive CMV identification in lung tissue should be treated with anti-CMV therapy using ganciclovir or foscarnet (📖 Chapter 44, Opportunistic infections (OIs) p. 514). A role for CMV immunoglobulin is not proven in the HIV setting.

Mediastinal and hilar lymphadenopathy

Patients with HIV-related persistent generalized lymphadenopathy have sub-diaphragmatic lymphadenopathy but do not have significant hilar or mediastinal node enlargement. Hilar or mediastinal adenopathy implies significant pathology. The differential diagnosis includes:
- lymphoma
- Kaposi's sarcoma
- TB
- MAC
- fungal disease.

May occasionally be seen in active PCP, but other pulmonary radiological abnormalities will be present. A careful search for peripheral lymphadenopathy, skin lesions, and other abnormalities that could be subjected to histological and microbiological examinations should be sought.

Pulmonary vascular disease

1° pulmonary hypertension can occur as a consequence of HIV infection. IDUs may develop pulmonary small vessel obstruction due to injection of particulate material or may suffer recurrent pulmonary emboli.

Intense fatigue, breathlessness, and faintness on exertion are features of severe pulmonary hypertension. Clinical features of right ventricular hypertrophy include a heave, prominent A wave in the jugular pulse, and a third heart sound. Should be considered in unexplained shortness of breath.

Diagnosis

- ECG: RV strain, RBBB, right axis deviation
- Echocardiography
- Ultrasonography of the deep veins
- Pulmonary angiography
- Right heart catheterization

Management

Anticoagulants and pulmonary vasodilators. HAART may improve mortality and morbidity.

HIV: neurological disorders

Introduction

HIV enters the central nervous system (CNS) soon after 1° infection, either carried by infected mononuclear cells or by cell-free transfer across the blood–brain barrier. Infected monocytes then differentiate into macrophages, and produce virions that can infect astrocytes and microglia (brain macrophages). Neurons are not infected, but they are lost and become dysfunctional in HIV brain disease.

Neurological disease is common and may be the presenting clinical syndrome in 30% of HIV infections occurring at any stage, but most often presents following seroconversion or with severe immunodeficiency. Neurological features have been reported in 40–70% of patients with AIDS, ↑ to 90% at postmortem examination (Box 43.1). Abnormal cerebrospinal fluid (CSF) findings including ↑ lymphocytes, protein, immunoglobulin, and oligoclonal bands may be found in patients with no neurological symptoms or signs. The presence or absence of neurological disease is independent of CSF viral load.

Mechanisms of CNS injury and the spectrum of neurological disease vary with the stage of HIV infection and the degree of immune deficiency.

- At seroconversion—viraemia and inflammation resulting from the initial immunological response to HIV infection predominate, inducing aseptic meningitis, meningoencephalitis, ataxic neuropathy, Guillain–Barré syndrome, acute myelopathy, a multiple-sclerosis-like syndrome, acute brachial neuritis, Bell's palsy, and acute meningoradiculitis.
  ▶Patients presenting with these syndromes should have their HIV risk assessed and be offered HIV screening.
- In chronic HIV infection asymptomatic neurocognitive impairment can be found in 5–20% of patients. This tends to improve with HAART.
- As HIV progresses, altered CNS cytokine production and direct neurotoxic effects of HIV components (e.g. gp120) are pathogenic.
- With immunodeficiency, opportunist infections (OIs)/tumours and complications of treatment predominate.

HAART has changed the epidemiology of the neurological manifestations of HIV resulting in ↓ CNS OIs, ↓ incidence of HIV dementia complex, and improved prognosis for some infections which were previously difficult to treat, such as progressive multifocal leukoencephalopathy (PML). However, there has been ↑ occurrence of drug induced CNS and peripheral nerve disease.

Box 43.1 HIV-related neurological and neuromuscular disease may present with a number of symptom complexes

Headaches

May be an important symptom of neuropathology, such as primary or opportunist meningitis, intra-cerebral opportunist pathologies, or the side-effects of drugs such as zidovudine or co-trimoxazole. Non-HIV-related problems such as migraine or psychogenic headache may occur.

Altered peripheral sensation

May occur with or without motor abnormalities and is a significant symptom in peripheral neuropathy secondary to HIV, drugs or OI.

Leg weakness

May result from muscular weakness due to myopathic processes but intrinsic or extrinsic spinal cord disease should be considered and sensory levels searched for.

Seizures

↑ risk. First seizure is a presenting manifestation of an HIV-associated disease in ~20% of patients. Seizures may result from:
- metabolic encephalopathy
- cerebrovascular disease
- OIs such as toxoplasmosis, cryptococcosis, and PML
- CNS lymphomas.

Focal neurological signs and symptoms

Particularly with cerebral toxoplasmosis, 1° cerebral lymphoma, and PML.

Cerebral disorders

HIV-associated dementia complex

Prior to HAART dementia was a common cause of morbidity and mortality, seen in up to 50% of patients before death. Pathogenesis may include altered cytokine levels, free radicals, and the neurotoxic effects of gp120. Histological abnormalities include perivascular infiltrates, microglial nodules, multinuclear giant cells, and pruning of dendritic processes in the white matter and subcortical grey matter with relative sparing of the cortex.

Presentation

Poor concentration, impaired short-term memory, and slowed thought and reaction times. Clumsiness and gait disturbance may follow with cortisospinal tract abnormalities. Psychiatric illness and personality change may also be presenting features. Depression, effects of substance abuse, cerebrovascular disease, and neurosyphilis should be excluded.

Diagnosis

MRI (preferred option) or CT brain scan reveal cerebral atrophy with abnormality of the periventricular white matter. Neuropsychological examination reveals ↓ thought processes and ↓ short-term memory. CSF should be examined to exclude other pathologies and OIs. Electroencephalogram (EEG) may reveal encephalopathic changes. Blood and CSF serological tests for syphilis should be carried out and vitamin B₁₂ deficiency excluded. Other conditions such as CNS infections (TB, toxoplasmosis, cytomegalovirus encephalitis), PML, lymphoma, and toxic metabolic states (e.g. alcoholism, adverse medication effects, drug interaction, recreational drug use) should be excluded as dictated by the clinical presentation.

Management

HAART, if possible including zidovudine (proven efficacy) or other drugs that cross the blood–brain barrier, can produce marked improvement in intellectual function and return to independent living. The patient may require psychological and social support.

Viral encephalitis

Varicella zoster virus (VZV) is a rare cause of meningoencephalitis and is seen when CD4 count <50 cell/μL. It is due to direct CNS infection rather than reactivation of dormant virus as is the case with shingles. The pathological process is large- and small-vessel vaculopathy leading to ischaemic and demyelinating lesions. 33–50% of patients do not have the typical rash. CT or MRI may show necrotizing encephalitis and help differentiate from toxoplasmosis and PML, but changes are not specific. CSF should be examined by PCR (highly sensitive and specific). Treatment with aciclovir 10mg/kg 8 hourly should be given for at least 14 days.

CMV encephalitis occurs in advanced immunodeficiency and may be suspected when there is evidence of CMV disease in other organs or blood and CSF PCR is positive. Herpes simplex virus (HSV) is an uncommon cause but diagnosis should be considered in patients with meningo-encephalitis, aseptic meningitis, myelitis, or polyradiculitis. DNA detection in the CSF is very useful because of its high sensitivity and specificity.

Progressive multifocal leukoencephalopathy (PML)

Unlike other OIs, the prevalence of PML has not significantly declined with HAART. It is a demyelinating disease caused by reactivation of the Creutzfeldt–Jakob (CJ) papovavirus (polyomavirus) and occurs in 4–8% of patients with advanced HIV infection. Fulminant disease with dementia and coma can occur, but the usual picture is of subacute or chronic progressive disease with focal deficits. These include personality change, aphasia, hemiparesis, dizziness, gait disturbance, visual field defects, and seizures. CT or MRI scans usually reveal lesions (single or multiple) without mass effect in the white matter, particularly in the parieto-occipital region (Plate 20). CSF CJ PCR is +ve in ~60% of cases and ↑ CJ VL associated with poorer prognosis.

Prognosis is poor, especially without HAART. HAART leads to significant improvement in ~10%, but 33% still die within 2 years. Some individuals, especially those with very low CD4 counts, can develop IRIS with worsening of PML or new-onset PML after the initiation of HAART. Treatment trials with cidofovir, interferon α, and topotecan were inconclusive.

Cerebral toxoplasmosis (*Toxoplasma gondii*)

The most common cause of mass lesions in HIV prior to the introduction of 1° PCP prophylaxis which has ↓ incidence. Results from reactivation of a previously acquired infection when CD4 declines (<200 cells/µL). All patients should be tested for toxoplasma IgG. If –ve should be advised to eat meat only if well cooked, avoid cats and dogs, and wash hands carefully after gardening or contact with excrement.

Presentation

Typically includes confusion, headache, personality change, hemiparesis, focal sensory disturbances, fits, and fever.

Diagnosis

MRI or CT scanning reveal ring-enhancing lesions, usually multiple, particularly in the cortex and deep grey matter. The differential diagnosis, particularly if lesions are single, includes 1° cerebral lymphoma, cryptococcal cerebritis, and tuberculomas. CSF changes are non-specific. Positive toxoplasma IgG in 90%. CSF PCR is helpful if +ve (sensitivity 50%, specificity 100%).

Management

Standard therapy for cerebral toxoplasmosis is sulfadiazine 100mg/kg/day in divided doses and pyrimethamine 200mg loading dose followed by 50–100mg/day with folinic acid to reduce bone marrow toxicity. High-dose clindamycin 1.2g IV four times daily if allergic to sulfonamide. Neuro-imaging should be repeated after 2 weeks followed by brain biopsy to exclude other pathologies if no improvement. Secondary prophylaxis should be given until immune reconstitution with HAART (CD4 >200 cells/µL for >6 months). Primary prophylaxis as for PCP.

Meningitis

Cryptococcal meningitis

Cryptococcus neoformans (an encapsulated yeast)—most common fungal pathogen in the CNS. Usually when CD4 <100 cells/μL.

Presentation

Usually as subacute meningitis (but symptoms may initially be surprisingly mild) with headache and fever. Evidence of meningism occurs in only 30%. A high index of suspicion must be maintained to avoid delays in diagnosis. Other presentations include acute confusional state and cranial nerve palsies.

Diagnosis

CSF pressures can be markedly raised but pleocytosis may be absent and protein and sugar levels normal. The organism may be visualized by India ink staining but this is relatively insensitive. Mainstay of diagnosis is detection of CSF and serum cryptococcal antigen, which is highly sensitive. Neuro-imaging is usually normal but cryptococcomas can occur, usually in the basal ganglia.

Management

Daily lumbar punctures may be required until CSF pressures normalize to avoid cranial nerve lesions. If CSF pressure does not ↓ with LPs, a lumbar drain may be used. Antifungal therapy with IV amphotericin β 1mg/kg/day IV in combination with flucytosine 100mg/kg/day or liposomal amphotericin 3mg/kg/day plus flucytosine for 2 weeks followed by fluconazole 400mg daily. A test dose of amphotericin 25mg should be given before commencing full therapy to detect hypersensitivity. Renal function should be monitored. Ongoing suppressive therapy with fluconazole (superior to itraconazole) is required to minimize significant relapse rates. Continue until immune reconstitution is achieved with HAART.

Aseptic meningitis

Most commonly presents at seroconversion but may be recurrent or become chronic. Usually presents with headache. Cranial nerve palsies and altered mental state can occur. Lumbar puncture, following neuro-imaging when focal deficits are present, needed to exclude other pathologies. Mildly ↑ CSF lymphocyte counts and protein level with normal glucose are typical findings.

Autonomic neuropathy

Evidence of autonomic dysfunction can be found at various stages of HIV infection. Measurement of pulse rate variation in response to standing, deep breathing, Valsalva manoeuvre, and cold exposure reveal autonomic dysfunction in ~15%. Frequency related to the level of immune function but, unlike sensory neuropathy, not the use of nucleoside reverse transcriptase inhibitors. Symptomatic autonomic neuropathy occurs in advanced immunodeficiency and may result in severe postural hypotension and syncope. Cardiac denervation may lead to serious cardiac dysrhythmias. Those developing postural dizziness or syncope should have postural blood pressure recordings, tests of autonomic function, and assessment of sodium intake. Adrenal insufficiency should be excluded by carrying out a short Synacthen® test. Therapy with mineralocorticoid (fludrocortisone 50–200mcg daily), sodium supplements, compression stockings, and α-adrenergic agents, such as midodrine, may reduce postural blood pressure falls and alleviate symptoms. There may be improvement in autonomic function with HAART.

Spinal cord disease

Vacuolar myelopathy

Post-mortem studies have shown vacuolar myelopathy in up to 30% but clinically it is far less common. Pathological mechanisms are probably the same as in HIV dementia complex. It is often associated with dementia but may be isolated when the clinical picture mimics that of vitamin B_{12} deficiency spinal cord disease.

Presentation

Typically with subacute progressive motor and sensory deficits with paraesthesiae, but brisk tendon reflexes. Uncharacteristic findings may occur if there is concomitant peripheral neuropathy or other cause.

Diagnosis

Investigations should include measurement of vitamin B_{12} level and radiological imaging to exclude structural lesions. Areas of ↑ T2 signal may occasionally be seen on MRI scan. CSF may be normal or show only non-specific abnormalities such as low-level pleocytosis or mildly ↑ protein levels.

Management

Spasticity may require anti-spasmodic therapy such as baclofen 10–30mg three times daily and dysasthesia may require amitriptyline or gabapentin. Physiotherapy and occupational therapy input may be valuable. Improvements in function may occur with HAART.

HTLV1-associated myelopathy

In patients from areas of significant risk for human T lymphotropic virus type I (HTLV1) infection, such as Japan, the Caribbean, and parts of Central and Latin America, subacute myelopathy may result from HTLV1 infection and anti-HTLV1 antibodies should be assayed.

Acute myelopathy

Acute spinal cord disease may occasionally occur as a seroconversion event. Other important causes are spinal cord compression from lymphomatous metastases, tuberculous or bacterial abscesses, and acute infections with VZV.

Presentation

Typically rapidly developing neurological deficit, such as leg weakness and sphincter disturbance, with evidence of a sensory level.

Diagnosis

Emergency investigation required with spinal MRI or CT. In the absence of compression CSF and/or biopsy of compressive lesion, patient should be examined for evidence of infectious and neoplastic causes including viral PCR and cytology.

Management

Supportive with specific treatment directed at the identified cause.

Peripheral nerve disease

Neuritis

Herpes zoster (shingles)

May occur at any stage of HIV infection with a typical distribution and course. Atypical multi-dermatomal involvement, viraemic dissemination of lesions, and recurrences more common as CD4 counts ↓.

Presentation

Frequently prodromal pain of dermatomal distribution followed by an erythematous maculopapular eruption evolving into vesicles which then pustulate and crust. Bullous haemorrhagic and necrotic lesions may occur. Lesions will be at various stages at any one time. Pain during the acute phase can be severe, and disabling post-herpetic neuralgia may follow.

Diagnosis

Clinical picture is usually characteristic. Varicella zoster virus (VZV) can be detected in vesicular fluid by immunofluorescence.

Management

Pain often does not respond well to conventional analgesics and adjuvants. Amitriptyline 25–150mg/day or gabapentin up to 2.4g/day in divided doses may be required. Begin antiviral therapy with IV aciclovir 10mg/kg 8 hourly as early as possible (most effective within 24 hours but useful even if given later in immunocompromised) and switch to oral famciclovir 500mg three times daily or valaciclovir 1g three times daily when lesions cease to progress for a total course of at least 7 days or until all lesions have dried and crusted. Ophthalmology review if ophthalmic branch of trigeminal nerve affected (forehead and inside of nose).

Mononeuritis multiplex

Usually occurs in patients with advanced HIV disease. Typical presentation is with subacute onset of multifocal or asymmetric sensory deficits. Nerve conduction studies show demyelination and axonal loss. May be associated with cytomegalovirus (CMV) infection in advanced immunodeficiency. Differential diagnosis includes nerve compression in severe wasting syndrome, neoplastic infiltration, and neurotropic viral infections (e.g. VZV). Consider treatment with ganciclovir or foscarnet if circumstantial evidence of CMV infection (e.g. positive blood PCR).

Neuropathy

Drug toxicity

The toxicity of therapeutic drugs, notably didanosine, zalcitabine, and stavudine, is responsible for ↑ proportion of neuropathy.

Distal symmetric polyneuropathy

Occurs in ~35% of patients with advanced HIV disease. ~15% of those with asymptomatic HIV infection have abnormal nerve conduction studies. Typical symptoms are tingling, numbness, and burning pain beginning in the toes or plantar surfaces, often ascending over time. Involvement of hands is rare. Examination shows ↓ ankle jerks, vibration sense, appreciation of temperature, and fine touch. Unexpectedly brisk reflexes should raise the question of additional spinal cord or brain disease. Differential diagnosis includes effects of alcohol, drug toxicity, and vitamin deficiency. Treatment is directed towards controlling neuropathic pain with drugs, such as amitriptyline 25–150mg daily or gabapentin starting at 300mg 8 hourly and titrating to a maximum of 2.4g daily.

Inflammatory demyelinating neuropathy (Guillain–Barré syndrome)

May occur with seroconversion or during late stages of HIV infection. Manifestations as in non-HIV status with progressive symmetric weakness in the limbs and loss of tendon jerks, but CSF pleocytosis may occur. Treatment is immunoglobulin 400mg/kg/day for 5 days or plasmapheresis up to six exchanges over 2 weeks. Patients with the chronic form may need monthly cycles of treatment until stabilization.

Progressive lumbosacral polyradiculopathy

Caused by CMV infection in patients with CD4 counts <50cells/μL. Evidence of CMV disease elsewhere. Bilateral leg weakness progresses over several weeks, sometimes to flaccid paraplegia. Sphincter disturbance is common and sensory loss combined with painful dys-aesthesia is usual. Sensory symptoms differentiate this from myopathy, and sphincter disturbance with sparing of the upper limbs distinguishes it from other forms of neuropathy. Cord compression should be excluded by imaging. CSF usually has a cell count >500 × 10⁶/L with 40–50% neutrophils, ↑ protein content, and low glucose. CSF PCR for CMV is positive and the patient should be treated with ganciclovir or foscarnet.

Miscellaneous

Cerebrovascular disease

Strokes and transient ischaemic attacks are reported in 0.5–8% of HIV-infected patients. Prevention should include attention to vascular risk factors such as smoking, hypertension, and hyperlipidaemia. Cocaine use and alcoholic binges may lead to thrombotic strokes. Embolic strokes may result from cardiac or carotid artery disease. Cardiogenic emboli may result from infective or non-infective endocarditis following myo-cardial infarction or from dysrhythmias. Cerebral vasculitis, particularly due to VZV or syphilis, may cause cerebral thrombosis. The hyper-coagulable state that may occur with HIV may contribute. Haemorrhage may complicate VZV cerebral vasculitis and thrombocytopenia, rarely due to metastatic Kaposi's sarcoma or as a result of an incidental cerebral aneurysm.

Neurosyphilis

Can affect most parts of the nervous system (📖 Chapter 6, Clinical features—late syphilis p. 118).

Neoplastic disease

Kaposi's sarcoma, although the most common systemic neoplasm in HIV infection, rarely involves the nervous system. The CNS may be invaded by non-Hodgkin's lymphoma, leading to malignant meningitis and compressive symptoms requiring intrathecal cytotoxic therapy and radio-therapy. 1° cerebral lymphoma occurs in patients with advanced immunodeficiency and presents with confusion, lethargy, personality change, focal neurological deficits, seizures, ataxia, and aphasia. On MRI or CT scanning lesions are ring-enhancing, and about 50% are associated with cerebral oedema and mass effect..The finding of a single lesion favours the diagnosis of lymphoma over cerebral toxoplasmosis. +ve EBV PCR is suggestive but not diagnostic of 1° cerebral lymphoma. Treatment for toxoplasma empirically may be considered with brain biopsy if no clinical response after 2 weeks. Cerebral radiotherapy may improve survival. Prognosis very poor with 3 months median survival.

HIV: disorders of the eye

Introduction

Ocular manifestations have been reported in up to 60% of those infected with HIV, ↑ in frequency as the CD4 count ↓. Patients with CD4 count <200/μL should be closely examined for signs of ocular disease which may be asymptomatic in the early stages. Close cooperation with ophthalmology is essential to ensure timely therapeutic interventions to ↓ risk of visual impairment and blindness. Widespread use of HAART has dramatically altered the incidence and natural history of many opportunistic eye infections.

HIV-related vasculopathy (retinopathy)

70–80% of patients with advanced HIV disease have asymptomatic transient microvascular changes which may occur simultaneously in the conjunctiva and retina.

Conjunctival changes are found near the limbus and are only detected by slit-lamp examination. Features include vascular narrowing, dilatation, and microaneurysms.

Retinal changes are detected by fundal examination. Cotton-wool spots (infarcts of nerve fibre layer) are the most common feature of retinal vasculopathy. they are differentiated from early CMV lesions by their small size, superficial retinal location, and transient nature with less frequent retinal haemorrhages and microaneurysms. No treatment is needed.

Iridocyclitis

Seen in association with toxoplasmic, syphilitic, bacterial, and fungal retinitis. Drugs such as rifabutin (especially with concurrent azole and macrolide use) and cidofovir are frequent causes. Diagnosed by slit-lamp examination.

Treatment

Treat underlying infection(s) and/or ↓ or discontinue implicated drug(s). Topical steroids may be used but not if there is active infection.

Neurological eye manifestations

Occur in 10%. Most common features include papilloedema, cranial nerve palsies, ophthalmoplegia, and visual field defects. Caused by lymphoma and any CNS infection, most frequently cryptococcal meningitis, neurosyphilis, and toxoplasmosis. HIV encephalopathy and progressive multifocal leukoencephalopathy may have similar complications.

Investigate by MRI and lumbar puncture (CSF—cell count, cytology, culture, and serology).

Immune recovery uveitis

Mainly involves anterior uveal tract and vitreous. Commonly associated with a marked disturbance of visual function due to macular oedema and epi-retinal membrane formation. Believed to be a consequence of the marked reconstitution of immune function induced by HAART. Marked cellular infiltration of the vitreous (in the absence of an active retinal or chorioretinal lesion) is a hallmark of this phenomenon. Responds well to systemic steroids.

Opportunistic infections (OIs)

Cytomegalovirus (CMV) infection

CMV retinitis results from reactivation of infection acquired in childhood or early adult life. Prior to HAART it was the most common eye OI, occurring in 30–40% of those with a CD4 count <50cells/μL. Bilateral in 30–50% of cases with optic nerve papillitis in 5%. Serious visual complications can be avoided by detection of its early features with regular dilated examination of the fundi for those at risk (CD4 <100cells/μL).

Clinical features

Symptoms depend on site and extent of retinal involvement. Peripheral retinal lesions are asymptomatic. Earliest and most common symptoms are multiple floaters due to inflammatory cells in the vitreous attempting to contain the infection. Other symptoms include blurring/loss of central vision, flashing lights, and scotomata. Initial focus of retinal inflammation expands peripherally inducing retinal necrosis.

Early active lesions appear as multiple granular white dots with occasional haemorrhages. With further progress areas of retinitis enlarge by following the vascular arcades, resulting in an arcuate or triangular zone of infection. Areas of active infection may also be linear, following the retinal vessels or nerve fibre layer into the periphery. Early CMV lesions may be confused with cotton-wool spots (due to HIV vasculopathy) which may coexist. Serial drawings or retinal photographs are helpful in differentiation. Continuing activity of the necrotic process results in atrophic features with thinning of the retina, resulting in visualization of the underlying choroid. Other features of CMV retinitis include vascular attenuation, vessel occlusion, vitritis, and anterior uveitis (Plate 21). May be complicated by retinal detachment and cataract.

Occasionally it may be difficult to establish the cause of retinitis.

Diagnosis

Usually clinical. Confirmed by obtaining a vitreous sample for CMV using PCR testing. CMV viraemia may be a useful predictor of CMV disease. A rising CMV viral load detected by PCR is associated with ↑ eye and other organ disease.

Treatment

- HAART ↑ response to treatment, prognosis, and ↓ relapse rates.
- Oral valganciclovir 900mg twice daily for 3 weeks followed by 900mg once daily produces blood levels comparable to IV ganciclovir. Main side-effects are bone marrow suppression and GI upset.
- Intra-vitreous ganciclovir implant is very effective but needs to be replaced after 6–9 months and does not give protection to the other eye or protect against systemic disease.
- IV ganciclovir given as an induction course for 2–3 weeks (5mg/kg body weight 12 hourly) followed by maintenance therapy (5mg/kg body weight 7 days a week or 6mg/kg body weight 5 days a week). Side-effects include rigors and neutropenia that may require discontinuation of treatment or the use of granulocyte colony-stimulating factor.

Oral ganciclovir (1g three times daily) may be given in place of IV formulation once retinitis has remained stable for at least 3 weeks.

- IV foscarnet given as an induction course for 2–3 weeks (60mg/kg body weight 8 hourly) followed by maintenance therapy (90–120mg/kg body weight once daily). Given when ganciclovir not tolerated because of its toxicity. Side-effects include nephrotoxicity, convulsions, meatal ulceration, and electrolyte disturbance. Has ↑ infusion time and requires an infusion pump.
- IV cidofovir (3–5mg/kg body weight once a week) given with probenecid (2g orally 3 hours before the cidofovir infusion followed by 1g for 2 hours and 8 hours following its completion) and fluids. Effective in ganciclovir-resistant CMV but highly nephrotoxic and myelo-suppressive.

Prognosis

Response to therapy achieved in 80–90%. Without immune reconstitution, the median time to relapse is 50–120 days using standard anti-CMV treatment. Maintenance therapy can be stopped once immune reconstitution is achieved.

Varicella zoster virus (VZV) infection

Ophthalmic herpes zoster results from involvement of the ophthalmic division of the trigeminal nerve and is recognized by characteristic vesicular eruptions. Involvement of the nasociliary nerve (indicated by skin lesions at the tip of the nose) makes eye involvement highly likely. VZV may be associated with blepharitis, conjunctivitis, keratitis, and uveitis. Complications and post-herpetic neuralgia ↑ in the immunosuppressed.

VZV is the most common cause of necrotizing retinitis which may occur at same time or follow recent herpes zoster. Early retinal lesions similar to CMV, but rapidly progressive, deep, and multifocal with ↑ risk of bilateral disease and retinal detachment which may lead to blindness in days without prompt treatment.

Diagnosis

May be made clinically. Vitreal biopsy and VZV PCR establish diagnosis.

Treatment

Oral valaciclovir (IV aciclovir if extensive lesions, posterior eye or nerve involvement) in addition to topical steroids. In the absence of anterior uveitis, mydriatics (e.g. 1% atropine) also required.

Herpes simplex keratitis

HSV eye infection causes keratitis or rarely acute retinal necrosis. Keratitis leads to corneal ulcers, diminished corneal sensation, and ↑ intra-ocular pressure. Corneal ulcers are usually painful and have a dendritic appearance. Difficult to treat and relapses are frequent.

Treatment

Oral aciclovir (400mg five times daily) or famciclovir (250–500mg three times daily).

Acute retinal necrosis

Commonly caused by VZV and HSV but CMV and other viruses may be implicated. Presents with eye pain associated with scotomata progressing rapidly to visual loss. The other eye is involved in one-third of cases. Detailed fundal examination reveals peripheral white lesions that progress to widespread necrosis over a few days. May be complicated by proliferative retinopathy and retinal detachment.

Treatment

Responds poorly to antivirals but IV ganciclovir should be started immediately combined with laser therapy to prevent retinal detachment.

Toxoplasma retinochoroiditis

Rare, accounting for 1–2% of retinitis with 30–50% of patients having CNS involvement. Characteristically causes bilateral multifocal retinochoroidal lesions that invade the vitreous in the later stages. Majority of patients do not have pre-existing eye lesions.

Diagnosis

Fundal examination reveals characteristic extensive fluffy areas of retinal whitening with accompanying vitritis, but unlike CMV infection retinal haemorrhaging is less likely. Toxoplasma serological tests unreliable, but absence of toxoplasma IgG antibodies makes its diagnosis less likely.

Treatment

Pyrimethamine in combination with sulfadiazine or clindamycin. Equally good response may be obtained with atovaquone. Long-term maintenance treatment with clindamycin and pyrimethamine usually required.

Candidal eye infection

Infection of the anterior segment of the eye results in superficial keratitis. Posterior segment infection seen in advanced HIV disease and presents as multiple, often bilateral, white fluffy retinal lesions that may extend into the overlying vitreous. Majority of patients have systemic candidal infection. Culture and sensitivity of the causative yeast provides the best outcome on which to base therapy. Superficial keratitis responds well to topical antifungals. Systemic antifungals are needed for posterior segment infection (e.g. voriconazole and liposomal amphotericin).

Kaposi's sarcoma (KS)

Up to 20% of patients with skin KS have eyelid and conjunctival lesions recognized by their characteristic appearance, although conjunctival lesions may resemble traumatic haemorrhages.

Treatment

Options include surgical removal, cryotherapy, and intra-lesional vinblastine. Systemic chemotherapy is given if there are associated skin lesions. Radiation is effective but may be complicated by loss of eyelashes and conjunctivitis.

HIV: dermatological disorders

Introduction

Skin conditions are extremely common and may occur at any stage of HIV infection. Pre-existing skin conditions may worsen after its acquisition. Appearance of certain skin conditions should alert physicians to possibility of undiagnosed HIV infection. Immunodeficiency is associated with atypical presentations, severe manifestations, and a poor response to treatment. In general, improved immunity with HAART resolves or improves them.

Infections

Viral infections

Acute seroconversion (acute retroviral syndrome)

Skin rash occurs in up to 70% cases. It is often part of an infectious mononucleosis-like illness. Typically symmetrical and non-itchy, extending over the trunk and upper limbs, and macular or maculopapular in appearance, although it can be vesicular, pustular, or urticarial. May be associated with oro-pharyngeal (highly suspicious of seroconversion illness) and genital ulceration. Resolves spontaneously within 1–2 weeks.

Herpes simplex virus (HSV)

1° and recurrent HSV present with genital and orofacial clusters of vesicles that ulcerate, crust, and heal within 2–3 weeks during the early stages of HIV infection. With advanced disease, ulcers become atypical or chronic and may coalesce to form large painful crusted lesions commonly seen peri-anally but may involve the peri-oral and rarely the peri-ungual region. Though dissemination is rare, lesions may be auto-inoculated to distant sites. HSV infection rarely presents with necrotizing folliculitis (difficult to diagnose without biopsy).

Swabs for viral culture and immunofluorescence usually confirm the diagnosis. Polymerase chain reaction (PCR) testing of skin lesions is very sensitive and specific but not widely available. Viral culture can be performed on skin biopsy from the edge of the lesion when swab is not conclusive. Histological examination may provide a rapid diagnosis by demonstrating multinucleated giant epithelial cells.

Treatment (🔲 Chapter 21, Management p. 268; Chapter 40, Anal diseases p. 470)

Varicella zoster virus (VZV) infection

Those with no previous exposure to VZV develop chickenpox which may be severe and associated with visceral involvement. Most adults have been infected by VZV and so present with herpes zoster. Usually affects multiple dermatomes, commonly the thoracic and the trigeminal nerves. Vesicular eruption is normally preceded by tingling and a burning sensation. Individuals with more advanced HIV disease tend to have painful bullous haemorrhagic necrotic lesions that may persist for several weeks and heal with severe scarring. Recurrences and dissemination ↑. Disseminated disease is characterized by dermatomal and non-dermatomal eruptions.

Rarely VZV presents with chronic widespread ulcers or hyperkeratotic lesions (if infected with aciclovir-resistant VZV).

Clinical diagnosis is usually accurate in typical dermatomal involvement but skin biopsy is required for atypical, chronic ulcerative, and hyperkeratotic lesions.

Prompt treatment with high-dose aciclovir ↓ risk of dissemination and shortens its course. Clinical presentation and degree of immune deficiency determine mode and length of therapy, which is usually continued until lesions start to crust.

• IV aciclovir (10mg/kg body weight three times daily) for disseminated infection, CD4 count <200cells/μL, and with involvement of the ophthalmic division of the trigeminal nerve. May be replaced with oral aciclovir once lesions start to crust.
• Famciclovir (500mg three times daily, usually for 10 days) and valaciclovir (1g three times daily, usually for 7 days) have better bio-availability than aciclovir.
• Oral aciclovir (800mg five times daily) may be given to those with limited disease and preserved immune function.

Skin care with bathing with water and mild soap is helpful. Analgesics for pain control.

Molluscum contagiosum

Caused by a pox virus and when widespread is a marker of advanced HIV disease. Lesion is typically a flesh-coloured, 2–3mm domed, umblicated papule with a faint whitish core. Those with relatively preserved immune function may have mollusca on the groin, which may be chronic. With advanced HIV disease, lesions may reach 1cm in size and may be widespread involving the face, trunk, eyelids, and rarely the mucous membranes (conjunctivae and lips). Mollusca are commonly seen on the beard area (related to trauma of shaving) where they are difficult to treat.

Treatment is given for cosmetic reasons as no cure is available. Usual treatment is cryotherapy. Curettage is effective for recalcitrant cases.

Human papilloma virus infection (warts)

Widespread, resistant, and recurrent warts which may have atypical appearances are seen more frequently in those immunosuppressed. Facial involvement, otherwise rare, is well recognized in HIV infection.

Principles of therapy are as for those not infected by HIV. Ablative treatment is used depending on morphology, location, and number.

Bacterial infections

Staphylococcal skin infection

Staphylococcus aureus nasal carriage is common explaining ↑ rates of infection with this organism. *Staph.aureus* skin infection presents as:

• folliculitis: commonly in the hirsute areas, e.g. groin, axilla, face (especially ♂), and trunk; infection may involve deeper tissues, forming abscesses
• hidradenitis-like plaques: many adjacent follicles infected forming large discoloured lesions several centimetres deep
• bullous impetigo: commonly seen on the groin and axillae as superficial vesicles or ulcers with yellow crusts

- ecthyma: an eroded or ulcerated lesion with an adherent crust covering an abscess
- scalded skin syndrome: part of systemic *Staph.aureus* infection.

Superficial infection responds to standard anti-staphylococcal antibiotics (e.g. flucloxacillin 500mg four times daily for 7–10 days).

Deep infection may require abscess drainage and prolonged courses of combined antibiotics based on bacterial sensitivities. Washing the area with antiseptics helps by removing crusts and ↓ bacterial concentration.

Bacillary angiomatosis

Caused by *Bartonella henselae* and *Bartonella quintana*, small Gram-negative aerobic fastidious bacilli. In addition, *B.henselae* causes cat scratch fever and *B.quintana* causes trench fever. Angiogenic lesions are most often recognized in cutaneous or subcutaneous tissues and can be difficult to differentiate from Kaposi's sarcoma (KS). *B.henselae* causes lesions in lymph nodes, liver (peliosis hepatis), and spleen. *B.quintana* has a predilection for subcutaneous deep soft tissues and bones.

Clinical presentation

- Bacilliary angioma: friable, easy bleeding hyperpigmented papules, nodules, or plaques but in the early stages may be purplish to bright red in colour, up to several centimetres in diameter. Lesions solitary or multiple and widespread on the skin. Need to be differentiated from KS and pyogenic granuloma.
- Bacteraemia presenting as pyrexia of unknown origin.
- Organ involvement (e.g. liver, spleen, brain, and lymph nodes).

Diagnosis

- Abnormal vascular proliferation and a mixed inflammatory infiltrate on histological examination of tissues.
- Special stains (e.g. Warthin–Starry, Steiner and Steiner) required.
- Electron microscopy.
- PCR of tissue and blood samples.

Serological tests are not reliable in HIV infection.

Treatment

Prolonged course of antibiotics, e.g. erythromycin 500mg four times daily, doxycycline 100mg twice daily, or azithromycin 0.5–1.0g daily, until lesions heal.

Mycobacterial infection

1° mycobacterial skin infection is rare. Skin may be involved in up to 10% of disseminated *Mycobacterium avium* complex infection, typically when the CD4 count is <50cells/μL. Most frequent presentations are chronic sinuses overlying an infected lymph node (scrofuloderma) and chronic skin ulcer. Rare presentations include violaceous nodules, necrotic papules, plaques, panniculitis, and erythema nodosum.

Mycobacterial infection should be considered in any chronic non-healing skin ulcer. Diagnose by demonstration of acid-fast bacilli in smears and by culture. Typical histological feature of caseating granuloma is usually absent.

Treatment (📖 Chapter 42, Tuberculosis p. 492; Chapter 46, *Mycobacterium avium* complex p. 532).

Fungal infections

Cutaneous candidiasis

Skin infection with *Candida* spp occurs in different forms including tinea unguium (leuconychia, nail ridging, flaking, onycholysis, and atrophy), acute paronychia (tender fluctuation of the nailbed), chronic paronychia, and intertrigo (an erosive painful erythematous rash on flexures associated with satellite pustules). Acute candidal paronychia must be differentiated from that caused by HSV infection using appropriate tests.

- Tinea unguium requires prolonged systemic antifungals (e.g. itraconazole).
- Acute paronychia and intertrigo respond well to topical antifungals (e.g. miconazole).

Dermatophytosis

Very common in HIV infection. May be atypical and extensive and may mimic inflammatory skin conditions such as seborrhoeic dermatitis or psoriasis.

- Tinea pedis: usually presents with interdigital maceration and scaling of the soles, rarely with hyperkeratosis of the soles. Usually associated with tinea unguium. Caused by *Trichophyton rubrum*. 2° bacterial infection common and may result in cellulitis.
- Onychomycosis: results in subungual hyperkeratosis and toenail atrophy.
- Tinea cruris: symmetrical, erythematous scaling rash with central clearance on the groin, sometimes extending to buttocks and thighs. In advanced HIV disease, it may resemble seborrhoeic dermatitis because of absence of central clearance.
- Tinea corporis: annular scaling plaques with central clearance.
- Tinea capitis: localized scaling discoid patch or generalized scaling resembling seborrhoeic dermatitis.
- Tinea faciale: differentiated from seborrhoeic dermatitis by asymmetrical distribution and well-demarcated edge.

Apart from tinea pedis, which can be treated with topical antifungals, other forms need systemic antifungals such as terbinafine (250mg daily for several weeks) or a triazole (e.g. fluconazole 50mg daily).

Cryptococcosis

Skin involvement occurs in up to 20% of systemic cryptococcal infection. Most common skin manifestation is a nodule or papule with central umbilication resembling molluscum contagiosum, usually on the face. Plaques and tender subcutaneous lesions are rare. Diagnosed by skin biopsy.

Treatment

Patient should be evaluated for systemic and neurological cryptococcal infection and managed accordingly (📖 Chapter 43, Meningitis p. 504).

Penicilliosis

Endemic to Southeast Asia. Caused by *Penicillium marneffei*. Presents with fever, skin lesions, anaemia, lymphadenopathy, and hepatosplenomegaly. Skin lesions resemble haemorrhagic molluscum contagiosum. Diagnosed by culture of blood, bone marrow, and skin scrapings. Responds well to liposomal amphotericin and itraconazole but relapses are common and long-term prophylaxis with itraconazole is recommended.

Histoplasmosis

Cutaneous histoplasmosis has been reported in up to 10% of patients with systemic infection, which usually occurs in endemic areas. Diagnosis by biopsy of papules, nodules, or ulcers. Treat with liposomal amphotericin or high-dose itraconazole followed by itraconazole maintenance.

Scabies

In advanced HIV disease crusted (Norwegian) scabies may occur, characterized by widespread scaly erythematous lesions on the face and scalp together with hyperkeratotic lesions on the hands and feet giving the characteristic 'breadcrumb' appearance. Highly infectious because of heavy infestation.

Treatment (📖 Chapter 26, Management p. 312)

Patients with crusted scabies must be barrier nursed and in addition to topical treatment may be given (ivermectin 200mcg/kg as a single dose). Topical steroids may be needed for eczematous nodules.

Inflammatory conditions

Seborrhoeic dermatitis

Occurs in up to 85% and may be a first indicator of HIV infection. Severity and recurrences ↑ with ↓ CD4 count. Related to infection with *Pityrosporum* spp, ↑ sebum production, and a genetic predisposition.

Presents as an itchy erythematous rash with a yellow greasy scale, but in severe cases plaques and hyperkeratotic lesions occur. Usually has a butterfly distribution but may involve eyebrows, post-auricular areas, and scalp. May also affect intertriginous areas and chest. Severe cases may resemble psoriasis. Facial lesions must be differentiated from lupus erythematosus and rosacea.

Treatment

* Topical antifungals and steroids (e.g. miconazole and hydrocortisone).
* Scalp lesions: tar-containing shampoos, selenium sulphide, salicylic acid, and ketoconazole.
* Severe disease responds well, but only temporarily, to systemic triazoles such as itraconazole.

Psoriasis

A chronic disease characterized by erythematous plaques or papules covered by silvery adherent scales. May appear for the first time or pre-existing disease may become worse with HIV infection. Psoriatic arthritis (📖 Chapter 50, Inflammatory arthropathies/Psoriatic arthritis p. 556) ↑. Several forms of psoriasis may coexist.

* Chronic plaque psoriasis classically involves elbows, knees, and scalp, and may be associated with nail dystrophy.
* Flexural psoriasis affects axillae, groins, and intergluteal cleft; more common in advanced HIV disease.
* Guttate psoriasis presents with widespread raindrop-size lesions.

Treatment

* Mild to moderate disease can be treated with a regular emollient plus moderately potent topical steroid, calcitriol, tar-containing ointments, or dithranol.
* Severe disease can be treated with methotrexate (especially in the presence of psoriatic arthritis), acitretin, ciclosporin, or hydroxycarbamide.

⚠ Beware of effects of these drugs (apart from acitretin) on the immune system.

Eczema

Seen in up to 30%. Severity and frequency ↑ as CD4 count ↓. Xerosis (dry skin) is a common complaint and may be associated with an itchy papular scaly rash on the arms and legs. Skin may be damaged as a result of excessive scratching, resulting in excoriation, lichenification, eczematous changes, and discoloration.

Treatment

Treatment includes topical steroids and emollients.

Pruritic follicular and papular eruptions

Pruritus is a common occurrence. 1° follicular, papular, or nodular lesions may be altered by excoriation and lichenification.

Eosinophilic pustular folliculitis

Chronic intensely itchy follicular rash affecting face, upper trunk, and extensor surfaces of the arms. Usually seen when CD4 count <200cells/µL. Sterile papular, papulo-pustular, or urticarial papules centred around hair follicles found. May be ↑ IgE with eosinophilia.

Treatment

Responds best to phototherapy. Emollients for eczematous lesions. Antihistamines not usually helpful. HAART may produce some improvement.

HIV-associated pruritus

Diagnosis of exclusion of other causes of pruritus. No 1° lesions. Clinical features 2°to scratching—excoriation, linear lesions, lichenified eczematous changes, and post-inflammatory pigmentation.

Treatment

Regular emollients, topical steroids for eczematous changes, and anti-histamines.

Malassezia furfur folliculitis

Yeast overgrowth producing folliculitis through production of fatty acids and scale formation blocking follicular ostea. Presents with chronic or relapsing pruritic follicular-centred papules on the scalp, flexures, upper trunk, and face.

Treatment

Oral itraconazole (preferred option) 200mg daily for 7 days. If patient has AIDS, maintenance (200mg once or twice daily) or intermittent 'pulse' therapy should be considered. Other options are oral fluconazole and 2% ketoconazole cream. Scalp relapses are best treated with intermittent ketoconazole shampoo.

Neoplasia

Kaposi's sarcoma (KS) (📖 Chapter 52, Kaposi's sarcoma p. 567)

Incidence ↓ since the introduction of HAART. Human herpes virus-8 (HHV-8) identified in 1994 as the causative agent. Although the skin is usual site, KS may develop in visceral organs.

Typically, KS lesions appear on the nose and hard palate, but may arise anywhere on the skin. Disease usually has an insidious course with new lesions appearing as existing ones enlarge. Rapidly aggressive disease may occur but is rare. Initially starts as a painless non-pruritic pink or red macule or a papule which gradually darkens to resemble a bruise. It is surrounded by a yellow halo due to extravasated red cells (Plate 22). May be dark and difficult to recognize in black people. KS lesions vary in size from a few millimetres to several centimetres. Extensive plaques with scaling can develop on the legs and may break down, producing local pain and oedema. Lesions on the soles may be particularly troublesome as they interfere with walking. Facial and genital KS is cosmetically unsightly. With treatment, the lesion becomes flat and the colour fades, but some pigmentation persists even in the absence of residual tumour.

Non-pitting oedema is commonly associated with KS, especially affecting the lower limbs. May be due to skin lymphatic involvement or 2° to vasoactive substances produced by KS. Degree of oedema occasionally disproportionate to size of KS lesions (i.e. feature of the disease itself rather than 2° to lymph node enlargement/lymphatic obstruction).

Diagnosis

Typical skin KS lesions are diagnosed clinically, but biopsy provides an absolute diagnosis in atypical lesions. Patients with symptoms or signs suggestive of other organ involvement should be evaluated by imaging techniques. Patients with severe oedema may require CT to exclude localized obstruction or accompanying pathology.

Treatment (📖 Chapter 52, Kaposi's sarcoma/Management p. 567)

Treatment for skin KS is for cosmetic reasons and to alleviate symptoms.

Lymphomas (📖 Chapter 52, Non-Hodgkin's lymphoma p. 570)

Extranodal cutaneous involvement occurs in up to 8% of those with B-cell non-Hodgkin's lymphoma. Presents with an enlarging violaceous nodule or plaque, which may ulcerate.

Cutaneous T-cell lymphoma presents as a scaly patch or plaque with erythema, hypo- or hyperpigmentation, and atrophy. It may be misdiagnosed as chronic eczema.

The skin may be involved when lymphoma (usually B-cell) involves an underlying lymph node.

Treatment (📖 Chapter 52, Non-Hodgkin's lymphoma p. 570)

The principles of management of non-Hodgkin's lymphoma are the same as for lymphoma elsewhere and chemotherapy is usually given.

Drug reactions

Cutaneous drug reactions ↑, as does the development of hypersensitivity reactions to previously tolerated drugs. Mild drug eruptions do not always necessitate the cessation of the causative drug, especially if it is the most effective agent and is given for a short time (e.g. co-trimoxazole for *Pneumocystis jiroveci* (*carinii*) pneumonia). Desensitization may be possible for essential drugs. Cross-sensitivities may occur, e.g. between dapsone and co-trimoxazole.

Hypersensitivity reactions are common with certain antiretroviral drugs such as nevirapine and abacavir which may cause a fatal reaction. Special attention (with counselling) to patients on these treatments is important to ensure early recognition and prompt action.

- Morbilliform (erythematous maculopapular) drug eruption is common and may be associated with systemic symptoms. Most frequent causative drugs are amoxicillin and sulfonamides. Progresses in a caudocephalic direction, resolving within 3–5 days but occasionally persisting for weeks after its withdrawal. Many viral infections cause a similar rash.
- Erythroderma occurs when a morbilliform rash becomes confluent and involves the whole body. May result in hypothermia and shock.
- Erythema multiforme, Stevens–Johnson syndrome, and toxic epidermal necrolysis ↑ in HIV infection. Offending drug must be stopped. Patients best managed in high-dependency units where attention to electrolyte and fluid balance and skin care are of paramount importance.
- Nail and oral pigmentation 2° to zidovudine.
- Penile ulceration due to foscarnet.

HIV: pyrexia of unknown origin

Introduction

Pyrexia of unknown origin (PUO) was defined by R.G. Petersdorf and P.B. Beeson (*Medicine* 40, 1–30, 1961) as a temperature of >38.3°C on multiple occasions over a period of >3 weeks with failure to reach a diagnosis after 1 week of investigation.

HIV-related diseases are an important cause of prolonged fever and must be considered in patients with PUO. In patients with known HIV infection PUO may arise during follow-up. D.T. Durack and A.C. Street (*Curr Clin Top Infect Dis* 11, 35–51, 1991) produced a definition of HIV-associated PUO, including temperatures >38.3°C on multiple occasions over a period of >4 weeks for out-patients or 3 days for inpatients, with negative microbiological results after at least 2 days incubation.

PUO occurs predominantly in the late stages of infection with CD4 counts <100cells/μL and is less common in patients on effective HAART. In the general population, infections account for only 33% of PUO. However, infectious diseases are the predominant aetiology in HIV-positive patients, accounting for 80–90% with neoplasia, with drug reactions accounting for most of the others.

A cause can be found in 80%. In those with undetermined diagnoses fever may settle spontaneously. In the general population a single pathology is almost universal but two or more simultaneous pathologies may be found in about 20% of HIV-related cases. Even if patients are taking standard prophylaxis against agents, such as *Pneumocystis jiroveci (carinii)* or *Mycobacterium avium* complex (MAC), these cannot be excluded without appropriate investigation.

There are important geographical differences, e.g. tuberculosis and leishmaniasis are much more common in Europe than in the USA. It is also important to consider non-HIV-related causes and other infections (e.g. gonorrhoea), whose presentation may be modified by immunodeficiency. Strenuous diagnostic efforts are important in PUO as it may enable the diagnosis and treatment of infections before the onset of specific organ dysfunction (e.g. a *Pneumocystis jiroveci* infection). A careful history including sexual, travel, immunization, consumption and source of dairy products, family history, animal contact, and drugs (prescribed and non-prescribed) is mandatory.

HIV-related aetiology (data from Europe and USA)

- Mycobacterial infection
  - *Mycobacterium tuberculosis*: 7% (USA) to 37% (Europe). CD4 count may be normal
  - *Mycobacterium avium* complex: 12–31% (CD4 count <100cells/µL)
  - Others (e.g. *M.kansasii*, *M.genavense*): 1–5%
- Pneumocystis jiroveci: 5–13% (CD4 count <200cells/µL)
- Viral
  - Cytomegalovirus: 5–9% (CD4 count <50cells/µL)
  - HIV itself, herpes simplex virus, varicella zoster virus, parvovirus B19, adenovirus, hepatitis virus B and C: 2–7%
- Bacterial: 5–7%
- Fungal (cryptococcosis, candidaemia, disseminated histoplasmosis, aspergillosis, Penicillium marneffei): 2–8% (CD4 count <200cells/µL)
- Parasitic
  - Leishmaniasis: 0% (USA) to 12% (Europe)
  - Toxoplasmosis: 1–3%
  - Others (isosporiasis, cryptosporidiosis): <1%
- Neoplasia
  - Lymphoma: 5–10% (CD4 count may be normal)
  - Kaposi's sarcoma: isolated reports
- Drugs: <1%.
- Other unusual causes include Reiter's syndrome, non-specific hepatitis, Castleman's disease, and angiofollicular hyperplasia.

Diagnosis

Careful history-taking followed by examination especially for lymphadeno-pathy, hepatosplenomegaly, skin rash, and retinal abnormalities (through dilated pupils). All patients should have first level (non-invasive) investigation proceeding to second level (invasive) if diagnosis is not established.

First level includes

- Full blood count/differential white count, liver function tests, C-reactive protein, urinalysis
- Pulse oximetry
- Chest X-ray
- Repeated cultures of blood, sputum, urine, and faeces as indicated for bacteria, mycobacteria (requires specific mycobacteria culture bottles), and fungi
- Blood film examination
- Serum cryptococcal antigen
- Other specific serologies indicated by travel or exposure history

2nd level includes

- Abdominal and thoracic CT
- Exercise oximetry
- Gallium scan
- Bronchoscopy with broncho-alveolar lavage
- Biopsy (histology and microbiology): bone marrow (useful if significant immunosuppression, anaemia, or cytopaenia), liver, lymph node (including mediastinoscopic), skin, intestinal/oesophageal mucosa
- Lumbar puncture
- PCR for CMV

Causes of PUO unrelated to HIV must not be forgotten (Box 46.1) and may require other investigations e.g. auto-antibody screen and isotope-labelled white cell scan.

Consider serology depending on history, country of origin/travel, and examination for CMV, EBV, toxoplasma, parvovirus, coxiella, mycoplasma, chlamydia pneumoniae, influenza, adenovirus, enterovirus, syphillis, bartonella, brucella, rickettsia, leptospirosis, borrelia, histoplasma, cryptococcus.

Consider serum PCR for CMV (rising or high CMV PCR correlates with development of end-organ disease but not diagnostic), parvovirus (particularly if anaemic), EBV (may be positive in lymphoma), and HHV-8 (associated with Kaposi's sarcoma and Castleman's disease).

Management

Management depends on the underlying cause. Cases where no underlying additional pathology is found may respond to HAART. As in any fever, general measures, such as good hydration, antipyretics, and reassurance, are important. In patients with late-stage HIV disease and limited treatment options, palliation with steroids may be necessary. MAC infections and, less commonly, leishmaniasis often present with unexplained pyrexia without focal organ involvement. Other causes of HIV-related PUO which may present with clinical features specific to their 1° infection site are described elsewhere in this book.

Box 46.1 Non-HIV-related causes of PUO

Infection
Bacterial
- Site-specific:
  - abscesses, urinary tract infection, endocarditis, hepatobiliary infection, osteomyelitis.
- General:
  - syphilis, relapsing fever, Lyme disease, gonorrhoea, lymphogranuloma venereum, psittacosis, salmonellosis, Q-fever.

Viral
- CMV, Epstein–Barr virus, hepatitis viruses.

Fungi (usually only if immunosuppressed):
- Candidiasis

Parasites
- Malaria, toxoplasmosis.

Connective tissue/autoimmune diseases
- Rheumatoid arthritis, Still's disease, systemic lupus erythematosus.

Vasculitis
- Giant cell arteritis, polymyalgia rheumatica, polyarteritis nodosa.

Granulomatous diseases
- Sarcoidosis, regional enteritis, granulomatous hepatitis.

Neoplasia
- Lymphomas, Hodgkin's disease, leukaemias, solid tumours especially renal cell carcinoma, malignant histiocytosis.

Inherited diseases
- Familial Mediterranean fever.

Drugs
- Antibiotic reactions.

Endocrine
- Hyperthyroidism.

Factitious

Mycobacterium avium complex

Ubiquitous and frequently isolated from soil, food, and water. Infection usually affects those with CD4 counts <100cells/μL (median ≈ 10cells/μL). Any organ can be affected, most commonly lymph nodes, spleen, GI tract, lungs, and bone marrow, but most patients develop disseminated infection without prior localization. Symptoms may be severe.

Clinical features

Most common is pyrexia (in ~90%) with night sweats, fatigue, diarrhoea/abdominal pain/nausea and vomiting/weight loss, lymph-adenopathy, and hepato-splenomegaly.

Investigations and diagnosis

- FBC: anaemia (common and often severe)
- LFTs: ↑ alkaline phosphatase (common)
- Blood cultures (>95% sensitivity for disseminated MAC)
- Culture of material from bone marrow, lymph nodes, and liver
- Staining of material from bone marrow, lymph nodes (Plate 23), and liver for mycobacteria (marrow provides rapid diagnosis in ~30%).
- PCR testing of potentially infected material (if available)
- X-rays may show internal lymphadenopathy with a typical abscess pattern on CT

Management

Three or four drug regimens are recommended as multiresistance is usual.

A macrolide (clarithromycin 500mg daily twice or azithromycin 500mg daily) plus ethambutol 15mg/kg daily plus a rifamycin (rifabutin 450–600mg/day or rifampicin 450–600mg/day) and/or a quinolone (e.g. ciprofloxacin 500mg daily twice). Data to advise on the duration of treatment are lacking, but it should be a minimum of 12 months and until CD4 >100 cells/μL for 3–6 months. HAART should also be commenced, taking into account potential drug interactions. Steroids may be required to ameliorate severe fever.

1° prophylaxis is now rarely required because of the effectiveness of HAART, but may be considered for those with a CD4 count <50cells/μL. Effective drugs include azithromycin (500mg 3 days a week) or clarithromycin 500mg daily. Combination with rifabutin does not increase survival and leads to drug interactions, and is not recommended. Prophylaxis can be stopped once CD4 is >100 cells/L for >3–6 months on HAART.

Visceral leishmaniasis

Caused by *Leishmania* spp, protozoa transmitted by sandflies from rodents, small carnivores, dogs, foxes, and humans. Typically presents with fever, malaise, weight loss, hepatosplenomegaly, and lymphadenopathy. Pancytopenia may occur.

Diagnosed by identifying organism in tissue by microscopy (Leishman–Donovan bodies in macrophages), culture, or PCR. Fine-needle aspiration of spleen is most sensitive (about 98%), but bone marrow aspiration is safer with 54–86% sensitivity. Serology (immunofluorescent antibody test and direct agglutination test) is insensitive (up to 76%) unless high protozoal load.

Treat with sodium stibogluconate 20mg/kg/day IV/IM for 28 days or liposomal amphotericin B. 2° prophylaxis with amphotericin or sodium stibogluconate every 2–4 weeks is essential to prevent recurrence (occurs in 60–90% without prophylaxis). Daily itraconazole may be effective 2° prophylaxis.

HIV: endocrine and metabolic disorders

Introduction

Metabolic disturbances and alterations in endocrine functions occur at all stages of HIV disease. HIV may directly infect endocrine glands, but more commonly endocrine abnormalities are due to functional disturbances or 2° to drugs and intercurrent severe illnesses. The wide use of anti-retroviral drugs has resulted in a decline in endocrine gland infiltration but ↑ prevalence of metabolic complications including insulin resistance, dyslipidaemia, and abnormal body fat distribution.

Endocrine disturbances

Pituitary function

Panhypopituitarism is rare but selective failure can occur, e.g. gonado-trophins. Pituitary infarction is found in up to 10% of autopsies of AIDS patients. The pituitary may also be involved by opportunistic infection (OI) such as toxoplasmosis, cytomegalovirus (CMV), *Mycobacterium avium* complex (MAC), and *Mycobacterium tuberculosis*. Dysfunctions of the hypothalamic–pituitary–adrenal (HPA) axis have been observed—hypercorticolism in early HIV disease (stimulation by cytokines and gp120) leading to impaired adrenal function with advanced disease.

Thyroid disease

Autopsy studies have shown infiltration by lymphoma, Kaposi's sarcoma, and OIs such as MAC and CMV. These pathologies are not usually associated with abnormal thyroid function tests. Thyroid binding globulins are high and this should be taken into consideration when interpreting total thyroid hormone levels.

Thyroid dysfunction may occur in those with advanced HIV disease during intercurrent illnesses. Overt hypothyroidism is rare.

Gonadal function

Dysfunction occurs in both sexes, especially in the late stages of HIV disease and in those with weight loss. Sex hormone binding globulin levels are ↑ in 30–50%. Free testosterone levels are more reliable in the assessment of hypogonadism. Panhypopituitarism from hypothalamic and/or pituitary destruction causing gonadal failure is rare. The aetiology of gonadal dysfunction is often multifactorial. Severe systemic illness, OIs, malnutrition, weight loss, recreational drug use, chronic alcoholism, and abnormal levels of cytokines may be contributory. HIV-related gonadal failure results in loss of muscle mass, fatigue, sexual dysfunction, and ↓ quality of life. Unlike HIV-negative men there is no ↑ in fat mass.

Testicular function

Total testosterone levels may be elevated in the early stages of HIV infection but tend to decline with disease progression. Erectile dysfunction is common in AIDS. Low testosterone levels may be due to a functional disorder of the hypothalamus, 1° testicular failure, or a combination of both. Gonadotrophins (LH and FSH) should be measured if testosterone is low: ↑ LH/FSH likely to be 1° testicular failure; normal or ↓ LH/FSH likely to be 2° pituitary and needs to be investigated. Testicular function is affected by drugs such as:

- opiates—associated with hypogonadotropic hypogonadism
- ketoconazole—causes oligospermia and gynaecomastia
- megestrol acetate—inhibits gonadotrophin secretion

Testosterone replacement ↑ lean body mass, body weight, and well-being.

Ovarian function

Irregular periods, oligomenorrhoea, and amenorrhoea occur with ↑ frequency as HIV disease progresses. ↓ muscle mass is associated with androgen deficiency. Up to 67% of ♀ with AIDS wasting syndrome have ↓ levels of free testosterone. The mechanism of this is not known.

Adrenal function

The adrenal gland is the most commonly affected endocrine gland, leading to glucocorticoid and, less commonly, aldosterone deficiency. HPA axis abnormalities in HIV are usually due to medication, destruction of the adrenals or the anterior pituitary by OIs and malignancies, autoimmune adrenalitis, and abnormal cytokine levels.

Adrenals may be directly infected by HIV. CMV adrenal gland involvement (found in 40–85% of autopsies) may lead to acute adrenal insufficiency.

Features of adrenocortical disturbances found in HIV infection are:
- ↓ levels of dehydroepiandrosterone with ↑ cortisol
- low basal adrenal androgen levels
- ↓ adrenal responses to adrenocorticotrophic hormone (ACTH).

Drugs may also compromise adrenal function:
- megestrol acetate (used as an appetite stimulant) ↓ plasma cortisol level and may lead to acute adrenal crisis if stopped abruptly after prolonged use
- ketoconazole results in ↓ cortisol and testosterone levels
- rifampicin enhances hepatic cortisol metabolism and causes adrenal insufficiency in patients with Addison's disease who are on replacement therapy or in those with limited adrenal function.

Patients with fatigue, loss of weight, postural hypotension, hypo-natraemia, and hyperkalaemia should be assessed with a short synacthen test. 1° adrenal insufficiency can be identified by measuring ACTH simultaneously with serum cortisol. Any severe illness may disturb the HPA axis, resulting in minor abnormalities of adrenal function tests.

Aldosterone deficiency may occur (often with glucocorticoid deficiency), leading to persistent hyponatraemia, hyperkalaemia, and metabolic acidosis requiring replacement therapy.

Management

- Patients with glucocorticoid insufficiency should receive replacement therapy with hydrocortisone 30mg/day in divided doses.
- Patients with aldosterone deficiency should receive fludrocortisone 50–300mcg/day.

Pancreatic function

Both exocrine and endocrine functions are affected during HIV disease.

Pancreatic endocrine function

Insulin resistance occurs more frequently in HIV infection, especially in those treated with protease inhibiters (PIs) and those with wasting syndrome. Diabetes is more likely to occur in those with other predisposing factors (e.g. family history).

Pentamidine, used in the treatment of *Pneumocystis jiroveci* (*carinii*) pneumonia (PCP), is toxic to pancreatic β cells, inducing hypoglycaemia in 15–28% (2–3 times more common than in HIV –ve patients). The reason for this is unknown. Substantial destruction of β cells may later lead to diabetes mellitus. Management of diabetes should follow the same principles as for HIV –ve individuals.

Recurrent or severe pancreatitis secondary to drugs (e.g. DDI, D4T) may lead to insulin-dependent diabetes secondary to destruction of β cells.

Pancreatic exocrine function (□ Chapter 40, Pancreatic diseases p. 472)

Reduced exocrine pancreatic function is common in HIV infection and may be asymptomatic. Severe chronic pancreatic insufficiency results in malabsorption.

Metabolic disorders

Lipodystrophy syndrome

Lipodystrophy, dyslipidaemia, and hyperglycaemia (2° to insulin resistance) are often combined, although each component may occur in isolation. May arise spontaneously but much more commonly associated with the use of HAART, especially if containing PIs. Mechanism is unclear. PIs have molecular homology with LDL-related receptor. Nucleoside reverse transcriptase inhibitors (NRTIs) may contribute to insulin resistance through mitochondrial toxicity leading to liver steatosis and adipocyte malfunction. The frequency and severity depend on gender, genetic factors, age, ethnicity, duration of HIV infection, and length and type of antiretroviral drugs.

Lipodystrophy

Found in ~4% of those with untreated HIV infection. Rate for those taking HAART is difficult to determine because of inconsistent diagnostic criteria but ranges from 20% up to 75% (median development time—18 months after HAART). Magnitude varies with individual PIs. Prevalence also related to duration of NRTI use, especially thymidine analogues such as stavudine (D4T) and zidovudine. More common in Caucasians and almost twice as common in ♀.

Lipohypertrophy (especially associated with PIs)
- Dorsocervical fat pad—buffalo hump
- Increased neck circumference (by 5–10cm)
- Breast hypertrophy (♀ and ♂)
- Central truncal adiposity—pot belly due to ↑ intra-peritoneal fat.
- Lipomas occur in ~ 10% of these patients

Lipoatrophy (especially associated with NRTIs, particularly stavudine)
- Loss of subcutaneous fat from cheeks—emaciated appearance, can be disfiguring, may identify patients as having HIV infection and may affect quality of life and compliance with drugs
- Peripheral subcutaneous fat loss from arms, shoulders, thighs, buttocks

Dyslipidaemia
HIV infection may cause abnormalities in lipid metabolism which include:
- ↑ serum triglyceride
- ↑ total cholesterol, but high-density lipoprotein (HDL) may be elevated in early stages and ↓with advanced disease
- ↓ low-density lipoprotein (LDL)
- predominance of small dense LDL particles.

It is reported in up to 80% of those taking HAART and especially prevalent in those taking a PI-based regimen. Typical abnormalities:
- hypercholesterolaemia—mostly very-LDL but also intermediate density lipoproteins. HDL unchanged or ↑
- hypertriglyceridaemia.

More frequent and severe with ritonavir, lopinavir–ritonavir, followed by amprenavir and nelfinavir with indinavir and saquinavir having few effects, atazanavir has the fewest effects. The newer PIs tipranavir and darunavir have moderate effects on lipids.

NRTIs are much less likely to be implicated although stavudine is more likely to be associated with ↑ cholesterol and triglycerides unlike lamivudine, emtricitabine, tenofavir and abacavir which appear to have minimum or no effect on lipid metabolism.

All non-NRTIs can cause alterations in the lipid profiles but to a much lesser extent than PIs. Nevirapine produces marginally smaller changes than efavirenz. Lipid levels improve when switching to NNRTIs from PIs.

Raltegravir has a very favourable lipid profile.

Hyperglycaemia

New-onset diabetes mellitus, diabetic ketoacidosis, and exacerbations of pre-existing diabetes mellitus have all been reported with ↑ rates when there are other concomitant risk factors, e.g. family history, pregnancy. Diabetes is directly associated with HIV infection, reported in 3.3% although this ↑ to 5.9% with concomitant hepatitis C virus infection. The HIV-associated insulin resistance and glucose dysregulation may lead to atherosclerosis and coronary heart disease. Stronger link is observed with PIs; atazanavir is the least associated.

Assessment

Patients on antiretroviral therapy should have body weight, lipids, and blood sugar measured every 3–6 months. Clinical examination and self-reporting of body shape changes help detect early signs. Photographs may aid in the early recognition of facial lipoatrophy. Additional cardiovascular risks, such as lifestyle, smoking, hypertension, family history, and age, should also be assessed.

Management

- General advice
  - Nutrition: assessment, dietetic advice (low fat), possible benefit from dietary supplements (fibre, omega-3 fatty acids).
  - Exercise: ↑ physical activity and exercise to build muscles, improve abdominal shape and combat peripheral wasting.
- Start HAART before CD4 <200cells/µL or AIDS is diagnosed.
- Care with choice of initial regimen if possible:
  - avoid PIs and NRTI combinations with highest risk
  - use lamivudine or emtricitabine and tenofovir instead of stavudine.
- Switch to drugs with low or no association. Benefit of switching is inconsistent, as morphological changes are more resistant.
- Fibrates and statins—used according to lipid profile
  - Hypercholesterolaemia managed with low-fat diet and statins.
  - Hypertriglyceridaemia responds best to low-fat diet, fibrates, statins.
  - Pravastatin is the preferred statin as it is least likely to interact with PIs. Fluvastatin is an alternative. Atorvastatin must be used with caution. Simvastatin and lovastatin should be avoided because of substantial risks of PI. NNRTIs are enzyme inducers and higher levels of statins may be required.
  - Fibrates (gemfibrozil, bezafibrate, fenofibrate) are usually used in combination with statins as more effective than fibrate mono-therapy. Seek advice from lipidologist before starting. ↑ risk of rhabdomyolysis and hepatoxicity.

- Other drugs
  - Metformin (avoid if lipoatrophy) for insulin resistance, dyslipidaemia, and fat accumulation.
  - Growth hormone for fat accumulation.
  - Tesamoreline (a growth hormone-releasing hormone analogue) improves abdominal fat accumulation.
  - Glitazones for insulin resistance with weight loss.
- Invasive methods for lipodystrophy
  - Plastic surgery e.g. liposuction and breast reduction.
  - Polylactic acid (New-Fill®) and Bio-Alcamid™ injections for lipo-atrophy.

Electrolytes and water imbalance

Sodium and water

Hyponatraemia is a common finding in patients with advanced HIV disease. Up to 60% of hospitalized patients have low plasma sodium levels, mostly due to GI loss associated with hypovolaemia. Respiratory and CNS infections or certain drugs, e.g. antidepressants, may cause SIADH characterized by hyponatraemia, inappropriately ↑ urinary osmolality for the degree of serum hypo-osmolality and normal blood volume in the context of normal adrenal and thyroid functions. Severe hyponatraemia causes confusion, seizures, and coma.

Decreased water clearance from HIV-related nephropathy may exacerbate hyponatraemia. Hyporeninaemic hypoaldosteronism should be considered when hyponatraemia is associated with hyperkalaemia, provided that kidneys and adrenals are functioning normally.

Hyponatraemia may be caused by miconazole and pentamidine and hypernatraemia (and nephrogenic diabetes insipidus) by foscarnet.

Potassium

High-dose co-trimoxazole may result in hyperkalaemia especially with pre-existing renal impairment. Other causes include pentamidine-associated tubular nephropathy, HIV nephropathy, and 1° adrenal insufficiency.

Calcium and phosphate

Up to 20% of patients will have hypocalcaemia at some stage. Causes:
- HIV enteropathy (most common)
- vitamin D deficiency
- severe intercurrent illness
- drugs:
  - foscarnet binds calcium resulting in decreased ionized calcium.
  - ketoconazole inhibits vitamin D synthesis.
  - pentamidine causes renal loss of magnesium with 2° hypocalcaemia.

Hypophosphataemia is very common in HIV +ve patients, occurs in 10% of patients not taking HAART and in 20–31% of those on HAART. Main causes are malnutrition, GI losses, osteomalacia, hyperparathyroidism, alcoholism and intercurrent illness. Tenofovir can lead to hypo-phosphataemia as a result of effect on tubular function.

HIV-associated wasting syndrome

Defined by CDC as involuntary loss of >10% of body weight plus >30 days of either diarrhoea or weakness and fever in the absence of concurrent illness other than HIV infection. It is an AIDS-defining illness, less common since the introduction of HAART, when it accounted for up to 37% of AIDS diagnoses. Still a common problem independently associated with an increased risk of OIs, disease progression, and death. Weight loss is mainly due to muscle wasting and, to a lesser extent, loss of fat.

Additional factors that exacerbate wasting include:
• depression
• nutritional balance, e.g. anorexia, dysphagia, poor nutrient absorption
• OIs
• metabolism, e.g. increased resting metabolic rate, increased protein turnover, increased production of cytokines, and low testosterone.

Assessment
• Weight and body mass index at regular intervals help with early recognition and monitoring.
• Specialist nutritional review.
• Testosterone measurement.
• Measurement of body composition (bioimpedence analysis and anthropometry are useful in monitoring changes over time).
• Techniques such as dual energy X-ray absorptiometry (DEXA) scan, MRI, and total body electrical conductivity provide more accurate measurement of body composition.

Management
• Treatment of contributing factors.
• Improving food intake by appropriate strategies including dietary supplements, enteral and parentral feeding.
• Pharmacological agents
  • Testosterone may be considered to reverse muscle loss but there is concern about the adverse effects of long-term administration.
  • Megestrol—an appetite stimulant (side-effects include hypogonadism, adrenal insufficiency, deep venous thrombosis, and avascular necrosis).
  • Growth hormone administration results in increase in lean body mass, but is expensive and benefit may be lost after discontinuation.
  • Thalidomide results in significant weight gain but has strict prescribing guidelines and potential serious side-effects.
  • Anabolic hormones, e.g. oxymetholone, are beneficial but side-effects include liver toxicity. Nandrolone is effective in increasing lean body mass in both men and women but long-term side-effects are not known.

HIV: renal disorders

Introduction

Kidney disease was relatively common before the HAART era. Proteinuria may be found in up to 30%. Necropsy studies in the USA have shown renal pathological abnormalities in 3–7%. In the HAART era primary renal diseases, diabetes, hypertension, vascular disease, and drug toxicity (including antiretrovirals) are more common than HIV-associated nephropathy.

Initial presentation may be as acute renal failure, especially in advanced HIV disease, secondary to the following.
- Dehydration and electrolyte disturbances (e.g. following vomiting and diarrhoea)
- Acute tubular necrosis due to:
  - sepsis
  - hypotension
  - drug nephrotoxicity (e.g. tenofovir, adefovir, aminoglycosides, pentamidine, aciclovir, cidofovir, foscarnet, amphotericin B)
  - rhabdomyolysis which is increasing due to more frequent use of statins in combination with HAART
- Obstruction (secondary to nephrolithiasis and crystalluria):
  - indinavir— ~4% develop nephrolithiasis, prevented by ample fluid intake (>2L a day)
  - sulfadiazine and aciclovir—can cause crystalluria especially in high dosage and with dehydration.
HIV-related 2° infection (e.g. tuberculosis) can involve the kidney but HIV infection itself may cause 1° renal disease.

The general management of renal failure should follow the same principles as for HIV –ve patients, i.e. fluid/dietary restriction, renal replacement therapy, erythropoietin, vitamin D analogues, etc.

Assessment of HIV-positive patients for renal disease:

Address all risk factors such as smoking, hypertension, dyslipidaemia, hyperuricaemia, metabolic syndrome, vascular disease The following should be measured routinely.
- Dipstick for protein in urine and if + or greater quantify more accurately by 24 hour urine protein or urine spot sample for urine protein/creatinine ratio (uPCR). 24 hour urine collection may not be reliable.
- Serum creatinine should be complimented by an estimated glomerular filtration rate (eGFR) using MDRD or Cockcroft–Gault equations. If uPCR >45 or eGFR <60 → renal ultrasound and consider referral to nephrology; otherwise annual measurements.
- Urinary sediment microscopy annually.
- Patients at high risk for development of renal dysfunction, i.e. HIV VL >4000copies/mL, CD4 <200 cells/μL, black race, diabetes, HCV co-infection, or HBV, may need to have renal function monitored more frequently.
- Patients with persistently low or declining eGFR (<60mL/min/1.73m^2), proteinuria, or uPCR >100mg/mmol should be referred to a renal physician.

HIV-associated nephropathy (HIVAN)

First described in 1984. Studies from USA demonstated that it accounts for >50% of HIV-related renal disease. Renal glomerular and tubular epithelial cells have been shown to be infected by HIV, although the mechanisms of viral-induced injury are unclear.

Predominantly found in black ♂ of African origin and currently the third most common cause of end-stage renal disease (ESRD) in 20–64-year-old African Americans. Low incidence amongst follow-up patients (0.25/1000 patient-years) and higher (1%) in newly diagnosed Blacks.

Clinical features

Presents with nephrotic syndrome—proteinuria (>3.5g/day), hypoalbuminaemia, oedema, and hyperlipidaemia. Typically no cellular casts or hypertension. Leads to progressive renal insufficiency, which is modified with HAART.

Diagnosis

- CD4 count is usually <200cells/μL.
- Urinalysis shows leucocytes, hyaline casts, and oval fat bodies but no cellular casts.
- Renal ultrasound typically shows normal or enlarged renal size with ↑ echogenicity.
- Markedly impaired renal function
- Renal biopsy may be required if diagnosis in doubt (e.g. patient with other risk factors for renal disease or not responding to HAART). Definitive diagnosis is made by renal biopsy showing focal segmental glomerulosclerosis, collapse of glomerular tuft associated with tubular ectasia, and tubulo-interstitial nephritis.

Management

- HAART, with dose adjustment when GFR<50mL/min. Leads to ~21% increase in creatinine clearance. Reduces need for renal replacement therapy.
- Prednisolone (improves renal function by ↓ HIV-initiated inflammatory process).
- Angiotensin-converting enzyme inhibitors if initiated prior to severe renal insufficiency may offer long-term renal survival benefits. Angiotensin receptor blockers are alternatives
- Dialysis if needed.
- Transplant should not be withheld if clinically warranted.

Immune-mediated renal disease

Less common than HIVAN but reported as the main cause of HIV-related renal disease in non-black races. Found in 10–80% of autopsy and biopsy studies in HIV +ve patients from different European and Asian countries. Most common form is membranoproliferative glomerulo-nephritis. Membranous nephropathy, post-infectious glomerulonephritis, fibrillary glomerulonephritis, and IgA nephropathy (majority Caucasians and Hispanics) are other described forms of immune-mediated renal disease.

Hepatitis B virus (HBV) and hepatitis C virus (HCV), both more common in injecting IV drug users, are important co-infections and may individually cause renal disease.

HCV-associated cryoglobulinaemic glomerulonephritis is found in both HIV- and non-HIV-infected patients, but is much more aggressive in the former. Typical presentation includes purpura, arthralgias, and peripheral neuropathy in addition to renal insufficiency. Circulating cryoglobulins and ↓ complement levels may be found.

HBV, syphilis, and malignancy may all cause membranous nephropathy and are all found more frequently in those with HIV infection.

Clinical features

Slowly progressive and mild compared with HIVAN. Typical early features are asymptomatic proteinuria and microscopic haematuria, with mild renal insufficiency.

Diagnosis

- Detection of other infection(s), e.g. syphilis, HBV, and HCV
- Renal biopsy

Management

- Treat any co-infection or malignancy.
- HAART

Thrombotic microangiopathy

Appears to be the most common microvascular injury associated with HIV. Thrombotic thrombocytopenic purpura (TTP) and haemolytic uraemic syndrome (HUS) occur, characterized by microangiopathic haemolytic anaemia with renal insufficiency, thrombocytopenia, fever, and neurological changes. Mean age at presentation 35 years with 80% males. Poor prognosis in HIV, with mortality of 66–100%. Massive proteinuria is uncommon, unlike immune-mediated disease and HIVAN. HAART and plasmapheresis are the mainstay of therapy. Splenectomy may be helpful in refractory cases.

Interstitial nephritis

Not uncommon and may be associated with other renal pathology such as HIVAN. Equal prevalence in Blacks and Caucasians. May present with proteinuria, renal failure, or nephrotic syndrome. Acute interstitial nephritis 2° to allergic drug reactions presents with acute renal failure, skin rash, and eosinophilia. Non-steroidal anti-inflammatory drugs are a common cause.

Acute renal failure and HIV seroconversion

Acute renal failure and nephrotic syndrome may be presenting features of acute HIV seroconversion. Renal biopsy typically shows acute tubular necrosis and mesangio-proliferative glomerulonephritis, with tubuloreticular inclusions.

Drugs and renal disease

- The overall incidence of severe renal dysfunction in patients taking anti-retrovirals is <1%.
- Indinavir: nephrolithiasis ~12%, interstitial nephritis. Patients should be advised to drink at least 2L water per day. Nephrolithiasis reported with other PIs (e.g. amprenavir and atazanavir).
- Ritonavir: interstitial nephritis
- Tenofovir: renal tubular dysfunction with hypophosphataemia, normoglycemic glycosuria, and proteinuria. Fanconi's syndrome may develop. Overall incidence of renal dysfunction is no higher than other anti-retrovirals. Phosphate should be monitored monthly, then 3 monthly after 1 year.
- Dose adjustment is not necessary for PI and NNRTI, but most NRTI require dose adjustment with renal dysfunction and creatinine clearance <60mL/min

Other diseases (less commonly reported)

Minimal change disease, amyloidosis, and renal malignancy.

End-stage renal disease

Dialysis should be considered (haemodialysis is currently the preferred method). May only be required on a temporary basis until HAART is introduced. Cadaver renal transplantation has been performed in a small number of selected patients with no evidence of ↑ rate of opportunistic infections or rejection.

HIV: cardiovascular disorders

Introduction

Reports of the prevalence of cardiac involvement in patients with AIDS vary from 28% to 73%, with the first case of myocardial Kaposi's sarcoma (KS), found at autopsy in 1983. Since the introduction of HAART, a sharp ↓ in mortality and morbidity has been observed. New risk factors for coronary heart disease such as increased insulin resistance, dyslipidemia, and lipodystrophy syndrome, which are associated with HAART, may accelerate underlying arteriosclerosis in HIV-infected patients.

Pericardial effusion

Prior to the introduction of HAART, the frequency of this complication was estimated to be 5–46%, and fibrinous pericarditis has been identified at autopsy in 9–62% of deceased AIDS patients. It is often small with no haemodynamic consequences, although if large it may cause tamponade. It is associated with low CD4 count and reported causes include bacteria, especially *Mycobacterium* spp and also *Cryptococcus neoformans*, cytomegalovirus, tumours (lymphoma, KS). Clinically similar to non-HIV infected patients, and although usually seen in advanced HIV infection rarely causes death.

Myocarditis

Prior to HAART autopsy evidence was found in ~33% of those with AIDS, with a specific cause found in <20% (the most common being *Toxoplasma gondii*, *Mycobacterium tuberculosis*, and *C.neoformans*). HIV alone can probably cause myocarditis, as HIV or its proteins have been found in the myocardium of patients with or without cardiac disease. Myocardial biopsy may be indicated, especially if CD4 ↓.

Dilated cardiomyopathy

Prevalence in patients with AIDS is 10–30% by echocardiographic and autopsy studies. Associated with advanced disease. Several studies have supported a direct role for HIV-1 as the cause of cardiac injury, but the mechanism remains unclear. Other viruses such as group B coxsackie virus, CMV, or EBV have been implicated (found in >80% of heart histology specimens). The patient will present with shortness of breath, persistent tachycardia, and signs of heart failure. Echocardiogram is of use in diagnosis. The overall prognosis is poor.

Endocarditis

Non-bacterial thrombotic endocarditis

Friable fibrinous clumps of platelets and red blood cells adherent to cardiac valves (usually tricuspid in HIV infection) without an inflammatory reaction. Occurs in 3–5% of those with AIDS, usually aged >50 years. Associated with malignancy, hypercoagulable states, and chronic wasting disease. Emboli may occur in up to 42%, involving the brain, lung, spleen, kidneys, and coronary arteries. They are usually asymptomatic, but rarely may be fatal.

Infective endocarditis

Occurs most commonly in injecting drug users (IDUs), usually affecting the tricuspid valve. The main causative organisms are *Staphylococcus aureus* (75%) and *Streptococcus viridans* (20%). Usually presents with fever, sweats, weight loss, peripheral signs of endocarditis, and coexisting pneumonia and/or meningitis. A murmur is normally heard and may be TR in setting of IDU. Echocardiogram is important, followed by transoesophageal echocardiogram. ↑ mortality in advanced HIV.

Pulmonary hypertension

HIV is an independent risk factor for the development of pulmonary hypertension. The true incidence is not known, but reported incidence in symptomatic patients is 0.3–0.5%, i.e. more than 50 times that in the general population. The precise pathogenesis is unknown. The stage of HIV infection is unrelated to the development and progression of pulmonary hypertension and it may predate the diagnosis of HIV disease. Found most commonly in young ♂. Progressive dyspnoea followed by ankle oedema are the usual presenting features. Diagnosed after excluding other causes, e.g. thrombo-embolism, talc granuloma (particularly in IDUs). Echocardiogram may show RV dilatation and right heart vascular studies may be required to confirm the diagnosis. The response to pulmonary vasodilator agents, antiretroviral drugs, and anticoagulation therapy is variable. The prognosis is poor compared with 1° pulmonary hypertension. Inconsistent reports of improvement with HAART.

Venous thrombosis

↑ risk of venous thromboembolic disease leading to deep venous thrombosis and consequently pulmonary embolism. Related to changes in coagulation (📖 Chapter 51, Haematological disorders p. 562).

Cardiac neoplasia

Kaposi's sarcoma

In autopsy studies, mostly ♂ who have sex with ♂ (MSM) incidence of cardiac KS prior to HAART was 12–28% (usually part of disseminated involvement). Typical cardiac sites are the visceral layer of serous pericardium or sub-epicardial fat (especially beside a major coronary artery). Clinical features are often negligible. May cause pericardial effusion which can produce cardiac tamponade requiring emergency paracentesis. If suspected, diagnosis can be confirmed by biopsy through a pericardial window which also provides decompression.

Non-Hodgkin's lymphoma

Usually part of disseminated neoplasia rather than primary cardiac lymphoma (very rare). Typically high grade with spread often early in those with AIDS. Any heart chamber may be involved but right atrium is the most common. Usually no specific symptoms but may present with progressive congestive heart failure, pericardial effusion, cardiac arrhythmia, or cardiac tamponade. Nodular or polypoid lymphomas may appear, predominantly involving the pericardium with variable myocardial infiltration. Their removal may alleviate mechanical obstruction. Prognosis is poor, although clinical remission has been observed with combination chemotherapy.

Vascular disease

May be directly caused by HIV with infected monocytes and macrophages producing atheroma by adhesion or angiitis. HAART, especially containing protease inhibitors (PIs), except atazanavir, may cause hyperlipidaemia leading to atherosclerosis and thrombosis. Hyperlipidaemia is found to a lesser extent with the nucleoside/nucleotide reverse transcriptase inhibitors (especially stavudine) and the non-nucleoside reverse transcriptase inhibitors. Insulin resistance (associated with PIs) is an independent risk factor for myocardial infarction and death. The risk of myocardial infarction is ~3 times that of ♂ in the general population if PIs are used for ≥30 months. Abacavir and didanosine have also been associated with ↑ cardiovascular risk. Abacavir has been associated with a 1.9-fold increased risk from other NRTIs; this is enhanced in those with an already high cardiovascular risk. Other cardiovascular risk factors are important to consider, especially cigarette smoking as higher rates have been reported in MSM with HIV infection. Therefore advice on low-fat diets, regular exercise, blood pressure control, lipid-lowering drugs, and smoking cessation are important in patient care.

Drug-associated disorders

Cardiomyopathy may be caused by zidovudine (also myocarditis), doxorubicin, amphotericin B, and foscarnet, dysrhythmias by ganciclovir and α-interferon, and conduction defects by co-trimoxazole, pentamidine, and pyrimethamine.

HIV: musculoskeletal disorders

Introduction

Before the use of HAART, diseases characterized by CD8 expansion dominated, e.g. reactive arthritis, painful articular syndrome, diffuse infiltrative lymphocytosis syndrome (DILS), and psoriatic arthritis. With HAART, new phenomena emerged such as osteoporosis, immune restoration inflammatory syndrome, and metabolic abnormalities.

Musculoskeletal problems are commonly reported in HIV +ve patients, up to 65% in some sub-Saharan Africa cohorts. However, studies show that they are likely to be influenced by HIV risk factors:

- injecting drug users (IDUs) and haemophiliacs are more susceptible to septic arthritis and osteomyelitis
- ♂ who have sex with ♂ are more likely to develop sexually acquired reactive arthritis (SARA).

Joint symptoms may also be a feature of other conditions found more commonly in those with HIV infection, e.g. haemophilia (with haemarthrosis), syphilis, gonorrhoea, hepatitis B and C virus, and chlamydial infections. They may also be due to the side-effects of drugs used to treat HIV and related conditions.

Autoantibodies are commonly produced (though in low titres), except when CD4 counts are very low and may re-appear with immune reconstitution by HAART. When CD4 counts are >500cells/µL (early after seroconversion or immune restoration with treatment) autoimmune diseases may occur. Diseases reported include systemic lupus erythematosus, vasculitis, polymyositis, Raynaud's phenomenon, Behçet's disease, primary biliary cirrhosis, and Graves' disease. Immune complex vasculitis is associated with counts of 200–499cells/µL and spondyloarthropathy with counts <200cells/µL.

Pathogenesis of autoimmunity in HIV

Rheumatic diseases encountered in HIV correlate with the degree of immune suppression. T regulatory cells expressing CD4 are specifically depleted in HIV infection. They are responsible for the maintenance of self-tolerance and help protect against the development of autoimmunity. The death of T cells may release proteins that prompt formation of autoreactive CD8+ cells. Cytokine production is important in HIV pathogenesis, and possibly contributes to the development of autoimmune complications. During primary HIV infection, tumour necrosis factor, IL-6, Il-12, and interferon-γ can be detected. These cytokines are associated with chronic inflammation. Molecular mimicry similar to other virus-triggered/mediated autoimmune diseases may also occur.

Inflammatory arthropathies

Arthralgia

Most common joint manifestation occurring in up to 45%. Pathology is unclear but may involve cytokines or transient bone ischaemia. Can occur at any stage of HIV disease and may be the first manifestation, being reported in 50–70% of those presenting with 1° HIV infection. Usually mild to moderate in intensity.

In up to 10% of those with advanced HIV infection a painful transient articular syndrome, characterized by an acute onset of severe pain in up to four joints, has been described. Knee most commonly affected, with shoulder and elbow also involved. Symptoms may mimic acute septic arthritis, but no effusion, synovitis, or ↑ in joint fluid white cells. Radiology normal or may show periarticular osteopenia. Treat with standard analgesics/ NSAIDs, although narcotics may be required.

Diffuse idiopathic lymphocytic syndrome (DILS)

Similar to Sjögren's syndrome and found at any stage of HIV infection. Presents with salivary gland enlargement (parotid swelling may be massive), xerostomia, xerophthalmia, and arthralgia. The incidence of DILS has decreased since the introduction of HAART. Treat with artificial saliva and tears in addition to HAART.

Acute symmetrical polyarthritis

Presentation similar to rheumatoid arthritis (RA), with involvement of small joints of the hand leading to ulnar deviation of the digits and swan-neck deformities. May be differentiated from RA by acute onset and negative rheumatoid factor. Radiological appearances similar to RA with peri-articular osteopenia, joint-space narrowing, and marginal erosions. Patients with RA may go into remission when they become infected with HIV, but some progress to destructive disease despite having low CD4 counts. The emergence of immune-reconstitution inflammatory syndrome (IRIS) has been associated with new-onset RA. Respond to standard disease-modifying anti-rheumatic drugs (DMARDs). Gold treatment may be required. Immunosuppression may be relatively contraindicated.

HIV-associated arthritis

Asymmetrical oligoarticular arthritis. Possibly caused by effects of local infection (HIV detected in joint fluid). More common in ♂. Typically presents with sudden onset of severe pain, mainly affecting knees and ankles. Self-limiting, usually lasting from a few weeks to 6 months. Synovial fluid commonly contains up to 2500 white blood cells/µL. Radiology may show osteopenia but no erosions. A chronic mononuclear cell infiltrate is found on synovial biopsy. Treat with NSAIDs or intra-articular corticosteroid injections for symptomatic relief.

Hypertrophic osteoarthropathy

May appear as a complication of *Pneumocystis jiroveci* (*carinii*) pneumonia (PCP). Affects bones, joints, and soft tissues. Presents with severe pain in the lower limbs, arthralgia, non-pitting oedema, and finger clubbing. Skin over affected areas (ankle, knees, and elbows) is shiny, warm, and oedematous. Extensive periosteal reaction and sub-periosteal proliferative changes in the long bones of the legs are found on radiology, with bone scans showing ↑ uptake along the cortical surfaces. Usually responds to treatment of underlying PCP.

Reactive arthritis

Probably no more frequent in those with HIV infection but tends to be more severe. Lower limb peripheral arthritis predominates. Synovial fluid is inflammatory (a few thousand polymorphonuclear leucocytes per mL) and sterile with a glucose level at least 66% of the serum level. Treat initially with NSAIDs (as in HIV −ve patients). Other drugs may be required, e.g. phenylbutazone, gold, methotrexate (with caution as immunosuppressive), and other disease-modifying agents. HAART is likely to be beneficial.

Psoriatic arthritis

More common and severe than in HIV −ve individuals. Usually poly-articular and asymmetrical. Extra-articular manifestations occur in ~50%. Usually insidious with the appearance of bone erosions within weeks or months. Radiological findings of the distal interphalangeal joints are pathognomonic. Joint and tendon involvement in HIV-associated psoriatic arthritis tends to be less responsive to NSAIDs (still 1st line therapy). Methotrexate and azathioprine are effective but require careful monitoring because of myelosuppression. Sulfasalazine may be helpful but skin rash occurs in 30%. Low-dose systemic corticosteroids are ineffective and high doses may produce many side-effects. Gold, retinoids, phototherapy, ciclosporin, and zidovudine reported to improve the skin and joints in some.

Osteonecrosis (avascular necrosis)

Result of direct damage to the vascular supply, leading to death of subchondral bone. Additional risks are prior use of corticosteroids, testosterone, or anabolic steroids, hyperlipidaemia, hypercoagulability, sickle cell disease, alcohol abuse, and smoking. Most common site is femoral head followed by humeral head, with bilateral involvement in 40%. May be asymptomatic or cause severe disabling deep pain. As plain x-rays may be normal MRI is recommended. In early stages rest may be adequate, but in advanced disease joint replacement or other surgery may be required.

Infections

Septic arthritis

Usually mono-articular, with the hip being most frequently affected, although in IDUs there may be sternoclavicular joint involvement. *Staphylococcus aureus* followed by *Streptococcus pneumoniae* are the most common causative organisms. If CD4 count <100cells/μL multiple joint involvement and associated skin infection may occur with opportunistic infections (e.g. *Mycobacterium avium* complex, cryptococcosis, sporotrichosis). Diagnosed by Gram stain and culture of synovial fluid. Blood cultures may be positive before synovial cultures. Treat with appropriate antibiotics (usually IV) and monitor inflammatory markers.

Osteomyelitis

- Septic osteomyelitis: may follow direct extension or haematogenous spread from an infected joint. Suspect if septic arthritis fails to respond despite adequate treatment.
- Tuberculous osteomyelitis: develops from the haematogenous spread of an acute or reactivated infection. The spine, especially the thoracic and lumbar regions, is most commonly affected, starting in the vertebral body and spreading to the adjacent disc spaces. Vertebral wedging leads to gibbus formation. In addition to antibiotics, surgical intervention with irrigation and debridement may be required.

Bacillary angiomatosis due to *Bartonella henselae* may cause osteomyelitis. Occurs in the immunosuppressed and is characterized by vascular proliferation involving the nervous system (aseptic meningitis, intra-cerebral mass lesions), liver (peliosis hepatitis), lymph nodes (adenitis), and bone.

Osteopenia and osteoporosis

HIV infection is associated with ↓ bone mineral density (BMD) determined by measurement of X-ray absorption, e.g. dual-energy X-ray absorptiometry (DEXA) scan. A DEXA scan T-score (number of standard deviations from the mean value in young, healthy individuals) is diagnostic. Scores between −1 and −2.5 indicate osteopenia (pre-symptomatic) and −2.5 or less indicates osteoporosis. Osteopenia is found in up to 65% of those with HIV infection and osteoporosis in up to 25%. Duration of infection is significantly associated. Other factors are HIV wasting, low body mass index, malnutrition, immobilization, hypogonadism, menopause, steroids, alcohol excess, and smoking. HAART, especially with protease inhibitors, has been suggested as a contributor, but evidence is conflicting. Tenofovir leads to ↓ BMD when compared to D4T; hypophosphataemia may be a contributing factor.

Occur mainly in the vertebrae, lower arms, and hips. Osteoporosis is often asymptomatic but may cause pain (low back, neck, hip), loss of height, kyphosis, and fractures. Bone metabolism should be assessed (serum calcium, phosphate, and alkaline phosphatase). Management should include advice on diet and exercise, and avoidance of alcohol/nicotine. Osteopenia can be managed with vitamin D (400–800IU daily) and calcium supplements (calcium-rich diet or calcium tablets 1.2g/day). Osteoporosis should be treated with bisphosphonates (with additional vitamin D and calcium supplementation).

Neoplasia

Non-Hodgkin's lymphoma

1° or 2° bone involvement occurs in 20–30%. May present as a pathological fracture, especially of the lower limbs. Radiology shows an area of osteolysis with cortical destruction. A periosteal reaction and soft tissue mass may also be present. Findings similar to bacterial osteomyelitis, therefore biopsy recommended. Treated with chemotherapy, radiation, and possibly surgical debridement.

Kaposi's sarcoma

Rarely reported and usually associated with widespread dissemination. Frequently asymptomatic, otherwise bone pain, with radiology either normal or demonstrating lesions usually lytic, occasionally sclerotic. Diagnosis by biopsy. Radiotherapy may alleviate bone pain.

Muscle disease

1° myopathy is uncommon and a polymyositis syndrome occurs very rarely. The most important cause of 2° myopathy is prolonged zidovudine therapy, associated with ↑ creatinine kinase level in 16% and symptomatic weakness in 6%. Zidovudine-associated myopathy is less frequent with HAART. It is probably caused by mitochondrial dysfunction because of the inhibition of mitochondrial DNA γ-polymerase by zidovudine. Muscle weakness and wasting is proximal with preserved reflexes and sensory function. Electromyographical evidence of myopathy is found in >90%. Ragged red fibres (due to the accumulation of abnormal mitochondria) may be seen on muscle biopsy. Treatment involves discontinuation of the drug and NSAIDs, but some patients may require prednisolone (starting with 60–80mg daily, reducing over several months) to restore muscle strength.

Rheumatic disease in HAART era

A new spectrum of disorders has appeared, e.g. osteonecrosis, rhabdomyolysis, and IRIS. The frequency of reactive arthritis and psoriatic arthritis ↓ in HAART era.

Rhabdomyolysis is more frequently a complication of anti-lipid drugs, e.g. when PIs are combined with statins. Adhesive capsulitis, Dupuytren contractures, tenosynovitis, and temporomandibular joint dysfunction have been reported as a consequence of indinavir treatment. Osteopenia and osteoporosis occur in the treatment naive but ↑ in those on HAART.

↑ prevalence of avascular necrosis of the bone in treatment-naive patients, but may be increasing after the introduction HAART. The most common presenting symptom is pain on weight-bearing, although pain can also occur at rest. Avascular necrosis can be asymptomatic in some patients, and be an incidental finding in radiological studies. Surgical stabilization of the affected bone may be required.

Hypergammaglobulinaemia, positive rheumatoid factor, antinuclear antibodies, cryoglobulinaemia, and anticardiolipin antibodies (low titres), all previously common, are less frequent with HAART.

Immune reconstitution inflammatory syndrome (IRIS)

Unexpected exacerbation of inflammatory disease and atypical clinical features that resemble the symptoms of autoimmune disease can arise as part of IRIS. Autoimmune diseases such as Graves autoimmune thyroiditis, pulmonary sarcoidosis, systemic lupus erythematosus, RA, and polymyositis may occur. Most cases arise *de novo*, but ~20% are flares of pre-existing diseases (often mild) that were in remission due to immunosuppression 2° to HIV.

HAART should be continued with IRIS as most symptoms will resolve. However, if the inflammatory process involves certain areas, e.g. CNS where damage is likley to occur, HAART should be stopped and steroids considered.

HIV: reticulo-endothelial disorders

Haematological disorders

Common haematological abnormalities may lead to consideration of HIV as the cause. Direct effect of HIV itself or 2° to concurrent infection, malignancy, and therapeutic agents. Common findings are ↓ haemopoiesis, altered coagulation, and immune-mediated cytopenias with ↓ bone marrow cellularity and dysplasia.

Anaemia

Most common form of cytopenia and an independent prognostic factor. Usually due to ↓ erythropoiesis, but other mechanisms (e.g. infection, drug toxicity, malignancy, dietary deficiencies, alcohol abuse, blood loss) may contribute. Chronic anaemia causes fatigue, exertional dyspnoea, and a hyperdynamic state which, if severe, may lead to angina, congestive cardiac failure, and confusion.

Diagnosis and evaluation

Examine and test for iron, vitamin B_{12}, and folate deficiencies, haemolysis, and blood loss according to red cell indices. Eliminate possible causes by excluding infection and malignancy and reviewing drug therapy. Bone marrow examination may be required.

- HIV-related: normocytic normochromic anaemia ↑ in frequency and severity as HIV progresses. May be a direct effect of HIV on bone marrow progenitor cells, ↓ erythropoietin production, and ↑ cytokines (inhibit haemopoiesis). Improves or normalizes with HAART provided that drug effects do not supervene.
- Drug toxicity
  - Macrocytosis and normal haemoglobin—typical with zidovudine (AZT).
  - Macrocytic anaemia—caused by AZT and stavudine. AZT exerts broader myelosuppressive effects, more frequent in patients receiving higher doses (in ~1% receiving 500mg a day) and those with advanced disease. Anaemia may require blood transfusion following discontinuation of AZT. In patients with a low level of endogenous erythropoietin (<500IU/L), recombinant human erythropoietin may resolve anaemia, thereby ↓ need for transfusion.
  - Normocytic normochromic anaemia—associated with normal or ↓ reticulocyte count, 2° to bone marrow suppression. Causes include anaemia of chronic infection and drugs (e.g. ganciclovir, co-trimoxazole, amphotericin, and interferons).
  - Haemolytic anaemia—features are macrocytosis, ↓ haptoglobin, and ↑ lactic dehydrogenase, indirect bilirubin, and reticulocyte count. Common causes include drugs, e.g. dapsone (with methaemoglobinaemia), ribavirin, and primaquin. Glucose-6-phosphate dehydrogenase (G6PD) deficiency predisposes to dapsone and primaquin haemolysis. Autoimmune haemolytic anaemia (AIHA) with positive Coombs' test also occurs.

- Bone marrow infiltration (usually causes pancytopenia)
  - Opportunistic infection (OI)—most commonly *Mycobaterium avium* complex (also tuberculosis and cytomegalovirus).
  - Tumours—lymphoma and rarely Kaposi's sarcoma.
- B19 parvovirus infects erythroid precursors. In immune deficiency persistent infection may result in severe chronic normocytic normochromic anaemia. Diagnosed by detecting B19 parvovirus antibodies and DNA (by polymerase chain reaction) in serum and/or bone marrow. Responds well to high-dose IV immunoglobulins (0.4g/kg/day) which contain parvovirus antibodies, but may require repeated blood transfusions.

Thrombocytopenia

Occurs in up to 30%. May be result of drug toxicity, immune and non-immune destruction, or defective platelet production. Commonly an isolated haematological abnormality with ↑ levels of antiplatelet immunoglobulin. HIV-related immune thrombocytopenia is frequent early finding, tending to deteriorate as HIV progresses. Results from clearance of immunoglobulin-coated platelets by reticulo-endothelial system.

Diagnosis and evaluation

Exclude underlying causes, e.g. drug toxicity, liver disease, alcoholism, and lymphoma. In their absence the presence of normal or ↑ megakaryocytes on bone marrow examination is sufficient to diagnose HIV-induced thrombocytopenia.

Treatment

- Mild and asymptomatic—HAART, switch/discontinue implicated drugs.
- Symptomatic or before surgical procedures—IV immunoglobulins, steroids, and HAART.
- Substantial bleeding—packed red cells and platelet transfusion.

Thrombotic thrombocytopenic purpura

Rare, of unknown aetiology, usually seen in early stages of HIV infection. Characterized by hyaline microvascular deposits. Clinical features include fever, renal impairment, neurological deficit, and microangiopathic haemolytic anaemia. Mortality rate ~65% without treatment. However, good response to plasmapheresis, steroids, HAART, and antiplatelets (e.g. aspirin).

Neutropenia

HIV directly implicated, especially in advanced stages. More commonly due to drug toxicity, associated infection, and bone marrow infiltration. Risk of bacterial infection ↑ significantly when absolute neutrophil count <500cells/μL. Drugs causing neutropenia include AZT, ganciclovir, co-trimoxazole, pentamidine, α-interferon, and chemotherapeutic agents.

Diagnosis and evaluation

Careful review of medication. Withdraw offending drug(s) if absolute neutrophil count <500cells/μL. If cause uncertain, consider bone marrow examination.

Treatment
- HAART: variable response.
- Granulocyte colony-stimulating factor:
  - HIV-induced
  - drug-induced (if implicated drug cannot be reduced or stopped).

Coagulation disorders

↑ risk of thrombotic disease associated with low CD4 counts, OIs, neoplasms, and HIV-associated autoimmune disorders.
- High inflammatory state; increased D-dimer and cytokines are proposed factors in advanced disease.
- Lupus anticoagulant may be detected with thromboembolic disease.
- ↓ levels of active protein S frequently found, although not associated with immune suppression.
- Contributing prothrombotic factors include ↓ plasminogen activator inhibitor level, abnormal platelet aggregation, and ↑ von Willebrand factor.

Persistent generalized lymphadenopathy

Generalized lymphadenopathy involving ≥2 extra-inguinal sites persisting for more than 3 months. Of no prognostic significance, but other causes of generalized lymphadenopathy should be excluded. Occurs in up to 70% of patients within 1 year of seroconversion but may coexist with other manifestations of HIV infection. Lymph nodes usually symmetrical, >1cm in size, rubbery, and non-tender. May be accompanied by hepatosplenomegaly. Mediastinal lymphadenopathy usually has other causes.

Important diagnoses to consider in HIV-associated lymphadenopathy

- Persistent generalized lymphadenopathy
- Bacterial infections (including mycobacteria)
- 2° syphilis
- Lymphoma
- Histoplasmosis
- Multicentric Castleman's disease

HIV: malignancies

Introduction

The overall incidence of many malignancies ↑ in patients with HIV. The incidence increases as the CD4 count falls below 500cells/μL. Certain malignancies occur more frequently in HIV infection, especially when immunosuppressed, and are often associated with other viral co-infection.

The following are designated as AIDS-defining illnesses:
- Kaposi's sarcoma
- high-grade B-cell non-Hodgkin lymphoma
- invasive cervical carcinoma (ICC).

Other associated malignant conditions include squamous cell carcinoma (anogenital, conjunctival, labial, and glossal), multicentric Castleman's disease, testicular tumours (seminomas), melanomas, Hodgkin's disease, multiple myeloma, leiomyosarcoma in children, colon cancer, breast cancer, and lung cancer.

The following viral infections contribute to the induction of malignant disease in the immunosuppressed.
- Human herpes virus 8 (HHV-8)—KS and body cavity lymphomas.
  Found in ~100% of multicentric Castleman's disease.
- Human papilloma virus (HPV)—anogenital and occasionally oral carcinomas.
- Epstein–Barr virus (EBV)—non-Hodgkin lymphoma.
- Hepatitis B and C viruses—hepatocellular carcinoma.

Other factors such as specific sexual practices and cigarette smoking may play a part.

Overall risk of malignancy is doubled in an HIV-infected population. Natural history of malignancy may be altered in HIV infection with advanced rapidly progressive disease more likely. Treatment may be made difficult because of ↑ sensitivity to side-effects of chemotherapy if immunosuppressed and ↓ bone marrow reserve. HAART has had a dramatic effect on the incidence of some tumours, particularly 1° cerebral lymphoma.

Kaposi's sarcoma (KS)

Initially described in 1872 by Moritz Kaposi and rare before HIV epidemic. There are four different types.

- Classic—usually elderly ♂ from eastern Mediterranean/Europe. Causes multiple skin lesions of lower limbs.
- Endemic—children and young ♂ in equatorial Africa. More virulent than classic, often affecting lower limbs.
- Acquired—people on immunosuppressant therapy. Resolves when drugs stopped.
- Epidemic—associated with HIV infection. Variable but generally more aggressive than other types.

Caused by HHV-8 (found in >90% of KS lesions) spread sexually, by mother-to-child contact and organ transplant. High viral levels in saliva suggest oral contact as a route of transmission. In ♂ who have sex with ♂ (MSM) new HHV-8 infection is associated with an HIV +ve partner. No evidence to support transmission by semen (HHV-8 rarely detected) and conflicting data on the role of rimming.

Epidemic KS

Most common malignancy associated with HIV infection. Before HAART, it was the AIDS-defining disease in 15–20% of MSM (found in up to 50% of patients with AIDS by mid-1980s). The incidence of KS started to decline prior to HAART introduction, but substantially so afterwards. Predominantly found in MSM and rare among IV drug users, haemo-philiacs and ♀ (where more aggressive and usually associated with HIV acquisition from bisexual ♂). KS found more commonly in those with advanced disease but may occur with preserved CD4 count. Rarely sole cause of death unless there is pulmonary involvement when respiratory failure may supervene. Prevalence of KS in different HIV populations reflects the background seroprevalence for HHV-8.

Clinical features

Skin lesions

May occur on any part of the body but facial involvement common (margin of nostrils, tip of the nose, and eyelids) (Plate 22). Typical pigmented macules, papules, plaques, and nodules ranging in size from several millimetres to many centimetres. Colour varies from pink to deep purple with a yellow or green halo (extravasated erythrocyte pigments) characteristically surrounding them. Colourless subcutaneous nodules may also be found. In dark-skinned people the lesions are dark brown or black. Ulceration of nodules may lead to bleeding or infection. Large painful plaques may appear, especially on thighs and soles of feet. Pain suggests more progressive disease.

Oral lesions

Found in ~33% of those with epidemic KS, usually affecting hard palate (also gingiva, tongue, uvula, tonsils, pharynx, and trachea). Often asymptomatic, although may cause local symptoms related to their site and extent. Usually appear as focal or diffuse red/purple plaques which may become nodular and ulcerate. May indicate more extensive mucosal involvement.

Others

- GI tract: prior to HAART found in up to 40% patients with skin and nodal KS. Unless symptomatic their presence does not influence prognosis. May occur without skin lesions and may cause GI bleeding or obstruction.
- Respiratory: may involve lung parenchyma, bronchial tree, and pleura, leading to large blood-stained pleural effusions. Usual symptoms dyspnoea, haemoptysis, cough, and wheezing. Radiology often shows ill-defined nodules or areas of infiltration.
- Lymph nodes: modest lymphadenopathy common. Rarely massive lymphadenopathy (possibly without KS elsewhere) necessitating diagnostic biopsy. Extensive lymphadenopathy may suggest Castleman's disease.
- Lymphoedema: non-pitting, most commonly affecting feet and legs and may be complicated by ulceration and infection. May result from direct KS dermal lymphatic involvement.
- Hepatic, splenic, cardiac, pericardial, bone marrow involvement all rarely reported, usually at autopsy.

Social/emotional implications

Lesions often obvious and disfiguring, acting as a constant reminder and leading to isolation, anxiety, and depression.

Diagnosis and assessment

- Cutaneous KS is diagnosed clinically. If biopsy taken lesions can be graded into patch, plaque, or nodular.
- Dependent on symptoms and signs: appropriate investigations can be organized (e.g. radiology, scan, endoscopy).
- Biopsy is not always necessary, but should be done where diagnosis is not clear.
- HHV-8 antibody and viral load (VL) tests, but clinical implication unclear. VL ↓ when KS treated with chemotherapy and HAART.

Staging based on distribution of KS, CD4 count, and other HIV-associated symptoms/opportunistic infections (OIs) to determine level of risk for disease progression. Patients with localized disease, CD4 >150cells/μL and no systemic symptoms have good prognosis. Poor prognosis if both extensive tumours and systemic illness.

Management

HAART often significantly improves KS (in up to 80%) without further intervention. HAART should be offered to all patients. Additional treatment options depend on site, KS extent/activity, CD4 count, presence of systemic symptoms, and other OIs, past or present. These therapeutic interventions have been shown to improve survival and prolong time to KS treatment failure.

No interventional treatment

Consider if few skin lesions and no additional problems. Disfiguring lesions can be cosmetically camouflaged.

Local therapy

- Cryotherapy—small flat lesions on thin skin (e.g. face, genitals). Repeat treatment usually required. May leave hypopigmented scar.
- Radiotherapy—for lesions that are painful, causing lymphatic obstruction, oropharyngeal, or ophthalmic. Side-effects include local erythema, hair loss, mucositis, and pigmented scarring. Reported response rate is 74–91%. Despite initial response to irradiation, regrowth was common in the pre-HAART era.
- 9-*cis*-retinoic acid (alitretinoin) 0.1% gel: not licensed in Europe.
- Intra-lesional vinblastine, vincristine, or interferon α—limited mucocutaneous disease. Painful injections causing inflammatory response before lesions shrink or disappear leaving a scar. Repeat injections required and relapse within 6 months is common.

Liposomal chemotherapy

Patients with features suggesting poor prognosis should be given HAART in addition to liposomal daunorubicin ($40mg/m^2$ every 2 weeks) or pegylated liposomal doxorubicin ($20mg/m^2$ every 3 weeks). Those with good prognostic features can be given HAART alone. Liposomal doxorubicin and liposomal daunorubicin now standard of care for KS where treatment indicated. Preferentially absorbed by vascular KS lesions, producing targeted chemotherapy with ↓ side-effects. Main side-effects are bone marrow suppression (occurs in 50%, neutropenia can be treated with granulocyte colony-stimulating factor (G-CSF)), alopecia, and vomiting.

Paclitaxel (a taxane)

Second-line chemotherapy at a dose of $100mg/m^2$ every 14 days plus HAART. Main side-effects are bone marrow suppression, myalgia, alopecia, and allergic reactions.

▶ Prophylaxis against *Pneumocystis jiroveci* (*carinii*) pneumonia (PCP) should be provided during chemotherapy because of 2° immunosuppression.

Interferon α

Rarely used in the era of HAART. May have a place in those with residual KS after immune reconstitution. Main side-effects are flu-like symptoms, depression, and neutropenia (ameliorated by G-CSF although this ↑ constitutional symptoms).

Non-Hodgkin's lymphoma (NHL)

NHL is the second most common HIV-associated malignancy. First cases were reported in MSM in 1982. Prior to HAART it accounted for 2–3% of AIDS-defining illnesses, with haemophiliacs and those with other clotting disorders having the highest incidence. The incidence of AIDS-related NHL has decreased since the introduction of HAART, although the percentage as first AIDS-defining illness has increased.

Most NHLs are clinically aggressive monoclonal B-cell lymphomas, especially diffuse large B-cell lymphomas (DLBCL) and Burkitt's or Burkitt-like lymphomas (BLs). Other much less frequent subtypes of HIV-related lymphomas include primary CNS lymphomas (PCL), primary effusion lymphomas, and plasmablastic lymphomas. More common in σ and Caucasians. EBV episome is found in 40–50% overall, ranging from ~100% of PCL to 20% of DLBCL.

Systemic lymphoma

Wide range of CD4 count at presentation including normal levels, but median is 100cells/μL. Typically presents with lymphadenopathy, fever, weight loss (>10%), and night sweats. Extra-nodal disease (any site) usual, with GI tract, CNS, bone marrow, and liver being frequently affected. GI presentation most common, and NHL should be considered if suspicious symptoms (e.g. dysphagia, GI bleeding/pain).

Diagnosis and staging
- Biopsy of 1° lesion.
- Staging by CT/MRI scanning, presence of type B symptoms (fever, sweats), and bone marrow aspiration and trephine.
- Prognosis depends on a number of factors and is poor if >60years old, CD4 <100cells/μL, ↑ LDH, lymph node involvement above and below diaphragm, extra-nodal involvement, and/or poor function. Failure to attain complete remission is associated with a poor prognosis.

Management
- Multidisciplinary team including oncology.
- Diffuse large B-cell lymphoma: chemotherapy (improved tolerance if CD4 count >200cells/μL), usually cyclical. PCP prophylaxis should be taken as treatment causes immunosuppression. Regimen examples include the following.
  - HAART+ CHOP (cyclophosphamide, hydroxydaunomycin [doxorubicin], oncovin [vincristine], prednisolone) should be given full dose where possible (reduced dose CHOP ↓ remission rate). Addition of G-CSF reduces neutropenia. Reported complete remission 48%
  - HAART+ infusional chemotherapy (e.g. EPOCH (etoposide, prednisolone, vincristine, cyclophosphamide, and doxorubicin) or CDE (cyclophosphamide, doxorubicin, and etoposide).
  - Rituximab (monoclonal antibody causing B-cell lysis): may improve efficacy in combination with above regimes, but not recommended if CD4 <50/μL because of ↑ OI. More data needed.

- Previously responding patients should be considered for high-dose chemotherapy and stem-cell transplant if they relapse.
- Burkitt's lymphoma: poorer response seen with above chemotherapy. May require more aggressive regime such as the following.
  - Cyclophosphomide, vincristine, doxorubicin, methotrexate/ ifosfomide, etoposide, and cytarabine (CODOX-M/IVAC).
  - Cyclophosphomide, vincristine, doxorubicin, dexamethasone, methotrexate, and cytarabine (hyperCVAD).

Primary CNS lymphoma (PCL)

- These are DLBCL or immunoblastic lymphomas confined to the CNS with no systemic involvement. It is EBV induced, and is 1000× more frequent in those with HIV infection. Significantly lower incidence in the HAART era.
- Survival better with PCL and has ↑ since the introduction of HAART, although its optimal use during chemotherapy has not been established. Generally continue HAART (with close monitoring)—risk of ↓ drug levels (with indinavir, didanosine, efavirenz, nevirapine) and ↑ side-effects.
- Associated with very low CD4 count (<50cells/μL in 75%) and history of OIs. Usually presents with confusion, amnesia, and lethargy. In addition focal symptoms may appear (e.g. seizures, hemiparesis, cranial nerve palsies and aphasia).

Diagnosis

Difficult to distinguish from cerebral toxoplasmosis.

- CT/ MRI: single (~50%) or multiple lesions (former suggests PCL as only ~20% of those with toxoplasmosis have a single lesion).
- Fundal and slit-lamp examination (20% have ocular involvement).
- Lumbar puncture for:
  - lymphoma cells
  - EBV DNA using PCR +ve in ~90% of CNS lymphoma.
- Toxoplasma serology (toxoplasma unlikely if negative serology).
- Combined EBV detection in CSF and hyperactive lesion on single-photon emission CT (SPECT) has a very high sensitivity and specificity. If available makes brain biopsy unnecessary.
- Brain biopsy confirms the diagnosis.
- Failure to respond to 2 weeks anti-toxoplasma treatment equates to a presumptive diagnosis of primary brain lymphoma.

Management

- Initially consider anti-toxoplasma therapy in any space-occupying lesion.
- HAART ↑ survival but much inferior to that of other lymphomas.
- Whole-brain radiotherapy (usually with short-term dexamethasone to reduce oedema) for symptomatic palliation.
- Combined radiotherapy and chemotherapy, e.g. high-dose methotrexate and other agents that cross the blood–brain barrier.

Prognosis still poor and partly dependent on control of OIs.

Primary effusion lymphoma (body cavity lymphoma)

Accounts for 5% of HIV-associated lymphoma. Usually seen in MSM and associated with HHV 8 and co-infection with EBV in >50%. Characteristic features include involvement of the pleural, pericardial, and abdominal cavities as lymphomatous effusions in the absence of a solid tumour mass.

Treat with chemotherapy (similar to systemic lymphoma) but poor prognosis (2–5 months).

Multicentric Castleman's disease

Induced by HHV-8 in HIV infection. Characterized by recurrent lymphadenopathy, multiple organ involvement, hepatosplenomegaly, systemic symptoms, effusions and sometimes KS. Histological examination confirms the diagnosis and HHV-8 viral load is helpful.

Ideal treatment strategy unclear. Treat with chemotherapy (e.g. CHOP or single-agent chemotherapy), interferon α. Anti-CD20 monoclonal antibody (rituximab) may also be used as first-line therapy, for relapse, or following chemotherapy. Addition of HAART improves survival.

Hodgkin's disease

Although not an AIDS-defining illness, incidence is increased 10–20-fold compared with HIV-negative population. Tends to be more aggressive, with the mixed cellularity subtype predominating. Associated with EBV infection, usually developing with CD4 counts of 200–300cells/μL.

Presents with lymphadenopathy (glands often very large), Pel–Ebstein fever, anaemia, and systemic symptoms. Diagnosed by lymph node or bone marrow histology (Reed–Sternberg cells). Must have full staging assessment and bone marrow biopsy.

Treatment
- HAART
- First-line chemotherapy is ABVD (doxorubicin, bleomycin, vinblastine, and dacarbazine).

Prognosis

HAART combined with chemotherapy improves prognosis: disease-free survival and complete remission rates approach those of HIV-negative patients.

Invasive cervical carcinoma (ICC)

Added to the AIDS case definition in 1993 following reports showing ↑ prevalence of cervical dysplasia with HPV infection and immuno-suppression (usually severe). Cervical intra-epithelial neoplasia (CIN) is more common and recurs more in HIV-positive ♀ especially if CD4 <200/μL. However, no substantial clinical evidence demonstrating ↑ incidence of ICC in ♀ with HIV not explained by other risk factors. May be due to the possibility of longer latency, improved screening and treatment to those at risk, and improved immunity with HAART.

Newly diagnosed HIV +ve ♀ should have a baseline colposcopy followed by annual cervical smear. The age range for cervical smear should be the same as for HIV −ve individuals. ICC should be managed as for ♀ without HIV infection. Abnormal cytology should be investigated by colposcopy with biopsy of suspicious areas. Mild dyskaryosis (CIN I) should be followed every 3–6 months as spontaneous regression is common. Standard treatment for moderate/severe dyskaryosis (CIN II and III) consists of lesional ablation, excision, or hysterectomy.

Anal carcinoma

Anal cancer is more frequent in HIV +ve individuals and in MSM. However, the excess risk amongst HIV +ve MSM is difficult to quantify as anal receptive sexual intercourse is a strong independent risk factor for the two conditions. Similar to cervical cancer, high-grade HPV is an important aetiological factor. Prior to the HIV epidemic the relative risk of anal carcinoma in MSM was estimated to be 80× higher than in heterosexual controls. Recent data suggest that HIV-infected individuals with anal HPV infection are significantly more likely to develop high-grade dyskaryosis or anal carcinoma if they acquire other local infections (e.g. gonorrhoea, syphilis, HSV).

Screening for anal intra-epithelial neoplasia

Similar to the female cervix, the anal canal has a transformation zone (TZ) at the junction of the anal squamous and rectal columnar epithelia. HPV infection of metaplastic cells ↑ tendency to oncogenic transformation in the anal TZ and thus the development of cancer.

Similar to cervical cancer, anal cancer is preceded by pre-cancerous changes referred to as anal intra-epithelial neoplasia (AIN). The role of anal cytology and anoscopy to detect pre-cancerous changes is not yet decided. Patients should be encouraged to report any anal symptoms and be clinically examined and referred to local specialists units as appropriate. Annual anal digital examination, especially for homosexual men, should be considered. HAART does not appear to alter AIN progression or the incidence of invasive cancer.

Anal carcinoma is treated as for those without HIV. Limited data are available on management of anal dyskaryosis but current practice suggests that treatment (by excision or laser ablation) should only be considered if severe dyskaryosis (AIN3).

Leiomyosarcoma

↑ rate in children with HIV when, unlike in HIV uninfected children, tumours are induced by EBV.

Lung cancer

The incidence of non-small-cell lung cancer, and to some extent adeno-carcinoma, in HIV +ve individuals is higher than in age-matched HIV −ve controls. This difference is not explained by smoking alone. Compared with HIV −ve individuals, lung cancer usually occurs at a younger age and with advanced disease. Similar to HIV −ve individuals, it presents with cough, chest pain, haemoptysis, and dyspnoea. HAART does not improve survival; median time is 4 months. Patients with operable or locally advanced disease should be treated similar to HIV −ve individuals and HAART should be commenced if they are not already on it. Patients with metastatic disease may have palliative chemotherapy (poorly tolerated) and HAART interrupted.

Hepatocellular carcinoma (HCC)

Generally seen in context of HCV and/or HBV co-infection. Overall poor prognosis (28% 1 year survival) in HIV +ve patients. Presents at later stage and with more aggressive tumours than HIV −ve patients. If offered active treatment, survival approaches HIV −ve population. Screening for HCC should be used in specific groups (📖 Chapter 41). Solitary small lesions can be resected even if multiple. Liver transplant may be considered if cirrhotic. Ethanol injections and chemo-embolization may be used palliatively and lead to significant improvement in life expectancy.

HIV: management

Introduction

Highly active antiretroviral therapy (HAART) has produced dramatic improvements in the prognosis of HIV infection with ↓ rates of mortality and opportunist infections (OIs).

Important principles to consider in those under regular review are as follows.

- Treat before symptomatic disease or critical immunological damage.
- Avoid treating earlier than necessary to ↓ long term drug side-effects.
- Regimen choice must consider patient lifestyle, potential drug inter-actions, and side-effects while ensuring adequate antiviral potency.

Patient's commitment to starting treatment is essential. Pre-treatment adherence education is vital as adherence must be >95% to obtain both maximum magnitude and duration of antiviral effect. HAART rarely needs starting as an emergency.

Drug resistance should be assayed pre-treatment, ideally at diagnosis, because of possible resistant viral transmission.

When to start

Primary infection

Prime indication for treatment is severe symptoms (which may indicate risk of more rapid progression to symptomatic disease). These may resolve with HAART. Treatment duration is undefined and its influence on subsequent clinical course is uncertain.

Chronic infection

In the asymptomatic patient, the likelihood of developing clinical AIDS over a 3 year period can be predicted from a combination of viral load (VL) and CD4 count (Fig. 53.1). CD4 counts give the best indication of OI risk but high VLs are associated with more rapid rates of CD4 ↓.

HAART should be offered:

- if HIV-related symptoms (independent of VL and CD4 count) are observed
- if there is AIDS-defining illness regardless of CD4 count (except tuberculosis (TB) with a CD4 >350cells/μL)
- before CD4 counts have fallen <350cells/μL. The point of maximum 'cost-effectiveness' has not been defined by trial data, but the consensus is that treatment should be commenced with CD4 counts of 200–350cells/μL depending on:
  - rapidity of CD4 ↓
  - VL level
  - patient's preference
- patients with CD4 counts between 350 cells/μL and 500 cells/μL may be considered for treatment if:
  - HCV + ve and treatment delayed
  - HBV + ve requiring treatment
  - high cardiovascular risk
  - low CD4 percentage (<14%) or AIDS defining illness.

Other factors, e.g. older age (↑ speed of development of immuno-deficiency) should also be considered. In pregnancy, treatment may be given to ↓ risk of mother-to-child transmission when such therapy may not be indicated in the non-pregnant state.

Starting HAART at very low CD4 counts ↑ drug side-effects, although with nevirapine hepatotoxicity is ↑ by CD4 counts >250cells/µL. In patients with active OIs commencement of HAART should not be deferred for a long time. Where there are significant drug interactions such as in TB/HIV co-infection HAART can be delayed if CD4 >200 cells/µL until completion or simplification of treatment. Once started, treatment (except when given for fetal protection) should be continued indefinitely.

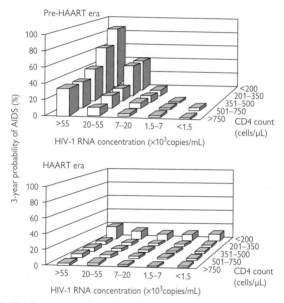

Fig. 53.1 Prognosis according to CD4 cell count and viral load in the pre-HAART and HAART eras. Reprinted from Egger M et al., Lancet **360**, 119–29, 2002.© 2002 with permission from Elsevier.

How to start

Initial treatment influences the pattern of resistance mutations. If it fails, the range of drugs available for 2nd-line therapy is restricted. Therefore the following are important aims for the first treatment.

- Maximize adherence—especially important for regimens containing drugs where resistance may be produced by single mutations (e.g. lamivudine and NNRTIs). Treatment based on a ↓ CD4 count should be continued long term. Intermittent therapy should only be considered in those achieving full viral suppression. For fully informed patients insisting on this option, the interruption of long-half-life drugs needs special care. If efavirenz is involved, NRTI backbone should be continued for 2 weeks at least after efavirenz cessation with or without a PI.
- Minimize drug reactions.
- Include drugs with good penetration to the central nervous system.
- Avoid toxicity/interaction. Toxicity of some antiretroviral drugs (e.g. stavudine causing lipodystrophy) makes them unsuitable as 1st-line therapy. Drug combinations with additive toxicity (e.g. didanosine + stavudine) and shared intracellular activation pathways (e.g. zidovudine and stavudine) should be avoided (📕 Antiretroviral drug combinations to avoid p. 585).

Drug interations between antiretrovirals and other drugs the patient is taking or is likely to take must be considered, all drugs should be checked against a reliable database.

Drug combinations in the treatment naive should take account of resistance testing, co-pathologies, risk factors for diabetes and cardiovascular disease, lifestyle, and informed patient choice.

Adherence

Essential for successful viral suppression. Stress importance prior to starting treatment and continually reinforce as adherence may diminish with time.

Sub-therapeutic drug levels select for HIV-resistant mutations arising from error-prone viral replication. Some regimens have a low genetic barrier to resistance. Investing in strategies that improve adherence is more cost effective than managing the consequences of poor compliance. Such strategies will also minimize the risk of transmission of drug-resistant virus which may adversely affect HAART response in the newly infected.

Factors influencing adherence

- Patient
  - Commitment
  - Religious/cultural/health beliefs
  - Poor diet (may be related to socio-economic difficulties)
  - Need to take medication (seen by family/workmates)
  - Drug and alcohol use
  - Psychological (depression associated with low adherence)
  - Presence of symptoms/side-effects (may encourage/discourage adherence, respectively)
  - Relationship with healthcare team
- Provider
  - Provision of adherence support services
  - Patient education
- Regimen
  - Lifestyle assessment and compliance with regimen
  - Dosing frequency, pill burden, and food/fluid requirements

How to improve adherence

A multifactorial approach should be adopted, taking account of the patient's perceptions of the benefits as well as the practicalities of treatment. The individual's commitment to taking drugs should be assessed before starting therapy and at regular intervals. Concerns about drug side-effects should be explored. Motivational techniques can help patients to strengthen their intentions and adherence behaviour. Psychosocial aspects including relationships, alcohol and drug use, housing, employment, and immigration status should be considered, with appropriate professional involvement. The following measures may improve adherence:

- Programmable wristwatches, text messaging, telephone reminders, pill diaries and charts, medication containers, and help of family and friends
- Input from nurses, health advisers, psychologists, and pharmacists
- Written information.

There is no ideal and accurate method of monitoring adherence. Self-reporting, pill counting, self-completed questionnaires, and drug levels have all been used with varying success.

What to start with

Current classes of antiretroviral drugs inhibit the virus at different stages of its cellular lifecycle (Fig. 53.2):
- interaction with CD4/chemokine receptors—fusion inhibitors/CCR5 inhibitors
- inhibition of reverse transcription (conversion of viral RNA to pro-viral DNA)
  - nucleoside–nucleotide reverse transcriptase inhibitors (NRTIs)
  - non-nucleoside reverse transcriptase inhibitors (NNRTIs)
- inhibition of protease processing of viral sub-units leading to assembly of infective virions—protease inhibitors (PIs).

Combination treatment

Triple combinations are the standard of care. The drug classes have differing side-effects, drug interactions, and impact on co-pathologies. Individual drugs, within classes, may have significantly better convenience, tolerability, or side-effect profiles than others, e.g. atazanavir (PI) ↓ effect on lipids and once-daily therapy.

Standard regimens for both asymptomatic and late diseases
- Two NRTIs (beware inadvisable combinations—📖 Antiretroviral drug combinations to avoid) plus an NNRTI.
- Two NRTIs plus a PI (usually boosted with low-dose ritonavir).
- Triple nucleoside analogue combinations are not recommeded as first line therapy.

	NNRTI	**PI**
Advantages	1. Low pill burden	1. ↓skin rash/hepatotoxicity
	2. ↓lipid abnormalities + central fat accumulation	2. ↓broad class resistance
	3. Once-daily dosage possible	3. High barrier to genetic resistance (e.g. Kaletra®)
Disadvantages	1. Class resistance with single mutations	1. Heavy pill burden (most)
	2. Ineffective against HIV-2 (inherent resistance)	2. Hyperlipidaemia, insulin resistance, lipodystrophy, central fat distribution if predisposed
	3. Low grade barrier to resistance	3. ↑ drug interactions
		4. ↑ food/fluid requirements/ restrictions especially when unboosted

Currently most treatment-naive patients are started on NNRTI regimens. Efavirenz and nevirapine have different side-effect profiles but are of equivalent potency. Nevirapine is associated with skin rash and hepatic reactions (↑ risk in women with CD4 >250 cells/μL and men with CD4 >400 cells/μL), and efavirenz with neuropsychological side-effects and potential teratogenicity.

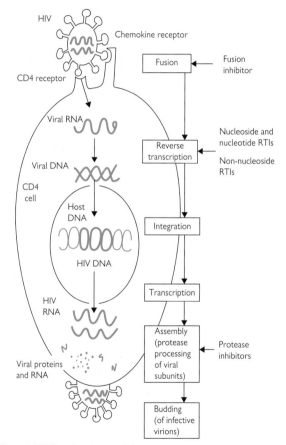

Fig. 53.2 HIV life cycle and points of drug action

NRTIs (nucleotide—tenofovir). All oral

Abacavir*(ABC)	300mg bd	Hypersensitivity (may be fatal) in 4% (associated with HLA–B* 5701, test prior to starting ABC and if +ve should not be commenced): fever, malaise, rash, GI. **Do not rechallenge**.
Didanosine†(DDI)	400mg if >60kg (or 300mg) daily	Take on empty stomach. Peripheral neuropathy, pancreatitis, nausea, diarrhoea. Rarely lactic acidosis, hepatic steatosis.
Emtricitabine(FTC)	200mg daily	Minimal. Rarely lactic acidosis, hepatic steatosis.
Lamivudine*(3TC)	150mg bd or 300mg daily†	Minimal. Rarely lactic acidosis, hepatic steatosis.
Stavudine*(D4T)	40mg if >60kg (or 30mg) bd	Peripheral neuropathy, lipodystrophy, pancreatitis, lactic acidosis, hepatic steatosis.
Zidovudine*(AZT)	250–300mg bd	Bone marrow suppression (anaemia, neutropenia), myopathy. Rarely lactic acidosis, hepatic steatosis.
Tenofovir(TDF)	300mg daily	Asthenia, headache, GI, rarely renal insufficiency (approximately 0.5%).

*Consistent CSF penetration.
†Reduce to 250mg when combined with TDF.

Combined preparations

Combivir®	1 tablet bd, contains AZT 300mg + 3TC 150mg
Trizivir®	1 tablet bd, contains AZT 300mg + 3TC 150mg + ABC 300mg
Truvada®	1 tablet daily, contains TDF 300mg and FTC 200mg
Kivexa®	1 tablet daily contains ABC 600mg and 3TC 300mg
Atripla	1 tablet OD, contains EFV 600mg and Truvada

NNRTIs. All oral and show evidence of consistent CSF penetration

Efavirenz (EFV)	600mg daily	CNS effects (advise take at night), hepatitis, contra-indicated in pregnancy
Nevirapine (NVP)	200mg bd or 400mg/day	Initially 200mg/day ↑ to 400mg/day after 2 weeks Rash, Stevens–Johnson syndrome, hepatitis
Delavirdine (DLV)	400mg tid	Diarrhoea, itching, and rashNot routinely available in the UK
Etravirine (ETV)	200mg bd	May be used following resistance with other NNRTIs (requires 3 mutations to confer resistance), rash, diarrhoea.

Boosted PI dosages with ritonavir (RTV), 100mg bd (except Kaletra® which already includes RTV) or 100mg daily with ATV. All oral. When boosted, food restrictions are not critical. Only IDV shows evidence of consistent CSF penetration

Atazanavir (ATV)	300mg daily	Indirect hyperbilirubinaemia, cardiac conduction defect (prolonged PR interval)
Darunavir	600mg bd	Take with food, lipodystrophy, GI
Fosamprenavir (FPV)	700mg bd (Sol^n 50mg/mL = 14mLs bd plus RTV Sol^n)	GI, rash, lipodystrophy (less than other PIs)
Indinavir (IDV)	800mg bd	Nephrolithiasis, GI, indirect hyperbilirubinaemia lipodystrophy. ↑ fluids by 2L
Kaletra®Lopinavir (LPV) 1 tab = LPV 200mg + RTV 50mg	2 tabs bd Sol^n: 5mL bd	GI, ↑ transaminases, asthenia, lipodystrophy, solution with food
Saquinavir (SQV)	1.0g bd	GI, headache, ↑ transaminase, lipodystrophy
Tipranavir (TPV)	500mg bd + 200mg RTV bd	Take with food, GI, lipodystrophy, hepatotoxity

PIs used without additional PI boosting. Both oral

Nelfinavir(NFV)	1.25g bd	Take with food
		Diarrhoea, transaminase, lipodystrophy
Ritonavir (RTV)	600mg bd	Take with food
		GI, parasthesia, hepatitis, raised
		↑ transaminase, pancreatitis, lipodystrophy

Fusion inhibitor (FI). Licensed for treatment failure. SC administration

Enfuvirtide(ENF)	90mg bd	Injection site reaction, ↑ pneumonia, hypersensitivity reaction (may recur on re-challenge)

CCR5 inhibitors, licensed for treatment failure

Maraviroc	150mg, 300mg, 600mg bd depending on interactions with other drugs in regime	Do viral tropism test (VL needs to be >1000) prior to starting. Not effective against CXCR4-tropic virus. Cough, fever, URTI, rash

---

Integrase inhibitors, licensed for treatment failure

Raltegravir	400mg bd	Abdominal pain, constipation, itching

Antiretroviral drug combinations to avoid

- D4T + AZT: thymidine analogues compete for the same intracellular enzyme plus antagonistic effect
- FTC + 3TC: cytosine analogues—no additive activity;
- ABC + 3TC + TDF: ↑ virological failure.
- DDI + TDF + EFZ: ↑ virological failure in treatment-naive patients.
- ETV + TPV/r or unboosted PI—↓ of ETV level, ↑ PI level.

Caution

- DDI and D4T: ↑ peripheral neuropathy, lactic acidosis, and acute pancreatitis, especially in pregnancy
- EFV + r/ATV or LPV/r—monitoring of PI levels may be needed.
- EFV + maraviroc—use 600mg bd of maraviroc
- Boosted PI (excl. fosamprenavir/tipranavir) + maraviroc +/– EFV—use 150mg bd of maraviroc.
- FPV or tipranavir and maraviroc—use 300mg bd of maraviroc.
- ETV + boosted ATV or FPV—decrease AZT level, increase FPV.

Monitoring therapy

Side-effects are very common with HAART, although most resolve spontaneously after a few weeks. Patients should be asked to report side-effects and be given written information about serious complications, e.g. abacavir hypersensitivity reactions. Consideration should be given to providing anti-emetics and anti-diarrhoeal agents for the common early GI symptoms. Sedatives may be needed for severe EFV-associated insomnia/vivid dreams.

Routine tests

- Full blood count, liver /renal function tests—should be checked 2 weeks into treatment and then at subsequent clinic visits. Patients who develop abnormal LFTs or a significant anion gap should have plasma lactate level checked.
- VL—the rate of fall on therapy is a useful prognostic indicator. Whatever the pre-treatment VL, suppression to a level of ≤1000copies/mL is achievable in most patients by 4 weeks. When not attained, associated with longer-term failure. The success of a treatment combination can be judged by achieving VL <50copies/mL within 3–6 months, which is then maintained for 48 weeks.
- CD4 count—usually ↑ with viral suppression initially as a result of recirculated existing reserves. Further ↑ and maintenance of continuous production of CD4 cells depends ability of thymus to produce new T cells. Complete restoration does not occur in most chronically infected patients, but immune reconstitution occurs to varying degrees even in those who achieve limited viral suppression. Prophylaxis against PCP can be discontinued in those responding to therapy (CD4 count >200cells/µL for at least 3–6 months).

Both CD4 and VL should be checked and repeated at 4 weeks and 12 weeks into therapy and then at 3 monthly intervals if virological control is achieved.

- Lipid profiles should be checked 3 monthly and major abnormalities addressed. Monitor for the development of lipodystrophy and consider early treatment switches if apparent. Elevated random lipids should be remeasured while fasting. Calculate cardiovascular risk. Patients with high risk or major abnormalities should be referred or treated.
- Blood sugar levels should be monitored, particularly with PI therapy. Fasting blood sugar should be measured if random level elevated.
- Creatinine clearance and urine protein/creatinine ratio (using a formula, e.g. MDM) should be done 3 monthly–yearly.

Adherence reinforcement should be undertaken at each visit. Risk of acquisition of co-infections and STIs should be assessed and tested for when appropriate.

Specific tests

- Tenofovir—phosphate should be measured pre-treatment and monthly for 1yr followed by every 3 months. Careful assessment for Fanconis syndrome and renal review should be undertaken for patients with CrCl <50mL/min or phosphate <1mg/dL.

- Abacavir—HLA B* 5701 (approx 5% of Caucasians, rare in sub-Saharan Africa) testing should be performed in all patients before starting. Patients +ve for HLA B* 5701 should not be started on abacavir. HLA B* 5701 has −ve predictive value for immunologically confirmed hypersensitivity of 100%.
- Maraviroc—Trofile™ assay should be performed, only patients with CCR5 tropic virus should be started on maraviroc.

Therapeutic drug monitoring (TDM)

Up to 35% of patients taking PIs have sub-optimal drug concentrations with ~50% developing virological failure. A fixed drug dose may not be appropriate for all patients. Measuring drug levels to determine therapeutic dose may help promote durable viral suppression and ↓ resistance. Dose–response and concentration–response relationships have been identified for PIs and NNRTIs (some data for NRTIs).

Potential use of TDM

Only of value if highly adherent (>95%) and at steady-state conditions (after at least 14 days of therapy). Blood samples should be obtained at the end of the dosing interval, as close to minimum concentration (C_{min}) as possible, to enable comparison with product monograph concentrations. TDM can be of benefit in the following.

- Pregnant ♀ and children—may have altered/highly variable pharmaco-kinetics.
- Highly adherent individuals who have poor initial or transient viral responses not explained by viral resistance. In these situations C_{min} values may assist in assessing genetically determined high hepatic metabolic rates, poor absorption, or drug interactions that prevent adequate drug levels. Adjusting antiretroviral doses to achieve C_{min} values within 30% of the mean/median value of the product monograph may ↑ likelihood of adequate therapeutic levels and viral response.
- Those on new drug therapy with unknown/potential drug interactions.
- Those on once daily PI—ensures adequate 24 hour drug concentration.

Major drug side-effects and interactions

See Table 53.1

Mitochondrial toxicity

A mechanism by which NRTIs may cause myopathy, peripheral neuropathy, hepatic steatosis, lactic acidosis, and, in infants, neurological disease. The link is strongest with lactic acidosis which has been reported in infants born to mothers receiving AZT or 3TC + AZT. D4T + DDI has been associated with lactic acidosis in pregnancy and should be avoided/switched. Caused by inhibition of mitochondrial γ DNA polymerase, the enzyme responsible for DNA synthesis, but effects on other mitochondrial enzymes may contribute. D4T and DDI inhibit γ DNA polymerase, whereas AZT inhibits other mitochondrial enzymes. Hence toxicity induced by D4T improves on switching to AZT or ABC.

Hyperlactataemia

Clinical significance of isolated hyperlactataemia (venous lactate between 2.5 and 5.0mmol/L) unknown. Routine measurement of venous lactate and anion gap in asymptomatic patients not recommended.

Lactic acidosis

Characterized by arterial pH <7.35 and venous lactate >5mmol/L (sample taken without tourniquet into tube containing fluoride-oxalate, transported immediately on ice to laboratory). Occurs most frequently with D4T and in ♀. Usually develops after several months of treatment. Main features are nausea, vomiting, weight loss, fatigue, abdominal pain, tender hepatomegaly, and respiratory failure. Laboratory findings:

- venous lactate >5.0mmol/L, metabolic acidosis, high anion gap (usually >18mmol/L)
- ultrasound and CT abdomen—hepatomegaly with fatty infiltration (microvascular steatosis found on liver biopsy)
- may find ↑ hepatic transaminases, creatine kinase, lactate dehydrogenase, and amylase.

Management

Diagnosis must be considered in any patient presenting with nausea, vomiting, abdominal pain, and abnormal LFTs. Essential to discontinue antiretroviral medication and exclude other causes. Supportive therapy required with fluid replacement, oxygen therapy, and, if necessary, assisted ventilation and haemodialysis. Benefit from carnitine, thiamine, co-enzyme Q, and riboflavin is limited.

Table 53.1 Important antiretroviral interactions with other drugs

Drug	Antiretroviral therapy	Effect	Action
Terfenadine	All PIs and NNRTIs	Dangerous arrhythmias	Use loratidine or cetirizine
Midazolam and triazolam	All PIs and EFV	Increased sedating effect	Use alternative sedative
Rifampicin	All PIs and NNRTIs	Complex effect on cytochrome P450	Use rifabutin instead
Rifabutin	SQV	↓ SQV by 40%	Do not use SQV unless RTV boosted
Rifabutin	RTV	↑ rifabutin 4-fold,	↓ rifabutin dose to 150mg/day, continue same dose of RTV
Rifabutin	Other PIs	↑ rifabutin level and ↓ PI level	↓ rifabutin to 150mg/day and ↑ PI dose as appropriate
Phosphodiesterase-5 inhibitors(used for erectile dysfunction)	All PIs	↑ blood levels andside-effects	Use smallest possible dose
Methadone	NNRTIs	↑ metabolism of methadone leading to withdrawal symptoms	↑ methadone dose
Simvastatin	All PIs and DLV	Large ↑ in simvastatin levels— myositis	Use pravastatin or low dose artovastatin

All PIs are substrate and inhibitors of cytochrome P450 (CYP450)—RTV is the strongest and SQV is the weakest.
NNRTIs NVP and EFV induce CYP450.
St John's wort (*Hypericum perforatum*) is a strong inducer of CYP450 and should not be used with PIs or NNRTIs.

Peripheral neuropathy

Risk of drug-induced peripheral neuropathy ↑ with HIV disease progression. Reported with NRTIs; more frequent with D4T and DDI. Presents with distal symmetric polyneuropathy (DSP), which may be difficult to differentiate from HIV-related DSP but tends to be painful, more sudden, and progressive. Discontinuation of the offending NRTI may result in improvement, but symptoms may deteriorate for several weeks. Pain relief may be obtained with acetyl-L-carnitine, tricyclic antidepressants, anticonvulsants (gabapentin and lamotrigine), and recombinant human nerve growth factor.

Abnormal liver function test and hepatotoxicity

Reported with all classes of antiretrovirals. ↑ in ♂ and those with other predisposing risk factors, e.g. excessive alcohol consumption, HBV and HCV infections. Abnormal LFTs graded from 1 (ALT 2–3 × upper limit of normal) to 4 (ALT >10 × upper limit of normal). Minor abnormalities do not require intervention apart from monitoring.

Abnormal LFTs found in those on antiretroviral treatment:

- NRTIs—commonly reported with DDI, D4T, and AZT. Hepatotoxicity— part of ABC hypersensitivity (usually associated with skin rash, fever, and eosinophilia)
- NNRTIs—8% with EFV and 15% NVP (hepatotoxicity in 4%). ♀ and those with higher CD4 count at ↑ risk.
- PIs—up to 30%, most frequent with RTV-containing regimens. Co-infection with HCV infection reported in most.

Avoidance and management

Careful history including alcohol intake. Screen for HBV and HCV. Important to measure LFTs before starting HAART. Asymptomatic ↑ of ALT (especially grade 1–3) does not normally require any action apart from close monitoring, exclusion, and treatment of underlying aggravating factors. Isolated hyperbilirubinaemia 2° to IDV and ATV not clinically significant.

Specific action required with:

- grade 4 ALT ↑—stop offending drugs
- symptomatic hepatotoxicity—stop all drugs until symptoms resolve; NVP should not be restarted if it was the cause
- symptomatic ↑ of ALT with hyperlactaemia—stop offending drugs
- ABC hypersensitivity reaction—stop immediately and do not re-challenge (fatal reaction).

Acute pancreatitis

Most commonly implicated NRTIs are DDI (up to 7%) and D4T. They should not be combined. Possibly caused by mitochondrial toxicity or direct toxic effect of the pancreas. Risk ↑ in ♀, especially with CD4 <200cell/μL, excessive alcohol use, and nutritional deficiencies.

Presents with acute abdomen ± nausea and vomiting. Differentiate from other causes of acute abdomen, e.g. cholecystitis and intestinal obstruction. Serum amylase usually ↑; may be normal (can also be ↑ in other causes of acute abdomen). DDI can ↑ salivary amylase, usually associated with sicca syndrome. Diagnostic accuracy higher if serum lipase also ↑. Ultrasound and CT scan of the abdomen may help to establish diagnosis, extent of disease, and complications, e.g. pancreatic abscess, pseudocyst.

Management

Monitor circulatory, renal, and liver functions (in a high dependency unit if necessary). Support with analgesia, fluid, and nutrition. Stop anti-retrovirals or substitute the implicated drug with TDF or a non-NRTI regimen.

Drug-related skin rash

Skin reactions are common. Most frequently found with NNRTIs (NVP 16%, EFV 4%) and ABC 8%. NVP-induced rash typically occurs in first 2 weeks of therapy. An induction dose of half the maintenance dose for 2 weeks minimizes this risk. Typically maculopapular, affecting the trunk. Systemic symptoms occur, with more severe reactions seen especially with ABC. Toxic epidermal necrolysis and Stevens–Johnson syndrome reported in 0.5%.

Management

Mild skin rash does not require intervention and will often settle spontaneously (with continuation of antiretrovirals). Antihistamines may be needed for symptomatic relief. More severe reactions need drug switching, e.g. EFV may replace NVP.

ABC hypersensitivity reaction

Occurs in ~4%, usually in the first 6 weeks of therapy (94%)—median 11 days. Normally presents with ≥2 of following features: GI tract (nausea, vomiting, diarrhoea, pain), headache, fever, malaise, maculopapular or urticarial rash, abnormal LFTs, myalgia, dyspnoea, cough, respiratory distress, and eosinophilia. Once suspected, ABC should be stopped promptly and supportive treatment instituted. Symptoms, except rash, resolve in 24–48 hours.
⚠ ABC should not be used again as mortality from re-challenge is 4%.

Lipodystrophy (📖 Chapter 47, Metabolic disorders p. 539.)

Immune reconstitution

CD4 count ↑ on HAART mainly due to CD4 memory cells in first 4 months then followed by ↑ naive cells associated with ↓ CD4 activation markers due to ↓ viral replication. Initial phase of CD8 ↑ followed by a second phase of ↓. Most studies demonstrate ↓ HIV-specific immune responses and ↓ CD8 responses towards HIV. This contrasts with ↑ immune responses against other pathogens. ↓ incidence of OIs in patients who have higher CD4 counts from HAART. HIV damages thymus and lymphoid tissue at an early stage and may ↓ immune recovery. ↓ immune response may be due in part to failure of the thymus, as demonstrated by ↓ thymus emigrants measured in peripheral blood. The lower the CD4 nadir, the slower and less complete immune reconstitution is likely to be.

Immune recovery inflammatory response (IRIS)

Inflammatory response induced by HAART occurring at sites of clinical and subclinical disease, usually seen in patients with CD4 count <100cells/µL at the initiation of therapy. The enhanced immunity is the likely mechanism converting a subclinical infection to an apparent symptomatic one due to the expansion of CD4 memory cells. Examples of IRIS include the following.

- Cytomegalovirus retinitis: 4–8 weeks after HAART. Immune recovery uveitis may occur in patients with previous CMV retinitis. Patients with active and subclinical infection and those with CD4 <50/µL are at special risk.
- HCV: restoration of HCV-specific responses occurs during HAART in patients with pre-existing HCV infection. Patients with negative HCV antibody but detectable HCV-RNA seroconvert with immune restoration. HCV-RNA levels ↑ with HAART, especially if treatment is started when CD4 count >350cells/µL. Accompanied by transient ALT ↑.
- *Mycobacterium avium* complex (MAC): presents with localized disease, e.g. painful lymphadenopathy or inflammatory masses associated with suppuration, unlike classical MAC where it is a disseminated infection. Due to the restoration of delayed hypersensitivity.
- Herpes zoster: ↑ by five times the expected rate, occurring in the first 4 months of HAART. Seen more frequently in those who develop a significant CD8 ↑.
- TB: paradoxical tuberculous reaction, e.g. ↑ in lymph node size, fever, and appearance of TB at other sites. Usually occurs in first 2 months (often 2–4 weeks) of starting TB therapy. Medication should not be routinely stopped. Steroids may be beneficial in controlling inflammatory process.
- Herpes simplex virus: more frequent and severe disease occurs in patients responding to HAART.
- Progressive multifocal leukoencephalopathy: may present for the first time or become worse in patients responding to HAART. Inflammatory brain changes (perivascular lymphocyte, macrophage, and plasmacell infiltrate) are more severe. CD8 seems to mediate the immuno-pathological process to JC virus.

Frequently asked questions

When do I start treatment?

Treatment is usually started when the CD4 level ↓, ideally below 350cells/μL and certainly before it reaches 200cells/μL. The aim of treatment is to suppress viral replication, measured by the viral load (VL), and this should later be followed by ↑ in CD4 count. A combination of three antiretroviral drugs is usually used termed HAART (highly active antiretroviral therapy).

What is drug resistance?

The HIV virus can develop resistance by mutating so that it can replicate despite the antiretroviral treatment. This most commonly arises when medication is not taken reliably. If a person is infected with a drug-resistant strain of HIV virus, their treatment options will be ↓ (sometimes severely).

Do I need to use condoms even if my partner is also known to be HIV positive?

Yes. It is important to practice safe sex to avoid superinfection (becoming infected with another strain of HIV) which may adversely affect the immune system and carry drug resistance.

Does it matter if I forget to take my medication for a few days?

Yes. It is very important that you take your anti-HIV drugs regularly. If doses are missed, the virus may not be suppressed and there is ↑ risk of viral mutations and drug resistance.

If my VL is undetectable, does it mean that I am no longer infectious?

No. An undetectable VL does not mean that there is no virus in the blood. It just means that there are too few particles to be detected by the test. There is still a risk of transmission with a low VL and so you must continue to practice safe sex.

When will I get AIDS?

Current therapy has had a dramatic effect in improving the wellbeing and life expectancy of people with HIV. Effective therapy makes HIV a chronic rather than a life-threatening infection. Therefore it is likely that you may not develop AIDS. Some people never need treatment, but if it is started it must be taken consistently and probably for life.

HIV drug resistance

May be intrinsic, e.g. HIV-2 resistance to NNRTIs, or acquired as a result of mutations in viral proteins targeted by antiretroviral agents. Two factors drive mutations: high rate of viral replication (10^{8-10} virions produced daily) and error-prone reverse transcription (1 base pair substitution, deletion, insertion, recombination for every genome transcription). Examples of resistance mutations are shown in Table 53.2

1° mutation predates antiretroviral treatment which selects for it. 2° mutation develops during HAART and may be additive to 1° mutation. HAART ↓ development of resistance by suppressing viral replication and thus generation of new variants. It can also suppress existing mutants if they are not resistant to all drugs in the regimen. However, resistance emerges if drug levels are insufficient to block viral replication but high enough to exert a positive selective pressure on these mutants. Even with undetectable VL, low-level replication may allow resistance to develop. Drug resistance has been demonstrated in up to 25% of patients on HAART. Compensatory (2°) mutation reverses ↓ viral fitness resulting from other mutations. Some mutations induce resistance to certain agents while simultaneously producing hypersusceptibility to others (e.g. M184V ↑ sensitivity to AZT).

Mutations

Many mutations ↓ viral fitness. However, resistance mutations confer a selective advantage by ↓ susceptibility to antiviral agents, thereby enabling the mutant quasi-species to proliferate under treatment with those agents. Resistance mutations are described using a number referring to the affected codon (group of three nucleotides coding for an amino acid). A letter may be added after the number to denote the amino acid in the mutant, e.g. 74V (**V**aline). This may be coupled with another letter preceding the number to show the wild-type amino acid, e.g. L74V (**L**eucine → **V**aline). Resistance develops rapidly (within weeks of commencing treatment) if only a single mutation is required e.g. M184V (3TC, FTC) and K103N (NVP). It evolves more gradually if multiple mutations are required, e.g. AZT, ABC, or PIs. Additional requirements may include a compensatory mutation, e.g. 30N (NFV).

K65R mutation (selected by TDF, ABC and DDI) confers resistance to TDF, ABC, and 3TC and ↑ susceptibility to AZT and D4T. This mutation develops rapidly when regimens combining TDF with two of ABC, DDI or 3TC are given to the treatment naive. Coexistence of K65R and M184V ↑ resistance to ABC and DDI but retains susceptibility to TDF, AZT, and D4T. Regimens with TDF must include AZT or a PI/NNRTI. Multiple mutations may interact. Resulting resistance patterns can be predicted by matching with resistance profile databases. This is provided by commercial resistance tests (e.g. *Virtual* Phenotype™).

Databases of resistance profiles are available at:
- http://hivdb.stanford.edu (Stanford Database)
- ℵ www.hiv.lanl.gov/content/index (Los Alamos Database)
- ℵ www.hivfrenchresistance.org (HIV-1 genotypic drug resistance interpretation's algorithms).

Table 53.2 Examples of resistance mutations (affected codons)

Nucleoside and nucleotide

3TC/FTC	184, 44, 118
ABC	65, 74, 115, 184
AZT/D4T	41, 44, 67, 70, 118, 210, 215, 219 (Thymidine analogue mutations—TAMs, now known as multi-NRTI associated—NAMs)
DDI	65, 74
TDF	65, ≥3 NAMs including 41 or 210
Multi-nucleoside	
'151 complex'	62, 75, 77, 116, 151
69 insertion complex	41, 62, 67, 69 (insertion), 70, 210, 215, 219

NNRTI

EFV/NVP single	103, 106, 188	
requiring 2	100, 181, 190, 230	
ETV †	*Mutation*	*Score*
	Y181V or Y181I	3.0
	K101P, L100I, Y181C, or M230L	2.5
	E138A, V106I, G190S, or V179F	1.5
	V90I, V179D, K101E, K101H, A98G, V179T, or G190A	1.0

† Viral response according to score: 0–2 = 74%, 2.5–3.5 = 52%, ≥4=38%.

Integrase inhibitor

Raltegravir	92Q, 138K, 148H/K/R, 155H, 47G, 66I/A/K

Protease inhibitors

	Major (primary)	*Minor (secondary)*
APV	50V	10, 32, 46, 47, 54, 73, 90
ATV	50L	32, 46, 54, 71, 82, 84, 88, 90
IDV	46, 82, 84	10, 20, 24, 32, 36, 54, 71, 73, 77, 90

Table 53.2 Examples of resistance mutations (*continued*)

	Major (primary)	Minor (secondary)
NFV	30, 90	10, 36, 46, 71, 77, 82, 84, 88
SQV	48, 90	10, 54, 71, 73, 77, 82, 84
DRV	11I, 32I, 33F, 47V, 50V, 54 L/M, 76V, 84V, 74P, 89V	

Susceptibility in treatment experienced according to number of DRV mutations: 0=72%, 1=53%, 2=37%, 3=29%, 4=7%.

TPV	10V, 13V, 20M/R/V, 33F, 35G, 36I, 43T, 46L, 47V, 54A/M/V, 58E, 69K, 74P, 82L/T, 83D, 84V	

>2 TPV mutations- reduced susceptibility.; >7 TPV mutations- resistance

RTV	82, 84	10, 20, 32, 33, 36, 46, 54, 71, 77, 90
LPV/RTV (4–6 required)		10, 20, 24, 32, 33, 46, 47, 50V, 53, 54, 63, 71, 73, 82, 84, 90
Multiple (if >4)	10, 46, 54, 82, 84, 90	10, 54

Persistence of mutation/resistance

When treatment that selected for resistant quasi-species is discontinued, wild-type virus usually becomes predominant within 2 months. Drug-resistant mutants occasionally remain dominant, e.g. 41L (zidovudine), but usually cease to be detectable by standard assay. However, they may still persist as minority quasi-species, e.g. 90M (PI), or latent integrated proviral DNA (archived resistance). Therefore standard assays may not exclude drug resistance if carried out >1 month after stopping a failing regimen. Interpretation of resistance mutations must take into account previous treatment history including evidence of viral persistence.

Resistance testing

Standard resistance assays require VL of ≥1000copies/mL and cannot detect minority species. Expert advice is needed to interpret the results.

Genotyping

Viral genes are sequenced to identify key mutations known to confer (alone or with others) resistance. Current methodology only detects viral mutants comprising at least 20–30% of the total population. Analysis is based on known correlation between genotype and phenotype from previous studies. Results are normally available in 2–4 weeks.

Phenotyping

Viral cell cultures are set up with increasing concentrations of anti-retroviral drugs to determine IC_{50}, the concentration of drug required to inhibit viral replication by 50%. Cut-off value indicates by what factor the IC_{50} of an HIV isolate can be ↑ while still being classified as susceptible (when compared with a wild-type control). IC_{50} above this value indicates resistance. Usually takes longer than genotyping.

Efflux pumps

P-glycoprotein (P-gp) and multidrug-resistance associated protein 1 (MRP1) are human cell membrane constituents known as efflux pumps. They are found in the lining of intestine, renal tubules, biliary canaliculi, capillaries in brain, testes, placenta, stem cells, lymphocytes, and macrophages. Their function is to protect tissues by actively transporting foreign substance out of cells. Cell membrane expression of P-gp/MRP1 and resulting activity of efflux pump vary depending on genetic polymorphism and induction or inhibition by various factors including HIV infection (↑ P-gp in advanced stage). PIs may be subject to efflux action resulting in ↓ absorption (intestinal P-gp) or ↓ levels in CD4 cells leading to ↓ response to treatment with ↑ likelihood of resistance mutations.

Clinical application of resistance testing

Now recommended soon after diagnosis of HIV infection. It is particularly required in the following situations:
- 1° infection (to identify transmitted resistance)
- pregnancy (to ↑ likelihood of viral suppression in the short time scale)
- virological failure of HAART (to guide choice of next regimen).

Studies suggest that HAART achieves better viral suppression when guided by resistance testing (with expert interpretation).

When to switch and options

Treatment switches may be required for intolerance, side-effects, metabolic disorders, or virological failure (defined as viral rebound or failure to achieve initial viral suppression).

In patients where new three-drug options (that are likely to fully suppress viral replication) are available, switches should be considered when there have been two or more consecutive viral loads >400copies/mL having excluded other explanations (e.g. intercurrent infection). Also important to exclude poor adherence or factors leading to ↓ drug levels before switching. Viral resistance testing should be done. Patients should always be switched onto at least 2 active drugs and where possible 3. Single drug switches can be made for drug-related problems (e.g. side-effects) if there is satisfactory viral suppression.

In the absence of resistance data, first treatment switches are influenced by initial therapy. First treatment failure options to consider:
- 2 NRTIs + PI regimens:
  - switch to two new NRTIs + an NNRTI;
  - if there is likely to be NRTI cross-resistance, switch to a new boosted PI + a NNRTI and a new NRTI.

Amprenavir may retain activity after other PI failures and boosted lopinavir, daranavir and tipranavir requires multiple resistance mutations to lose efficacy.
- 2 NRTI + NNRTI regimens—switch to a boosted PI and two new NRTIs.
- triple NRTI—switch to a PI + an NNRTI + a new NRTI.

Failing regimens may be continued if no viable treatment change possible. If viral load moderate and immune function stable, residual antiviral activity is likely to be beneficial.

Consequent failure

The following may be considered:
- Change regime—always give at least 2 effective drugs. There are a number of new treatment combinations available that may be considered. DRV and RTV and optimized background associated with very good response in treatment experienced. Etravirine may

be used in combination if resistance not induced by previous NNRTI use. Trofile™ should be performed and maraviroc may be used in combination. Enfuvirtide (T20 inhibitor)—a complex 36 amino acid peptide that inhibits HIV (syncytium and non-syncytium inducing) fusion to CD4 cells. Has low potential for metabolic complications or drug interactions because of extracellular site of action. Must be used in combination with other effective drugs

- Continue failing regimen—if no viable options. May be preferable to addition of single drug. If viral load moderate and immune function stable residual antiviral activity is likely to be beneficial. 3TC should be considered in these circumstances to maintain 184V and reduce viral fitness. Further drugs may be added if resistance pattern suggest hypersusceptibiity. Inadvisable to continue NNRTI as part of failing regimen as it may lead to resistance against newer NNRTIs.
- Structured treatment interruptions—not recommended associated with ↑ mortality.

Adjuvant therapy

Immune therapy

Pathogenesis of HIV is complex, involving interactions between virus and immune system. Precise immune control of HIV infection is not fully understood. HIV infection is characterized by ↑ production of certain cytokines (e.g. IL-1, IL-6, tumour necrosis factor) and ↓ production of others (e.g. IL-2, IL-12, and interferon γ).

HAART partially reverses some immune abnormalities, but most patients, even with full viral suppression, lack effective HIV-specific responses. Especially common if treatment commenced in advanced disease. Immune therapy may improve these responses.

Cytokine therapy

HIV infection results in gradual ↓ production and response to endo-genous IL-2. Synthesized by CD4 cells, it induces proliferation and differentiation of CD4 and CD8 cells. IL-2 given subcutaneously as an intermittent course produces ↑ CD4 count if given alone but more enhanced when combined with HAART. Viral load does not ↑, but long-term effects are unknown. Side-effects such as fever, tachycardia, hypotension, and respiratory failure, are typically dose dependent and can limit its use.

Immune stimulation

Endogenous antigens (structured treatment interruptions) or exogenous antigens (therapeutic vaccination) are other ways of stimulating immune responses. Remune (Th1 stimulant) and ALVAC vcp 1452 are examples of therapeutic vaccines which have shown immunological benefit.

Structured treatment interruptions

Failure of HAART to restore HIV-specific immune responses may be related to loss of antigen presentation. Viral rebound following treatment interruption presents fresh HIV antigens to the immune system, facilitating rapid response by resting memory cells. Structured treatment interruption allows for emergence of wild-type virus, which is more responsive to anti-retrovirals. It may be considered as a salvage therapeutic intervention for multidrug resistance. Main drawbacks are a rapid rebound of virus, re-emergence of archived drug resistant virus, ↓ CD4 count, and development of an acute retroviral syndrome.

Hydroxycarbamide

Acts by reducing cellular adenine (a nucleotide necessary for DNA synthesis) by inhibiting the enzymes needed for its production. It enhances antiretroviral activity (and toxicity) of adenosine analogues, such as DDI, and induces cellular kinases that phosphorylate NRTIs, ↑ their antiretroviral activity (and toxicity). Main side-effects are bone marrow suppression (dose dependent), pancreatitis, and liver toxicity. Optimum dose unknown (usually given as 500mg twice daily) and so far no major trial evidence of benefit.

Post-exposure prophylaxis (PEP)

Following occupational or non-sexual contact

A case–control study conducted by the US Centers for Disease Control (CDC) showed that zidovudine PEP given to those occupationally exposed to HIV was associated with an 80% ↓ in infection. Combination treatment, demonstrably more potent and less likely to be affected by viral resistance, is now recommended.

Therefore consider if contact with HIV likely through:

• percutaneous injury (e.g. from needles, instruments, bone fragments, bites which break the skin)
• exposure of broken skin (e.g. abrasions, cuts, eczema)
• exposure of mucous membranes (including the eye).

Average risk for HIV transmission after percutaneous exposure to HIV-infected blood in healthcare settings is ~3/1000 injuries. ↑ with large volumes of blood, deep injury, and high VL. After mucocutaneous exposure average risk is ~1/1000. No risk of HIV transmission if intact skin exposed to HIV-infected body fluids.

If HIV status of source is unknown, a designated doctor (not exposed worker) should obtain consent for HIV and other blood-borne virus testing.

Management

Wash skin or exposed wound with soap and water, without scrubbing and antiseptics. Bleeding of puncture wounds should be encouraged. Exposed mucous membranes, including conjunctivae, should be liberally irrigated with water before and after removing any contact lenses.

Following a discussion of risks and benefits, PEP should be recommended to HCPs if they have had a significant occupational exposure to blood or other high-risk body fluid from someone either known to be HIV infected or considered to be at high risk of HIV infection. PEP should be commenced as soon as possible after the event and should be continued for 4 weeks. UK Department of Health guidance states that PEP may still be worth considering even if 2 weeks have elapsed following exposure. However, studies suggest that delays >72 hours may render PEP ineffective.

Following sexual contact

Limited data, but reports from Brazil and South Africa suggest that PEP may provide some protection. Use of PEP following sexual exposure to HIV is only recommended within 72 hours of exposure (as early as possible).

Risk–benefit assessment should be made considering risk of transmission according to the coital act (Box 53.1) and the likelihood of the source being HIV +ve (📖 Chapter 35, Prevalence p. 414). Other factors to consider include the possibility of pre-existing HIV infection, and the ability to adhere to/tolerate the proposed antiretroviral regimen.

Box 53.1 Situations when PEP following sexual exposure is recommended (from BASHH guidelines)

- Unprotected contact with known HIV +ve individual:
  - receptive and insertive anal sex
  - receptive and insertive vaginal sex.
- Unprotected contact with unknown HIV status where prevalence is >10%:
  - receptive anal sex.

PEP regimens

- Combivir® (AZT 300mg + 3TC 150mg) twice daily + NFV 1.25g twice daily.
- Alternatives are D4T or TDF for AZT, and LPV/r (Kaletra®) for NFV.

PEP continued for 1 month. A negative antibody test 3 months after completing PEP confirms that infection has been avoided.

HIV: pregnancy

Preconception

Advise HIV-discordant couples wishing to conceive on maximizing the chance of conception while minimizing the risk of sexual transmission. Risk of transmission is likely to be lower on treatment with low viral load (VL), and higher during seroconversion and as disease progresses and CD4 ↓ with VL ↑.

♀ HIV +ve–♂ HIV –ve

Advise on how to perform artificial insemination at the time of ovulation, using quills, syringes, and gallipots.

♂ HIV +ve–♀ HIV –ve

- Transmission risk 1 in 500–10,000 per unprotected sexual act. Therefore after discussion of risk advise unprotected sexual intercourse around the time of ovulation. The risk is considered low if plasma VL is totally suppressed with HAART and intercourse at time of ovulation (although semen and plasma VL do not always correlate).
- Sperm washing, i.e. separation of spermatozoa from surrounding HIV-infected seminal plasma by a sperm swim-up technique, is available in a number of centres in the UK. Sperm obtained can then be used for intra-uterine insemination, *in vitro* fertilization or intra-cytoplasmic injection. To date, there have been no cases of HIV transmission to ♀ inseminated with washed sperm.
- If ♂ has low sperm count, intra-cytoplasmic sperm injection of ovum following sperm washing may be offered.

In vitro fertilization

Now considered ethically acceptable for subfertility because of vertical transmission rates of <1% and ↑ life expectancy for parents taking HAART. The effectiveness of pre-conceptual folic acid for those requiring such prophylaxis is unknown, although a higher dose (5mg) is recommended.

Contraception

See ▢ Chapter 33, HIV-positive women.

Mother-to-child (vertical) HIV transmission without intervention

Vertical transmission rates vary from 15% to 20% in non-breastfeeding European ♀ to 25–40% in African ♀ who breastfeed. Although transmission is associated with advanced HIV disease and low antenatal CD4 count, a high maternal VL is the strongest individual predictor. The presence of genital infections and more importantly genital ulcerative disease ↑ transmission risk.

In ♀ who do not breastfeed >80% of vertical transmission occurs late in the 3rd trimester (from 36 weeks), during labour, and at delivery, with <2% during the 1st and 2nd trimesters. The main obstetric risk factors are vaginal delivery with detectable viral load, vaginal ulceration, duration of membrane rupture >1 hour, chorioamnionitis, low birth weight, and preterm delivery. An undetectable VL significantly reduces transmission during uncomplicated vaginal delivery. HIV transmission may still occur in women with undetectable plasma viral load in the circumstances of premature rupture of membranes or preterm delivery. It is estimated that breastfeeding ↑ the mother-to-child transmission rate by 14% for ♀ infected with HIV before birth and by 30% in those infected postnatally.

In ♀ without advanced disease North American and European studies suggest no ↑ risk of accelerated immunosuppression during pregnancy. CD4 counts may fall but return to pre-pregnancy levels after delivery.

Frequently asked questions

Can I get pregnant?

It is possible for an HIV +ve ♀ to have a baby. The risk of vertical transmission is 15–40% but this is ↓ to <1% with anti-retroviral treatment, Caesarean section (if viral suppression inadequate), and avoidance of breastfeeding. Also the parents' life expectancy is ↑ with treatment if it is required. Artificial insemination techniques avoid the risk of transmission to an HIV –ve ♂ partner and sperm washing ↓ the risk of a positive ♂ infecting a ♀.

Can I have a vaginal delivery?

It is generally advisable to have an elective Caesarean section as it ↓ the risk of vertical transmission by 50%. However, if there is viral suppression vaginal delivery may be considered if there are no complications and delivery occurs within 1 hour of membranes breaking.

Can I breastfeed?

No. There is a high risk of mother-to-child transmission with breastfeeding.

Vertical HIV transmission with intervention

Transmission rate has been reduced to <1% by:
- antiretroviral therapy, given antenatally and intra-partum to the mother and to the neonate for the first 4–6 weeks of life
- delivery by elective Caesarean section
- avoidance of breastfeeding.

Management

▶ Guidance on the management of HIV infection changes rapidly with new evidence. Therefore it is important to consult contemporary guidelines (📖 Useful resources p. 615).

Identification

Routine antenatal HIV antibody testing should be advised and offered to all pregnant ♀ in early pregnancy (usually at booking). Midwives must be able to provide information on the benefits of early diagnosis, ensuring that an expert sees newly diagnosed cases promptly. Management during pregnancy should be multidisciplinary, involving an obstetrician, HIV physician, midwife, paediatrician, and appropriate others (e.g. social worker, psychologist). Partner notification should be managed with the ♀'s cooperation and support. However, in the absence of this, the ♀'s HIV status may be disclosed to an at-risk sexual contact (for his protection) although the ♀ must be informed and the clinician must be able to justify this action. Otherwise assurances should be given regarding confidentiality, especially relating to friends and relatives accompanying the ♀ who may be unaware of her HIV diagnosis. The HIV status should be clearly indicated in the woman's antenatal notes with a clear plan of management and what to do and who to consult in emergency.

Advice should be given about avoiding unprotected sexual intercourse both for the benefit of partner(s) and the safety of the ♀.

Assessment and screening

Repeat HIV antibody test to confirm and assess as for any newly diagnosed case (📖 Chapter 38, Assessment of HIV +ve patient p. 442) with regular and close monitoring of CD4 count and at least monthly plasma viral load (VL). A viral load should be obtained as close to the due date as possible.

HIV infection is associated with the presence of other STIs that may ↑ genital HIV VL potentially increasing the risk of vertical transmission. Screening should include:
- serological testing for syphilis (at booking and 3rd trimester), hepatitis B and C viruses (if not already done at booking)
- screening for STIs at booking and 3rd trimester; including specimens for *Chlamydia trachomatis, Neisseria gonorrhoeae, Trichomonas vaginalis,* and bacterial vaginosis
- baseline (at diagnosis) resistance assay.

Antiretroviral treatment

▶ Advised for all ♀ during pregnancy and at delivery.

The AIDS Clinical Trials Group protocol 076 (1994) demonstrated that zidovudine (ZDV) monotherapy, initiated between 14 and 34 weeks of pregnancy, intravenously during delivery, and to infants for 6 weeks, ↓ risk of HIV-1 infection if not breastfeeding from 25.0% to 7.6%. ZDV monotherapy does not fully suppress plasma viraemia, leading to ↑ risk of viral resistance. Therefore HAART, involving three or more drug combinations, should be used if the mother requires it for her own health as in the non-pregnant state (📖 Chapter 53). This can be delayed until after the first trimester. It should be considered early if the CD4 count ↓ <350cells/µL and immediately if CD4 count ↓ <200cells/µL . Prophylaxis against *Pneumocystis jiroveci* (*carinii*) should be considered for those presenting with a CD4 count <200cells/µL. First-line prophylaxis is co-trimoxazole, which is a folate antagonist. Therefore potential benefits have to be balanced against the risks of fetal neural tube defects. If used in early pregnancy folic acid supplements should be provided and ultrasound scanning arranged after the first trimester.

- Avoid:
  - combinations containing didanosine and/or stavudine unless no alternatives
  - nevirapine as part of regimen if CD4>250/µL (↑ risk of hepatitis) unless already on it
  - efavirenz in first trimester (more data needed).
- HAART used before conception can be continued (not advisable to change efavirenz if part of an ongoing regimen) unless failing.
- Boosted PI + Combivir® (ZDV+lamivudine co-formulated) appears to be a safe and effective combination

All ♀ who receive antiretroviral therapy in pregnancy should be registered prospectively with the Antiretroviral Pregnancy Registry (🖰 www.apregistry.com).

To prevent vertical transmission only (♀ does not require HIV treatment for own health)

UK (BHIVA) guidelines recommend starting treatment between 20 and 24 weeks if VL >10,000 copies/µL and up to 28 weeks if VL <10,000copies/µL. Options are as follows.

- Short-term antiretroviral therapy (START), especially with a high VL (>10,000copies/mL).
  - During pregnancy: HAART regimen (see above), if possible containing ZDV, which may be stopped shortly after pregnancy.
  - Pre-delivery: IV ZDV infusion, 2mg/kg for first hour reducing to 1mg/kg/hour until cord clamped.
  - Delivery: obtain VL at 36 weeks. If VL <50 copies/µL → trial of normal vaginal labour. If VL >50copies/µL → change therapy according to resistance test + Caesarian section at 38 weeks + IV AZT for 4 hours + PEP to newborn + single dose NVP to mother.
  - Neonate if mother had ZDV and VL <50copies/ml: oral ZDV syrup.

- ZDV monotherapy: option for ♀ with low VL (<10,000copies/μL) wild-type virus, and not requiring HAART in their own right or not wishing to take HAART during pregnancy but agreed to have a planned lower segment Caesarian section.
  - 300mg twice daily or 200mg three times daily by mouth: start at 24–28 weeks and stop immediately after delivery.
  - Pre-delivery: start (4 hours before delivery) IV ZDV infusion, 2mg/kg for first hour reducing to 1mg/kg/hour until cord clamped
  - Delivery: plan Caesarean section at 38 weeks.
  - Neonate: oral ZDV syrup.

Consensus appears to be moving away from monotherapy as combination treatment is more likely to suppress VL to undetectable levels with a ↓ risk of viral resistance. However, its use must be balanced against the risks to mother and fetus of exposure to multiple potentially toxic drugs. Preterm delivery is associated with HAART (especially <32 weeks). Data suggestive of PI-induced impaired glucose tolerance and pre-eclampsia are not consistent.

Women requiring treatment in their own right

Resistance testing should be performed before commencing HAART (see above). Treatment should start at 20–24 weeks if VL>10,000copies/μL and at up to 28 weeks if VL <10,000copies/μL. Treatment should be continued after delivery. A zidovudine-containing regimen (such as combivir) is recommended unless there is resistance or other contraindication (extensive safety data in pregnancy).

Measure VL regularly, at 36 weeks, and at delivery to ensure viral suppression. If not fully suppressed, change therapy according to resistance assay.

- At 36 weeks VL <50copies/mL: consider normal vaginal delivery at 39 weeks
- At 36 weeks VL > 50copies/mL: Caesarean section at 38 weeks + IV ZDV intra-partum and until cord is clamped + oral HAART to the neonate for 4 weeks.

Women conceiving while taking HAART

Continue regimen if effective viral suppression. If failing, consider changing therapy after first trimester following resistance testing.

Women presenting in late pregnancy or during labour

If immunological and virological assessment is not possible, HAART, including zidovudine (IV intra-partum), should be started. Continue HAART intra- and postpartum until the results of the CD4 count and VL are known.

Delivery should be by Caesarean section with consideration given to its timing to allow peak fetal concentrations. If this is not available a single 200mg oral dose of nevirapine can be given during labour and the neonate treated with nevirapine 2mg/kg 48 hours post-delivery.

⚠ Nevirapine monotherapy may lead to NNRTI-resistant mutations which could compromise future treatment options for the ♀ as well as ↑ risk of further transmission of resistant virus.

Options in countries with limited resources

- Zidovudine–lamivudine combination: from 36 weeks of gestation, intrapartum, and for 1 week postpartum—50% ↓ in vertical transmission for breastfeeding African ♀.
- Nevirapine (long half-life): single 200mg dose at onset of labour and 2mg/kg single dose to the neonate 48 hours post-delivery. Relative efficacy at 14–16 weeks is 47%.

Obstetric arrangements

Elective Caesarean section before labour or rupture of membranes

Overall provides 50% ↓ in vertical transmission persisting when antiretroviral treatment used. Effective even with low VL (1000copies/µL) but additional benefit uncertain in those taking HAART if VL <50copies/µL. BHIVA guidelines recommend planned lower segment Caesarean section if maternal VL near delivery is detectable. It should be timed to take place after 38 weeks of gestation. 'Bloodless' technique (using a staple gun) may further reduce transmission rates. Prophylactic antibiotics are recommended.

A zidovudine infusion should be started 4 hours before beginning the Caesarean section and continued until the umbilical cord has been clamped. Maternal VL should be checked at delivery. The cord should be clamped as soon as possible after delivery and the baby bathed immediately after birth.

Indications for Caesarean section

- ZDV monotherapy, plan at 38 weeks.
- HAART but VL detectable (>50copies/µL).
- HIV and HCV co-infection.
- Mothers preferred mode of delivery despite VL<50copies/µL. Plan at 39 weeks.

Vaginal delivery

If a woman chooses a vaginal delivery:
- membranes should be left intact for as long as possible
- fetal scalp electrodes and fetal blood sampling should be avoided
- emergency Caesarean section may be required for other obstetric reasons including prolonged rupture of membranes (in pre-HAART era transmission rate doubled after 4 hours).

The neonate

All infants born to ♀ who are HIV positive should be treated with antiretroviral therapy from birth. Treatment may be discontinued after 4 weeks.

ZDV monotherapy should be used if the infant's mother received ZDV antenatally or intra-partum, either as monotherapy or in a HAART regimen. Consider HAART for neonates if mother started antiretroviral therapy late in pregnancy, or mother had a high VL at delivery or complicated delivery. Preterm or sick infants may not tolerate oral therapy and ZDV is the only antiretroviral drug available as an IV preparation.

Maternal antibodies crossing the placenta are detectable in most neonates of mothers who are HIV-positive. In non-breastfed infants proviral DNA is the test of choice. Tests are carried out at birth, 6 weeks, and 12 weeks. Additional testing may be done at 2–3 weeks in infants at high risk. Blood sample should be taken from the mother at birth and amplified with day 1 infant sample to confirm that the primers used detect the maternal virus. Final confirmation is a negative HIV antibody test at 18 months of age, following decay of maternal antibodies.

Infant feeding

All HIV +ve mothers should be advised to avoid breastfeeding. Mixing breast with artificial feeding appears to ↑ risk of viral transmission compared with breastfeeding alone (African data).

Anti-retroviral drugs used in pregnancy with usual doses

Nucleoside reverse transcriptase inhibitors (NRTIs)

Recommended

- Zidovudine (300mg twice daily): preferred NRTI in HAART that usually includes two NRTIs with either an NNRTI or one or more PIs.
- Lamivudine (150mg twice daily): in combination with zidovudine recommended NRTI backbone for pregnant ♀.

Alternative

- Abacavir (300mg twice daily): in non-pregnant hypersensitivity 5–8%.
- Emtricitabine (200mg daily): another NRTI for dual nucleoside background although no data in pregnancy.
- Tenofovir (245mg once daily): NRTI backbone, no data in pregnancy.

Non-nucleoside reverse transcriptase inhibitors (NNRTIs)

Recommended

- Nevirapine (200mg daily for first 14 days then 200mg twice daily): caution in combination therapy if CD4 count >250cells/μL when initiating treatment in ♀. ↑ risk of potentially fatal liver toxicity, often associated with a rash. (Unclear if further ↑ risk with pregnancy.)

⚠ Avoid

- Efavirenz: reports of neural tube defects in infants when used in first trimester.

Protease inhibitors (PIs)

Recommended

- Nelfinavir (1.25g) twice daily.
- Saquinavir tablets (1g) boosted with ritonavir (100mg) twice daily.

Alternative

- Lopinavir (400mg) + ritonavir (100mg) twice daily: early studies suggest ↑ dose may be required during pregnancy, particularly in last trimester. Consider therapeutic drug monitoring.

Monitoring in pregnancy

Electrolytes and liver function tests should be performed every 2 weeks during the 3rd trimester in view of the potential risk of lactic acidosis and hepatic steatosis when using NRTIs.

HIV: travel

Planning

Travel, particularly to developing countries, may carry substantial risks of infection, e.g. malaria, salmonella, hepatitis viruses, and cryptosporidiosis. Infections, especially relevant for those with immunodeficiency, include leishmaniasis, *Penicillium marneffei*, coccidioidomycosis, histoplasmosis, and blastomycosis (the latter three are possible causes of cerebral abscesses). Many developing countries have high rates of tuberculosis.

Some countries have introduced HIV antibody testing for visitors (and demand their own test) or require a certificate of HIV antibody testing (done within 1 month of travel). Information by country is available at: ◐ www.aids.about.com/od/legalissues/a/traveldi.htm. Specific information should be sought from relevant consulates.

Travel risk in relation to degree of immune deficiency, range of potential pathogens, and availability of medical care needs to be discussed and evaluated with the patient. Medical costs must be considered and adequate insurance arranged, recognizing HIV status and immune function. A confidential letter containing essential medical information is invaluable if help should be needed. Adequate medication (which may require refrigeration) should be supplied with written confirmation of treatment needed to prevent problems with customs. Rehydration sachets and standby therapy for GI infections and malaria may be indicated. If travel crosses time zones, either remain on UK time for taking medication for the entire trip or adjust in 1 hour steps before/during travel.

Vaccination

Preparation for travel should include review and updating of routine vaccinations (Table 55.1). Special precautions are required for non-European areas surrounding the Mediterranean, Africa, the Middle East, Asia, and South America (details available at ◐ www.dh.gov.uk).

Table 55.1 Travel vaccination and HIV infection

Vaccine	Asymptomatic HIV	Symptomatic HIV
Polio (inactive)	Yes	Yes
Meningococcus (ACWY)	Yes	Yes
Hepatitis A	Yes	Yes
Hepatitis B	Yes	Yes
Rabies	Yes	Yes
Tetanus	Yes	Yes
Typhoid	Yes	Yes
Tuberculosis (BCG)	No (CD4 >200cells/μL)	No

There is no ↑ incidence of adverse reactions to inactivated vaccines although their protective efficacy may be ↓. Live vaccines may carry ↑ risks of adverse reactions and in general should be avoided (except for measles).

Yellow fever vaccine is a live attenuated vaccine with uncertain safety and efficacy in HIV infection. WHO recommends immunization for asymptomatic HIV-infected people travelling to endemic areas, but there is insufficient evidence to advise those with symptomatic infection. Those who become asymptomatic with CD4 >200cells/μL following HAART may be offered immunization (evidence supports safety and efficacy). A certificate of exemption is needed for those who cannot be immunized if travel is necessary, and advice should be given on the risk and methods to avoid of mosquito bites (vector of yellow fever).

Cholera vaccine has little protective value.

Food and water

Those with CD4 <250cells/μL are at ↑ risk from GI pathogens (cryptosporidiosis, salmonella, etc.). Particular care should be taken with raw fruit/vegetables, undercooked or raw seafood/meat, tapwater/ice, unpasteurized milk/dairy products, and food/ beverages purchased from street vendors. Safe products include thoroughly cooked food, fruit peeled by the traveller, bottled/canned drinks (especially carbonated), hot coffee/tea, or water brought to the boil and simmered for 1 minute. If local tap water must be used, and cannot be boiled, the use of a water filtration unit with added chlorine or iodine ↑ its safety. Water-borne infections (e.g. cryptosporidiosis, giardiasis) may also result from ingesting water during recreational water activities. Therefore swimming in contaminated water (sewage, animal waste) should be avoided.

Travellers' diarrhoea

Prophylactic antimicrobials against travellers' diarrhoea are not routinely recommended (side-effects/promotion of drug-resistant organisms) but if risk–benefit analysis favours their use, options include fluoroquinolones, e.g. ciprofloxacin 500mg daily and co-trimoxazole (trimethoprim–sulfamethoxazole) 960mg daily (resistance common in tropical areas). Antibiotics may be carried for empirical therapy if significant diarrhoea develops (e.g. ciprofloxacin 500mg twice daily for 3–7 days). Antiperistaltic agents, e.g. loperamide, are useful (except if diarrhoea is bloody or associated with pyrexia) but should be discontinued if symptoms persist >48 hours. Seek medical advice if failure to respond, blood in the stool, pyrexia/ rigors, or dehydration.

Other precautions

Advice should be given about other preventive measures for anticipated exposure, e.g. malaria prophylaxis and protection against arthropod vectors. Avoid direct soil and sand contact with skin by wearing shoes, protective clothing, and using towels on beaches to avoid hookworm, strongyloidosis, and cutaneous larva migrans. Avoid swimming in fresh water in areas of risk for schistosomiasis.

Recreational travel is commonly associated with sexual encounters. Newly acquired STIs, including HIV superinfection, can compromise the underlying HIV infection. A supply of condoms should be carried, as availability at the destination may be limited and of dubious quality.

Useful resources

Books

Cohen PT, Merle AS, Volberding PA (1999). *The AIDS Knowledge Base.* Lippincott–Williams & Wilkins, Philadelphia, PA.

Holmes KK, Mardh P-A, Sparling PF, Lemon SM, Stamm WE, Piot P, and Wasserheit JN (1999). *Sexually Transmitted Diseases.* McGraw-Hill, New York:.

McMillan A, Young H, Ogilvie MM, and Scott GR (2002). *Clinical Practice in Sexually Transmissible Infections.* WB Saunders, London.

Websites

International/national bodies
- Department of Health: 🖰 www.dh.gov.uk
- Medical Foundation for AIDS and Sexual Health: 🖰 www.medfash.org.uk
- National Institutes of Health: 🖰 www.nih.gov
- World Health Organization: 🖰 www.who.int
- Health Protection Agency (England and Wales): 🖰 www.hpa.org.uk
- Scottish Health Statistics: 🖰 www.isdscotland.org
- Centers for Disease Control: 🖰 www.cdc.gov
- Joint United Nations Programme on HIV/AIDS: 🖰 www.unaids.org
- National AIDS Trust, UK: 🖰 www.nat.org.uk

Colleges and faculties
- Royal College of Physicians (London): 🖰 www.rcplondon.ac.uk
- Royal College of Physicians (Edinburgh): 🖰 www.rcpe.ac.uk
- Royal College of Physicians and Surgeons (Glasgow): 🖰 www.rcpsglasg.ac.uk
- Royal College of Obstetricians and Gynaecologists: 🖰 www.rcog.org.uk
- Faculty of Family Planning and Reproductive Healthcare: 🖰 www. ffprhc.org.uk

Professional organizations
- General Medical Council: 🖰 www.gmc-uk.org
- British Medical Association: 🖰 www.bma.org.uk
- British Association for Sexual Health and HIV: 🖰 www.bashh.org
- International Union Against Sexually Transmitted Infections: 🖰 www. iusti.org
- British HIV Association: 🖰 www.bhiva.org
- International AIDS Society—USA: 🖰 www.iasusa.org
- Society of Sexual Health Advisers: 🖰 www.ssha.info
- Genito-urinary Nurses Association: 🖰 www.guna.org.uk

Management guidelines
- UK STI Management Guidelines: 🖰 www.bashh.org/guidelines/ceguidelines.htm
- Lazaro N (2006). *Sexually Transmitted Infections in Primary Care.* RCGP Sex, Drugs and HIV Task Group, BASHH. 🖰 www.bashh.org/documents/702/702.pdf

- US STI Management Guidelines: ℘ www.cdc.gov/std/treatment/rr5106.pdf
- UK HIV Treatment Guidelines: ℘ www.bhiva.org/guidelines/2003/hiv/index.html
- Other HIV guidelines (pregnancy, hepatitis B/C co-infection, TB, adherence) available at ℘ www.bhiva.org
- RCOG Management of HIV in Pregnancy Guidelines: ℘ www.rcog.org.uk/resources/Public/RCOG_Guideline_39_low.pdf
- US HIV Treatment Guidelines: ℘ www.aidsinfo.nih.gov/guidelines
- WHO STI Management Guidelines: ℘ www.who.int/reproductive-health/ publications/rhr_01_10/01_10.pdf
- WHO Medical Eligibility Criteria for Contraceptive Use: http://℘ www.who.int/reproductivehealth/publications/family_planning/9241562668index/en/index.html
- European STD Guidelines: ℘ www.iusti.org/guidelines.pdf
- National Institute for Clinical Excellence: ℘ www.nice.org.uk

HIV/AIDS information

- Medscape: ℘ www.medscape.com
- AIDSInfo—US Department of Health and Human Services (also HIV Management Guidelines): ℘ www.aidsinfo.nih.gov
- Johns Hopkins AIDS Service: ℘ www.hopkins-aids.edu
- AIDSmap: ℘ www.aidsmap.com
- AIDS Education Global Information System: ℘ www.aegis.com
- HIV i-Base: ℘ www.i-base.info
- HIV drug resistance
  - Stanford HIV Drug Resistance Database: ℘ www.hivdb.stanford.edu
  - HIV-1 Genotypic Drug Resistance Interpretation's Algorithms: ℘ www.hivfrenchresistance.org
  - Los Alamos-Database: ℘ www.hiv.lanl.gov/content/index.
  - Also at AIDSinfo: ℘ www.aidsinfo.nih.gov
- HIV Drug Interactions: ℘ www.hiv-druginteractions.org

Miscellaneous

- e-medicine: ℘ www.emedicine.com
- Chlamydia Professional: ℘ www.chlamydiae.com
- International Herpes Management Forum: ℘ www.ihmf.org
- National Electronic Library for Health: ℘ www.nelh.nhs.uk
- British National Formulary: ℘ www.bnf.org
- NHS Sexual Health Information: ℘ www.playingsafely.co.uk

Self-help

- UK Self Help: ℘ www.ukselfhelp.info
- Herpes Viruses Association: ℘ www.herpes.org.uk
- International Herpes Alliance: ℘ www.herpesalliance.org
- Vulval Pain Society: ℘ www.vul-pain.dircon.co.uk
- Sexual Dysfunction Association: ℘ www.sda.uk.net
- Terrence Higgins Trust: ℘ www.tht.org.uk
- +ve: ℘ www.plusve.org

Index

Italicised entries denote figures, tables or boxes.

Reference ranges (continued)

These figures are for guidance only as normal ranges vary between laboratories. Always check with your local laboratory. 📖 See also inside front cover pages.

Continued from inside front cover.

Biochemistry (all blood) continued	Your laboratory
Folate (plasma)	3.3–13mcg/L
Folate (red cell)	160–600mcg/L
Follicle stimulating hormone	
♂	1.3–9.2IU/L
♀ follicular	2–9IU/L
♀ luteal	1–10IU/L
♀ post-menopausal	>30IU/L
Gamma-glutamyl transferase	
♂	<70IU/L
♀	<50IU/L
Glucose (fasting)	3.5–5.5mmol/L
Lactic dehydrogenase	<215IU/L
Luteinizing hormone	
♂	3–13IU/L
♀ follicular	2–12IU/L
♀ luteal	1–12IU/L
♀ post-menopausal	>30IU/L
Oestradiol	
♂	<180pmol/L
♀ follicular	60–355pmol/L
♀ mid-cycle	250–1900pmol/L
♀ luteal	75–900pmol/L
♀ post-menopausal	<180pmol/L
Phosphate (inorganic)	0.8–1.44mmol/L
Potassium	3.4–5mmol/L
Prolactin	<450mIU/L
Prostate-specific antigen	<4mcg/mL